Classical Homoeopathy

Margery Grace Blackie
CVO, MD, FFHom

Homoeopathy, as formulated by Hahnemann, is the most scientific and the most successful system of medical treatment yet devised. Our responsibility for its pure and truthful presentation is great.

Margery Blackie

Edited for publication by
Charles Elliott, MB, BCh, MFHom
and
Frank Johnson, MB, BS, FFHom

Repertory compiled by
Dr Charles Elliott

BEACONSFIELD PUBLISHERS LTD
Beaconsfield, Bucks, England

First published in 1986

Reprinted 1990

British Library Cataloguing in Publication Data

    Blackie, Margery G.
      Classical Homoeopathy.—(The Beaconsfield
      homoeopathic library 6)
      1. Homeopathy
      I. Title   II. Elliott, Charles   III. Johnson, Frank
      615.5'32   RX71

ISBN 0–906584–14–0

Phototypeset by Prima Graphics, Camberley, Surrey
in 10 on 12 point Times.
Updated by Gem Graphics, Trenance, Mawgan Porth, Cornwall.
Printed in Great Britain at The Bath Press, Avon.

Preface

The material in this book is drawn from Dr Margery Blackie's teaching and writing over the whole span of her career. It encapsulates the warmth, enthusiasm, learning and clinical understanding of a remarkable person whose professional life was devoted to the practice and furtherance of homoeopathy. She was admired by her patients for her concerned approach, kindness, and skill. It is as a brilliant teacher, whose vivid descriptions of the various constitutional types of patients became engraved in the minds of her listeners, that she is remembered by her undergraduate and postgraduate students. It was this deep understanding of the characteristics of the individual remedy that formed the basis of her international reputation.

Margery Grace Blackie was born at Redbourn, Hertfordshire in 1898, the youngest daughter of Robert and Elizabeth Blackie and the niece of James Compton Burnett. She qualified in medicine at the London School of Medicine for Women in 1923, and in the following year joined the staff of the London Homoeopathic Hospital. Here she came under the teaching influence of John Henry Clarke, Charles Wheeler and Douglas Borland, himself a former student of James Tyler Kent. She obtained her M.D. from the University of London in 1928.

During her career she combined a busy homoeopathic general practice with her hospital work, which culminated in her appointment in 1966 as Honorary Consultant Physician to the Royal London Homoeopathic Hospital. She was Dean of the Faculty of Homoeo-pathy from 1965 to 1979. Appointed Physician to H.M. The Queen in 1968 she was admitted to the Royal Victorian Order in the rank of Commander in 1979. She died in 1981.

With few exceptions Dr Blackie prescribed only in the 10M and 6c potencies. Her use of high potency remedies derived from Dr Borland's visit to Chicago before the First World War to study under Dr Kent. She freely acknowledged her debt to Dr Borland for his influence on this and other aspects of her practice and teaching.

She prescribed a 10M potency if the remedy was clearly the patient's constitutional one – a choice implying that the selection each time was made with infinite precision. She divided the high potency into three doses to be taken at intervals of twelve hours, the purpose being to minimise the possibility of aggravation. On the few occasions that such occurred she subsequently prescribed the same remedy in the CM potency, or gave the 10M potency dissolved in a glass of water, to be taken in small sips as often as was necessary to control the symptoms. On some occasions she would repeat a 10M potency frequently for up to three days. The use of such potencies should be confined to the experienced homoeopath.

Dr Blackie normally used the 6c potency for essentially local conditions, to be taken three times per day until improvement. Occasionally she used 12c, 30c, 200c or 1M potencies.

C.E., F.J.

The Editors would like to record their appreciation to Beaconsfield Publishers Ltd for their diligence, care and sympathetic handling of the material in this text.

Champion of Homoeopathy, A Life of Dr Margery Blackie
Constance Babington Smith (John Murray, 1986)

Margery Blackie was the most dominant figure of her generation in the world of British homoeopathy – a world of men. Largely thanks to her initiative, homoeopathic treatment is becoming more widely recognised as a most valuable branch of medicine, the therapy of 'let likes be treated by likes'. In this account of her life the meaning and methods of homoeopathy are made clear, through illustrations of her practice, patients, teaching and campaigning.

Also by Dr Margery Blackie: **The Patient, Not The Cure**

Contents

Contents

Contents

Introduction

After being a houseman for eighteen months at the London Homoeopathic Hospital I decided I would like to put up my plate in South
Kensington. I thought I ought to know the neighbourhood a bit, so I
walked as far as the Fulham Road and then past the Royal Marsden
Hospital, still called The Cancer Hospital in those days and where I
had done six months training, and also the Brompton Chest Hospital.
I passed a chemist's and saw a notice on the back wall of the entrance,
painted out but still perfectly readable, which said, 'Homoeopathic
Dispensary, Monday, Wednesday and Friday from 6 p.m.–8 p.m.' I
went in and asked the chemist what this meant. 'Oh', he said, 'that's
been shut for twelve years', so I asked if he would like to open it again.
He took me to the first floor and showed me a good waiting room and
a smaller consulting room. This was on a Thursday. The next day I
papered the consulting room, had the necessary furniture sent in on
the Saturday, and arranged to start at 6 p.m. the following Monday.
When I arrived there were twelve patients waiting.

The Homoeopathic Approach

1

Hahnemann and the Discovery of Homoeopathy

Dr Compton Burnett went to the length of recommending an annual lecture on the life and work of Hahnemann for the benefit of successive generations, so that they might have a standard by which to measure the foibles of the hour . . . 'for the pigmies of the day are very apt to appear mighty giants unless the deeds of the great dead be present with us'.

Hahnemann was an outstanding man, apart altogether from his discovery of homoeopathy. No candid observer of his actions or writings would hesitate for a moment to admit that he was an extraordinary person, a genius and a scholar, a man of indefatigable industry and of dauntless energy. It appears that from an early age he determined to be a doctor, but parental opposition and poverty had to be overcome. To do this he supported himself through his student days by doing scientific translations. He had an extensive knowledge of eight languages and was a keen student of chemistry. By sitting up every third night doing translations he was able to keep himself and, at the same time, his knowledge of science grew, for he was no mere translator.

On qualifying he quickly rose to fame in the world of medicine and science. After twelve years of prosperous practice he came to the belief that medicine was not only no good, but that it was positively harmful and sometimes little short of murder. Medicine at that time consisted mostly of unscientific prescriptions, leeches and blood-letting. Other doctors were discontented too, but few gave up their practice and wealth because of the promptings of their conscience. Sir John Forbes wrote, 'in a considerable proportion of diseases it would fare as well or better with patients if all remedies were abandoned. Things have arrived at such a pitch that they cannot be worse, they must mend or end'.

He was asked to translate Cullen's *Materia Medica* into German. Cullen had practised in a swampy district, where the prevalent fever was known to respond to cinchona bark, and defended the old idea that the action of cinchona on the fever was due to its tonic effect on

1

the stomach. Not so, Hahnemann wrote to Cullen. From practical experience he knew that the strongest mixture of astringents and bitters had no effect on the fever, but that such things as coffee, pepper, ignatia bean and arsenic did. Cullen did not reply, but Hahnemann went on wondering how it acted and decided to take some cinchona bark himself.

He was amazed to find that he developed all the symptoms of the fever, but without the pyrexia. These symptoms disappeared when he stopped taking the bark. After an interval he tried it again and also on some members of his family. Everyone produced the same symptoms, varying only in degree. Here was a strange phenomenon – a remedy which was effective for disease induced the symptoms of that disease when given to a healthy person. Could there be some method of cure upon which he had stumbled? Hahnemann now started on his life's work.

He gave up his practice and to support his wife and family returned to translations. His great desire now was to find some system by which one could ascertain the exact properties of drugs and know beforehand in what diseases they would be applicable. 'Then', he said, 'the uncertainties of medieval practice would be removed and we might anticipate as great success in the treatment of all disease as in those for which we had specifics.'

It occurred to him that the effects of drugs on healthy persons might provide knowledge of their specific properties, and that their administration in cases with similar symptoms might be the law of specifics he was looking for. Being familiar with all the old medical writings through his translation work, he knew that the idea of homoeopathy had arisen in various forms from the time of Hippocrates. Frostbite had been treated with snow, and acidity by small doses of sulphuric acid. It was known that stramonium (the thorn-apple) could cause and cure cases of insanity and convulsions, and it had been noticed that when similars were administered the ailing patient returned to good health.

He now began his research to record the effect of a large number of substances on the human body. He gathered a band of helpers to whom he gave remedies, interrogating them daily on any special sensations experienced. He called these the 'provings' of the remedy. In this way he built up a materia medica consisting of symptoms which had been experimentally produced in healthy people. This materia medica represented a vast collection of accurate observations, which, when identified in a sick person, became the indication of the remedy which would cure when given homoeopathically.

He also found that after a small but material dose of the indicated remedy the symptoms were aggravated before any improvement started. However, by diluting and 'succussing' the remedy (by which he meant shaking it vigorously between each dilution), he found that the improvement usually started without any aggravation. This process he called 'potentisation'.

Dr Compton Burnett said that Hahnemann succeeded in formulating a law where other people merely observed the facts, because he possessed what they did not, namely the true spirit of philosophy, the requisite leisure, and a knowledge of the history of theories of drug action. That being so, all the influences of his early life were preparing him for his great discovery.

Having searched through medical literature and found corroborating evidence of his theory, he began to experiment upon himself, then on his family and friends. Between 1790 and 1805 he proved sixty drugs on himself, saying, 'When we have to do with an art whose end is the saving of human life, any neglect to make ourselves masters of it becomes a crime'. Then, when he was sure of the truth of the great principle he had discovered, he put it before the medical profession: 'I believe I have discovered a system which will render the practice of medicine certain and its success brilliant. I have laboured fifteen years to test my discovery. My own experiments and the testimony furnished by the records of medicine convince me of its truth. I lay it and them before you, my colleagues, and I conjure you in the name of truth and in the interests of humanity to investigate it candidly and without prejudice. If experience should show you that my method is the best, then make use of it for the benefit of mankind and give God the glory'.

How did they react? With bitter aspersions upon his personal character, and contempt and scorn on the system he had unfolded, without a single suggestion to investigate or put it to the test.

At this stage Hahnemann was suggesting nothing more startling than giving a single drug in a material though small dose, according to some rule, so it is difficult to understand why his contemporaries refused even to investigate it. They proved the truth of Plato's words: 'Nothing can be more repugnant to an ordinary mind than the thorough sifting of deep-seated, long familiar notions'. He went on with his provings and started medical practice again. He was more successful than before, and in a bad epidemic of scarlet fever his active and prophylactic treatment enhanced his reputation.

His colleagues had not been able to find any legitimate complaint against him but someone at last had an idea. Hahnemann gave his own preparations of medicines free of charge to his patients. The law said that practitioners must not compound and sell the medicines which they prescribed, so the apothecaries were incited to prosecute him on this score, winning their case in spite of the fact that Hahnemann was an experienced chemist and an appointed inspector of apothecaries. He had to leave his place of practice. He and his family set off with their worldly goods on a cart, for it was before the day of furniture removers, accompanied by a crowd of sorrowing patients. A few miles away the cart overturned going downhill, his goods were scattered, his son was fatally injured, his daughter's leg was broken and he, badly bruised and shaken, became a changed man.

Up till then he had been anxious to share his great discovery with his medical brethren. But from now on he became bitter against them and his language became strong, and who can blame him. He turned instead to the laity for recognition, publishing his articles in general literature. He wandered from place to place, eventually settling in Leipzig, where he was allowed to lecture at the University. His growing popularity with patients and students was again too much for his fellow practitioners – the apothecaries came to their rescue once again.

It is interesting to note that eight years after his death a costly bronze statue was erected to Hahnemann in this same town. The Leipzig Council officially celebrated the unveiling of this statue to what they termed one of Saxony's most illustrious sons. What an amazing life – over eighty years of industry, perseverance and devotion to service for the benefit of mankind while facing poverty, hardship and persecution almost to the end. His last words were, 'Have I ever rested? Forward, ever forward! By constantly curing you I will compel justice to be done to you and will call faithful disciples to your side. Hand on my traditions'.

2

The Organon

It seems strange that we should give serious consideration to a medical book published in 1810. We read it because Hahnemann, in ceasing to practice the orthodox medical procedures of his day and coming upon a strange phenomenon in his new occupation, found a better way. After twenty years of close observation, reasoning and experiment, he put his views into print in the *Organon*. There were five editions in his lifetime.

The concept of the time was that in disease there was an evil in the body that had to be removed by drastic means. Hahnemann had come to the conclusion that in man there was a balancing mechanism which kept him in perfect health in spite of all the stress of life, psychological, physical and atmospheric, provided that the stresses were not too great or prolonged, or the balancing mechanism itself, which he called the 'vital force', was not impaired. But if the stress was too great or the vital force impaired, unusual signs, sensations and symptoms would follow. These were the language of the sick body. This sick body could be restored rapidly to its original state of health by a remedy that had been found by experience to produce a similar condition in a healthy body.

'The physician's high and only mission', says Hahnemann, 'is to restore the sick to health, to cure, as it is termed. He is likewise a preserver of health if he knows the things that derange health and cause disease and how to remove them from persons in health. Useful to the physician in assisting him to cure are the particulars of the most probable exciting cause of the acute disease, as also the most significant points in the whole history of the chronic disease.'

'The apparent physical constitution of the patient is to be taken into consideration, as well as his occupation, his mode of living and habits, his domestic relations, his age, his sexual functions, and so on. The unprejudiced observer notices only those deviations from the former healthy state of the now diseased individual which are felt by the patient himself, remarked by those around him, and observed by the physician. All these perceptible signs represent the disease in its whole extent. That is, together they form the true and only conceivable portrait of the disease.'

He discusses the concept of health. 'In the rude state of nature but few remedial agents were required, and the simple mode of living admitted of but few diseases. With the civilisation of mankind, on the contrary, the occasion of disease and the necessity for medical aid increased in equal proportion.' I wonder what he would have thought of the torrent of new drugs that pour through our letter-boxes daily? Health seems no longer to be a natural, positive condition, but merely an absence of disease. I prefer the saying, 'Fundamental to health is the fact that only he is healthy who never thinks of his health'.

He continues, 'In the healthy condition of man there is a spiritual vital force that animates the material body and retains all the parts of the organism in admirable harmonious vital operation, with respect to both sensations and functions, so that our in-dwelling, reason-gifted mind can employ this living healthy machine for the higher purposes of our existence'. 'Incredibly great is this if our physicians but knew how to keep it right in days of health by a properly-regulated, wholesome regime.' The idea of the vital force is fundamental to the rest of his teaching. We have the same idea when we talk of someone being 'healthy' or 'delicate', or 'having no resistance' or even being 'accident-prone'.

'When a person falls ill, it is only this spiritual automatic vital force, everywhere present in his organism, that is primarily deranged by the dynamic influence upon it of a morbific agent inimical to life. It is only the vital force, deranged to such an abnormal state, that can furnish the organism with its disagreeable sensations and incline it to the irregular functions that we call disease.'

'How the vital force causes the organism to display morbid phenomena it would be of no practical utility to the physician to know, and therefore it would for ever remain concealed from him. Only what is necessary for him to know of disease, and what is fully sufficient for enabling him to cure it, has the Lord of life revealed to his senses.' 'The causes of our maladies cannot be material, since the least foreign material substance, however mild it may appear to us, is suddenly repelled like a poison by the vital force, or when this does not happen, death is the consequence. If even the minutest splinter penetrates a sensitive part of our organism, the vital principle everywhere present in our body rests not before it is removed by pain, fever, suppuration or gangrene.'

'Every agent that acts upon the vitality – every medicine – produces more or less change in the vital force, and causes a certain alteration in the health of the individual for a longer or shorter period. This is termed Primary Action. Although a product of the medicinal and vital powers conjointly, it belongs principally to the influencing power, and the vital force seems to conduct itself in a passive manner. The vital force then appears to rouse itself again to action and endeavours to oppose its own energy against the influencing power. This automatic reaction belongs to our preserving vital force and is termed Secondary Action. This reaction is equal and opposite to the Primary Action.'

'The noxious agencies, partly psychical, partly physical, to which our terrestrial existence is exposed, do not possess the power of morbidly deranging the health of man unconditionally. We are made ill by them only when our organism is sufficiently disposed and susceptible to the attack of the morbific cause that may be present – hence they do not produce disease in everyone, nor at all times. It is undeniably shown by experience that the living human organism is much more disposed to be excited and to have its health deranged by medicinal powers than by morbific noxious agencies and infectious miasms. Cure is only possible by a change of the health of the diseased individual to the healthy condition, and the curative power of medicines is due solely to this power they possess of altering man's health. A medicine must be sought which has the power and the tendency to produce an artificial morbid state most similar to that of the cause of the disease in question.'

Hahnemann stated, 'There is nothing morbid that is curable which does not make itself known to the accurately observant physician, by means of signs and symptoms. Whoever will take the trouble to select the remedy for the disease by the rule of the most perfect similarity will ever find it a pure and inexhaustible source whence he may derive the means of saving the lives of his fellow men. None but the careful observer can have any idea of the height to which the sensitiveness of the body to medicinal irritation is increased in a state of disease. It exceeds all belief when disease has attained a great intensity. An insensible comatose patient unroused by any shaking, deaf to all calling, will be rapidly restored to consciousness by the smallest dose of Opium, when in a million times smaller dose than any mortal has yet prescribed'.

He then gives many instructions on how to take the case. The chief one is to listen: not only to what the patient has to complain of, but also to what his friends have to say. Another one is not to interrupt: wait until he has finished before you ask how, why, when and where.

Then he deals with the remedies and how they are proved, and with potencies. When Hahnemann began to put his law to the test he had not thought of potency. He used crude drugs, using smaller and smaller doses, in order to find the smallest dose that would give the desired result without injuring the vital force. Finding that the small doses were more effective, he started potentising. At the time of writing the *Organon* he was proving with the thirtieth potency.

It is easy to get worried about the question of potency, some advocating high, some low. He said, sparing the feelings of no-one: 'The praise bestowed of late years by some few homoeopaths on the larger doses depends on this, either that they chose low dynamisation of the remedy to be administered, as I myself used to do twenty years ago from not knowing any better, or that the remedies selected were not perfectly homoeopathic'.

The rest of the book deals with acute diseases, epidemics and chronic disease, and goes into more detail on points already touched on in this chapter.

3

The Patient as a Person

When Hahnemann systematised the principles of homoeopathy he emphasised over and over again that the doctor must be particularly attentive to those symptoms which are peculiar to the patient and characteristic of the patient; that he should not be obsessed with the symptoms and characteristics that are common to the disease. After many years of experience, Dr Kent stated that he regarded this to be the most vital point in the practice of homoeopathic medicine.

As a rule there is not much difficulty in recognising the symptoms that are peculiar to the patient suffering from an acute disease. These usually appear in an ordinary manner, and the common or pathological ones are well known. However, in chronic diseases this is not so easy, and it may be very difficult to separate the symptoms peculiar to the patient from those that are common to the disease. In long-standing chronic cases the peculiar and characteristic symptoms may sometimes disappear, or may have been utterly forgotten, and so make our work of diagnosis much more difficult. Naturally, in analysing the symptoms which are specifically those of the patient, as opposed to those which are common to the disease, one has to be fully conversant with the latter.

We first take a careful history and make a thorough clinical examination, and seek to make a diagnosis and prognosis. The treatment, however, is not based so much on the diagnosis as on the patient's individual reaction to the disease, for having made your clinical diagnosis, you must forget both it and the prognosis. The latter is difficult at first, but is essential and becomes a habit. If not, would you ever tackle, or continue to treat with hope or confidence, a case that was hopeless? While the patient has enough life to produce symptoms, you can prescribe on them. 'Where there is life there is hope' is the motto of the homoeopath.

It is essential to record the case history carefully, to pay strict attention to what the patient has to say and to let him tell his story in his own way. When he has described his complaint it is necessary to

9

enquire into his family history and his own past history, including any hereditary or latent diseases which may have occurred. There are many other things that the doctor will want to know in order to get a picture of the whole patient. One has to find out about his appetite – is it good and has it varied recently? Does any food upset him? Does he dislike something particularly? Has he a special craving for sweets, salt, spicy foods, meat, fat, fish, eggs, milk? Is he thirsty for hot or cold drinks, and for how much at a time – a full glass at one go or just a sip? Does he prefer hot or cold food? Is he ever dyspeptic or flatulent after eating, or at any time of the day or particular hour?

Then there is sleep. Does he go to sleep quickly, or is his brain so active that he goes on working out things and does not relax? How much does he dream? Does he suffer from nightmares – occasionally or frequently; does he find himself awake and screaming? Is there any favourite position when sleeping – on his face or with his arms above his head, on one side rather than the other?

One invaluable general symptom is the effect of different temperatures. This will often help in deciding the remedy. To be of use, the patient must be very definite in his reply to a question on how he is affected by heat or cold. He may state that he cannot stand heat, but on asking further questions it is not surprising to learn that what he really means is that he cannot abide a stuffy room and that he hates the cold.

Then there are reactions which our homoeopathic materia medica takes into account, but which can be completely ignored by an orthodox consultant. A patient with arthritis told me that her pains were always worse in wet stormy weather. She was surprised that I was interested. She had seen a rheumatologist who had said, 'It's no good telling me things like that – weather does *not* affect rheumatism'.

The most important thing to the homoeopath is the totality of symptoms. Hahnemann stressed that the most important symptoms are not the pathology of the organs most affected, but the mental and general symptoms, and it is these which take priority in the selection of the remedy. Yet it is the search for these symptoms which can be the most difficult task of all. So many patients are diffident about telling their inmost thoughts, nor do they like to reveal their yearnings and hatreds, their motives and fantasies, despite the fact that they are generally much relieved after doing so.

The taking of the history is not merely the collection of facts. A new patient will often feel encouraged because this may be the first time a doctor has listened to him or her or has shown an active interest in the details of some strange symptom. Even with the consultation over, patients will often tell you strange facts that they think have nothing to do with their complaints. I always accompany the patient to the front door – you often get important symptoms on the doorstep. All these reactions are mirrored in the materia medica and will dictate the selection of a curative, rather than a suppressive, remedy.

Thus so many things that patients notice in themselves become valuable aids to treatment – and not manifestations of a neurotic temperament. By the same token, the so-called neurotics can be treated successfully. These are patients who have qualities which make the doctor refer to them as hysteric. They are likely to show an absence of relevant physical findings, the presence of a multitude of symptoms, and quite possibly some evidence of psychogenesis. This patient may also have certain personality traits, a tendency to seek more attention than he is thought to deserve, a tendency to play up or to exaggerate symptoms, extroverted manners and lively phraseology, self-pity and self-concern, dependency and immaturity, and a tendency either to over-reaction or indifference.

All these are noted automatically by the homoeopath as he builds up the patient's picture. He can start treating the patient immediately without waiting for the results of tests, and he can treat hopefully whatever the diagnosis, or even if no diagnosis can be made. He finds that he understands his patients and that they trust him, and in searching for the symptoms which lead to the remedy that will help so much, he finds a new and exciting approach to medicine.

4

Potency

What is our teaching about potencies? That there are two schools, one high, the other low, and that the inquirer should take his or her choice?

My modus operandi, working on what I understand to be Hahnemann's teaching, is to give a high potency (10M) of the remedy most similar to the reactions of the patient, taking into chief consideration the mental and general symptoms, that is, the symptoms produced by the reaction of the vital force. If there are only local and pathological symptoms I give what I think will help those, in low potency (6c), till the vital force again is spurred to action, maybe by some stress.

As a newly-qualified doctor I had the advantage of seeing the results of Sir John Weir and Dr Borland with high potencies, and also those of Dr Wheeler, who used mostly low. I felt convinced that there was a place for both high and low potencies, but the question was what was the place for each?

Dr Borland had studied under Dr Kent, and then did a busy general practice for years. No one knew more about the personalities of remedies than he did. He taught us to study our patients and to look at them in terms of remedies; and when we studied remedies to think in terms of people. We residents were all very keen, and when we came back from an evening at the theatre we would not discuss the acting, but the remedies that the characters in the play were needing! No one was safe from our homoeopathic analysis.

Dr Wheeler knew more about the theory and philosophy of homoeopathy than anyone else, and he used to keep us spellbound with his reminiscences of homoeopathy and homoeopaths as he had breakfast with us, having already done the ward round at 8 a.m. It was on pure symptoms and pathology that he prescribed, not on the personality. With him we saw nothing that compared with the results of high potency prescribing in acute cases, but we did see results in chronic conditions; in chronic bronchitis and emphysema, in old TB cases, and in arthritic joints.

To summarise: in chronic cases the high potencies should be tried. Old standing cases clear up and patients are often surprised and delighted that something which has troubled them for a long time, and which they have come to look upon as inevitable and never even mentioned, has cleared up too. A medicine case of low potencies is also necessary in the home. Chamomilla at teething time, Aconite when the child comes in from playing in a cold wind crying with earache, Spongia for the croupy cough waking him in the night, Arnica for all the bumps and bruises – all these given immediately will generally stop the trouble from developing.

Many old people today do more than they really should, and for the resulting tiredness, fretfulness, aching limbs and increased rheumatism and so on, I find low potencies of Arnica, Chamomilla, Nux Vomica and Rhus Tox., as well as others, quite invaluable in helping them to carry on, and in many cases to feel surprisingly better. In cases where illness has left some more or less permanent tissue damage, such as rheumatoid arthritis, cardiac conditions, emphysema, bronchiectasis and cancer, the high potency indicated will make the patient feel much better; but they still have their pain and coughs and local discomforts, and here I prescribe in low potency for the local condition.

In gardening terms I compare my high potency to a shower of rain, and my low potency to the watering can that I must use occasionally on some corner of the garden in order to weather a critical stage.

5

The Constitutional Remedy

The 'constitutional remedy' is a term peculiar to homoeopathy. The dictionary says that the original meaning of 'constitution' is 'the fundamental system of laws governing the body'. This is true of our material, physiological body, but beyond that we are individuals, each having our own personality and each acting in our own characteristic way. The constitutional remedy is a picture of the sum total of the strengths and weaknesses of the person, mentally, emotionally and physically. It is in the early undiagnosable stages of illness that we must find the constitutional remedy.

How often does a patient come to you saying apologetically, 'I am not ill doctor, but I have not felt well for the last two months'. Or a mother brings a child, saying, 'She is not ill, but she is not herself'. It is easier to assess the totality of the person in a child, because it is there for you to see. In the adult it is not so easy, as time, circumstances, education, opinions and self-control all enter in, and it sometimes needs extra stress before you see the real person.

I always make a point of fetching each patient from the waiting room, and it is astonishing what one can learn in doing so. It is essential to notice every detail. The things we see and note can so often be something that the patient himself may be unaware of, or something he thinks he has concealed. There are some which are obvious immediately, such as the woman who was so terrified of draughts that she kept an open umbrella over her head!

One notices the young adult who is patently very tense – his resentful expression surely means he has been forced to see a doctor. Or the two women sitting together in friendly conversation, both pleased to meet again. Or the teenage boy reading a book, to the utter exclusion of a boy of his own age seated next to him. The second lad has a frown and looks worried. This fact, and his rather detached attitude, makes one feel quite certain that after hearing his case history Lycopodium will be prescribed. Without saying a word the patients can tell so much to the experienced homoeopath.

14

One notices if the patient is well-groomed or untidy; the appearance of the skin and hair; a blotchy complexion, a tendency to skin eruptions, acne, cracks in the corners of the mouth or on the lips; whether the hair is fine or glints, is coarse or greasy; horny finger nails, cracked fingertips, crusted eyelashes, or even a slightly blue tinge in the sclerotics.

We also gain information from the way the patient gets up and walks. The deliberate walk of the man who has come to give his history and wants to get it over and done with. He is rather flushed as he enters the room and puts his briefcase down with a slight tremor, but he quickly goes quite sallow and has a rather greasy skin. He may also have an eruption round his hair line, and one thinks of Natrum Mur. before he even starts his history. There is the neat elderly patient who is nervous and very restless, who comes into the room alertly, extends a cold dry hand, quickly glances round and begins her history before there is time to write down her name and address. These characteristics suggest that she is going to need Arsenicum Album.

On shaking hands, there are important things to notice. The cold, damp hand of the Hepar Sulph. patient, frequently with split and overgrown nails. The cold, damp, limp, boneless-feeling handshake of the Calc. Carb., or the firm handshake of the Lycopodium, particularly firm if he is grateful for improved health. Is there profuse sweating of the hands? There was the typical case of a nineteen-year-old secretary whose hands dripped with sweat. She had to retype most of her work because the paper got so wet and smeared, and even had to wear a cotton apron under the back of her skirt, because she sweated so profusely that it soaked through. She was cured with Thuja.

By looking at children you will learn through experience how to classify them. The untidy, dirty Sulphur child who looks as if his clothes were dragged on, with red lips, nostrils and eyelids – slow, lazy, hungry and always tired. He hates a bath, because his skin is frequently affected with rashes, and is worse for one. He is often hungry in spite of being thin and scraggy, and usually craves for fat.

I remember watching a scruffy little boy at a garden party, standing near a vast table set out with chocolate biscuits, cream buns, scones, jam and everything that any seven-year-old would want. The boy approached the table, and after looking at it very carefully, stretched out his hand and drew a dish of butter pats towards him and proceeded to eat every one! These children are characteristically the ones whose health improves when given Sulphur. I also remember a doctor describing a case of a girl in bed. He had not been able to get good prescribing symptoms and she was not improving. He suddenly noticed safety pins all round the bed and asked why. The mother replied, 'You said she was to be kept warm but she would push her feet out, so I thought I'd keep them in this way'. Sulphur was given and a speedy cure the result.

There is the bright, intelligent, eager child who sometimes perspires, leaving beads of sweat on the upper lip and forehead because of nervousness at coming to a doctor, but who otherwise never perspires without reason. Who keeps his eye on you all the time and badly needs reassurance. The mother will most likely tell us that when the child is unwell he cannot lie on his left side, and that his most comfortable position is lying propped up with his head back. He will certainly need Phosphorus.

Silica is for the child who comes in nervously or who is dragged in. He is generally listless and uninterested, but not frightened; he just feels and looks poorly. When in good form he is delightful and friendly, but should he be mismanaged or unwell he can look belligerent and bad-tempered. Sometimes it is better to see him on his own. He has a pale, sickly face with an eruption around the eyes, rough, yellow nails and very cold feet, probably damp to the touch and frequently offensive to smell. He sits hunched up as if huddled against a chill, and yet starts to sweat, particularly round the head. Most prevalent – and a decisive factor in prescribing Silica – is a tendency towards skin eruptions which suppurate and are slow to heal.

When we see a child who is fat, fair, flabby and pale, who is often dumped into a chair and sits smiling round at everyone, not stirring and sweating quite profusely in a cool room, whose general aspect is one of being weak and heavy, then we feel that Calc. Carb. will very probably improve the condition. This is especially so when the parent tells us that at night the child's pillow is soaked because he perspires so much. As he gets older he usually becomes a worrier and is apt to have night terrors. At school this type gets a reputation for being slow. He cannot keep up with others of his own age, either in work or games, and is sensitive to criticism.

Psorinum works wonders on patients who are often greasy and dusky, with a dirty appearance, whose thin limbs are covered with a harsh, dry skin described in some books as 'unwashable'. Psorinum is also one of the rare remedies for certain asthmatic children. The type who, in trying to ease their breathing, lie flat on their backs with their arms stretched out from their sides. This patient very much resembles those who respond well to Sulphur, but is unlike them in one aspect – they suffer intensely from the cold.

A frequent patient among the young is the fair-skinned child, blond, blue-eyed, on the whole plump and engaging, who also likes fuss and being petted. For some reason she will come into the consulting room tearful and hiding behind her mother, and yet for no reason will then be laughing. This very changeable child may often go faint in a hot room and will certainly wilt in the first heat of summer. They are thirstless children who hate fat and like sweet things. Their eyes are often strained or weakened, making them subject to styes on the upper lids, and at night they will sleep with their arms above their heads. We treat these children, with their fluctuating temperaments and physiques, with Pulsatilla, 'the wind flower'. The flower, like the patient, is very changeable, and Pulsatilla is often referred to as the 'weather-cock remedy'.

Chamomilla, on the other hand, is known as the 'can't bear it remedy', and we prescribe it for sick children who are in a turmoil in their tempers. The infant who whines and howls and insists on being carried about. The moment Father puts his baby down, the infant begins again. He holds out his hands for things and is no sooner given them than he pushes them away in digust. This calming remedy brings peace to the household within minutes, and it is said that more fathers have been converted to homoeopathy by the use of Chamomilla than by any other remedy.

Many serious kidney troubles have signs and symptoms in common – dysuria, oedema and albuminuria, and we cannot determine the curative remedy from these alone. If, in addition, the patient has a strong craving for fat, powerfully odoriferous urine and a chilling sensation in passing urine, these may well indicate that Nitric Acid is the appropriate remedy.

Should the asthmatic patient try to find relief in his breathing by lying on his face, possibly the knee–elbow position, Medorrhinum will be necessary. The observation that the patient finds comfort in this position is the essence of the difference between noting the symptoms typical of a disease but prescribing for the individual who suffers from the disease.

It is instructive to compare the picture we expect to see in a Bryonia or Phosphorus in an acute influenza or rheumatic fever, or any other acute disease. You see the Bryonia patient lying in bed – not in the least pleased to see you, for he hates being disturbed in any way. He is heavy and drowsy, his face puffy and bloated, the fine features gone. The lips may be dry and cracked. He is anxious and worried, mostly about business. He must get back because he had left something unfinished. He shows his irritability when you examine him. Every movement brings on some symptom and he keeps all painful parts still, either by pressure or lying on them. He is hot and sweaty.

The Phosphorus patient is entirely different. She is delighted to see you. She is nervous alone, full of apprehension about her illness as well as other things and wants to be reassured. She is afraid something is going to go wrong – some friend on a journey will have an accident, or an inspector is coming and she knows he will find some fault. You see someone really alive even when very ill, and often the picture of activity, even to the glint in the hair. The face is brightly flushed, then will suddenly go pale. Her skin is dry and will only sweat on exertion, even mental exertion, either on telling you her symptoms or from fright. She likes to have things done to her and all her pains are relieved by rubbing. She lies on the unaffected side.

Once we have taken into account the symptoms that signify the patient, and those which identify the disease, we come upon another important division of symptoms – the distinction between the generals and the particulars. By the 'generals' we mean those symptoms which affect the patient as a whole and which are of the utmost importance in deciding on a remedy. The 'particulars' are those that affect a specific organ. In treating the patient one must pay strict attention to what he may say of himself. Beside giving details which signify the complaint from which he may be suffering, he will often give other bits of information, such as saying 'I am thirsty' or 'I am cold'. This shows that the whole of him is affected and not only one particular organ.

A patient may have a number of gastric ailments combined with headaches, a roaring sensation in the ears, an aversion to fat and butter – all these tend to aggravate his condition and can be treated with simple remedies. If, in addition, the person is suffering from night-time diarrhoea, a nausea that arises after a hot but not a cold drink, and has palpitation, these combined reactions strongly indicate the prescription of Pulsatilla.

Many mental states consistently call for the same treatment because the symptoms are so consistent. Those over-fastidious patients, those whom we dub 'the man with the gold-headed cane', can respond marvellously to a course of Arsenicum Alb. Frequently the use of Bryonia, Nux Vomica or Chamomilla calms those who suffer from extreme irritability. The gently lachrymous patient can become less tiresome after using Pulsatilla, and a prescription of Platina will often change a haughty personality to that of someone more affable and more approachable. There are those who when ill become withdrawn, ungrateful and tyrannical, and who have a complete volte-face when treated with Phosphorus or Sepia. Many a would-be suicide, after confessing to this deep distress, has taken on a new lease of life after taking Cinchona.

These in a way are simplifications, for mental states can vary in importance. The innermost workings of the mind are determined by attitudes of will and affection, and these determine desires and aversions. One has to enquire after the prevailing moods, fluctuations of temper, what makes the patient angry, how he may react to grief or disappointment, what he fears, and does he prefer solitude or company? Symptoms connected with intellect and memory are of some value, but less so than others. Sleep and dream patterns are of importance; those who suffer from a chronic grumpiness or aggravation on waking often need Lachesis or Sulphur. The opposite temperament – who are irritable due to loss of sleep, benefit from Cocculus, while a course of Phosphorus or Sepia will make others feel immeasurably well with the world after a good sleep. Some people who are plagued with recurring dreams of throwing themselves from great heights are relieved of their painful nightmares with Thuja.

The question of temperature occurs in a patient whose whole body is markedly sensitive to a specific temperature, while some definite part of him is sensitive to an opposite temperature. Some patients may feel extremely cold in an acute illness and yet be covered with cold sweat and find comfort in being fanned, and will ask to have the windows open in the coldest weather. Carbo Veg. is the answer in these conditions. Lycopodium is effective in curing those who are in discomfort whenever there is great heat, and yet complain of stomach troubles and rheumatic pains, both of which should be improved by warmth. Again, there are people who are only comfortable in what they describe as a medium temperature and who will suffer at either extreme of cold or heat. It is the definite answer to the definite question which we need to help us in finding the remedy. Easy perspiration does not necessarily indicate that the patient suffers in hot weather, for those who respond to Calc. Carb. are the very ones who are liable to sweat in a cold room and who by temperament generally feel very chilly.

A patient's skin condition reveals much. Someone with glowing red cheeks and dry, burning skin among his other symptoms is often best treated with Belladonna. This is very useful when administered early on, when they are acutely flushed and the skin is hot, red and dry with

19

throbbing sensations which are burning to the touch. The patient twitches in his sleep. Often, when ill enough to be delirious, he has to be held down and will quite literally spit at everyone around him.

The effect of weather on the complaint can provide hints that will suggest or reject a treatment. If wet weather does not affect a patient's rheumatism we can eliminate Calc. Carb., Rhus Tox., Mercury, Natrum Carb., Natrum Sulph. and Ruta.

We must take into consideration the reaction a patient may have to periods of, say, standing for a long while. If there is unusual fatigue or aggravation to the system after standing, which is peculiar to the patient, then Sulphur might be indicated. On the other hand, extended lying on the right side might further aggravate the symptoms and Mercury could well be needed. Different sides of the body call for different remedies – Apis, Belladonna or Lycopodium for the right side, or Argentum Nitricum, Lachesis or Phosphorus for the left side.

We must also consider how diseases are influenced by time – it is not unusual for symptoms to become more aggravated at regular intervals, and this can be a decisive factor in selecting the remedy. Chelidonium, Natrum Mur. or Nux Vomica are recommended when the suffering is most acute in the morning, whereas evening recurrences of symptoms may indicate Belladonna or Pulsatilla. Some symptoms which only occur every other day make us look to Cinchona, Sulphur or Lycopodium. Should the recurrence be, say, every two weeks then we must consider Arsenicum Album or Lachesis. These two might apply equally well where the periodic return of symptoms is an uncommon occurrence in disease.

Cravings for various food substances, and aversions to them, are general symptoms of importance. An aversion to fat is common in people who need Pulsatilla – if by chance they eat fat it disagrees with them to a marked degree. An inordinate desire for salt could mean a prescription for Natrum Mur. or Phosphorus, whereas we would give Argentum Nit. or Lycopodium to someone who constantly craves sweet things. These are examples of cravings which would indicate one remedy or another when the patient recognises these hungers as having no physiological basis. In line with this there are the reactions to meals. Is there a feeling of discomfort in the stomach after eating, or relief? We must take note when a patient is made better or worse in an area of the body having nothing to do with the stomach. If a pain elsewhere in the system should be relieved after a meal, perhaps the patient requires Natrum Carb. or Kali Bich.

The effect of special foods on the entire system as well as on a specific part of the body can be helpful. As a rule only the digestive organs are affected, in which case the symptoms are only particulars. The special senses are indicative of the whole man and give general symptoms, such as when he complains, for instance, that the odour of cooking food sickens him. But should he be offended by the smell of an open drain, or a disinfectant, this would be a particular symptom and as such, not so important. There is a very significant general symptom which reveals itself in the blending of the general and particular symptoms into a harmonious whole. When all these characteristics fall into a specific and consistent pattern, the condition assumes in our thinking the name of the remedy for the patient. Thus those whose suffering in mind and body is so frequently cured by the wonderful remedy Sepia are called Sepia patients, and when the homoeopath talks of a 'Sepia type' he has a definite picture in his mind.

There are three other points to notice. One of these is the occurrence of a group of symptoms which we classify as 'strange, rare and peculiar'. A good example is found in the patient with a temperature of 40°C who is nevertheless quite thirstless, in which case treatment by Pulsatilla or Antimonium Tart. might be indicated. The second is the alternating of complaints, such as a stomach disorder being succeeded by eye trouble. Sometimes it may be a mistake to treat the patient for his stomach and then to give him something to cure his eyes. Not infrequently the constitutional remedy for this particular person will cover all the symptoms displayed, and will result in the cure of all his ailments. Lastly, there are times when a patient, whose constitutional remedy is already clear to you, will be behaving in ways that do not correspond to the picture of that remedy. Under these circumstances it is necessary to prescribe on the symptoms and modalities of the moment, and in the appropriate potency. If the symptoms are severe one would give a high potency; if relatively mild, a low potency.

6

Acute Prescribing

Kent said that all acute diseases, no matter how painful and malignant they may be, may be aborted or cured by homoeopathy. Typhoid and whooping cough within ten days; acute bronchitis, pneumonia, scarlet fever, diphtheria and measles within a few days; specific fevers within a few hours.

How does one prescribe for acute cases in this busy life? Once again one must know about a dozen remedies to begin with, and know them backwards. For example: Arsenicum Alb., Bryonia, Causticum, Gelsemium, Kali Carb., Lachesis, Natrum Mur., Natrum Sulph., Phosphorus, Pulsatilla, Phytolacca and Sulphur. Dr Tyler, sometimes assisted by Dr Borland, published *Pointers to the Remedies*, wonderful for gaining the local modalities, and with these aids one will soon be able to prescribe for an acute case with high potencies as quickly as in any other way.

Dr Hughes taught that every remedy had an individual kind of action and a special centre upon which it acted. Many remedies might have the same action on an organ, but there was always that little characteristic that distinguished it, which in an individual you might call the 'trick-o'-the-voice' or the 'twitch of an eyelid'. It was necessary to know the pathology of a remedy, he said, because mere mechanical symptom-covering was as likely to miss the mark as to hit it.

In taking a case, the homoeopathic doctor is frequently surprised at how often the patient's complaints fit into a single remedy. Not long ago there was a man whose 'gammy' knee was causing him trouble, and quite sensibly we gave him Ruta 6c. Some time later he came in for more medicine to complete the cure and asked off-handedly, 'By the way these pills couldn't have helped my piles, could they? When I first came to see you they were giving me great trouble and now they are so much better'. Ruta is one of the best pile remedies, and it was just the remedy for his painful knee as well.

The experienced homoeopath will not necessarily have to go into every detail to find the right remedy. Just as the orthodox physician can spot a case of myxoedema or pernicious anaemia, so the homoeopath will be able to tell in an instant whether it is Phosphorus or Pulsatilla that the patient requires. Nor is he surprised when, as above, he is told that some other, hitherto unrevealed, symptom has been improved. The patient's story and mental and physical attitudes themselves will often point in the direction of the needed cure. This is easily confirmed by a few simple questions, always posed so that the prescriber does not suggest any ideas. It is essential in a busy clinic that he or she has a full knowledge of the homoeopathic materia medica, and this comes with experience. But even in the early stages it is possible to acquire a thorough knowledge of quite a small number of remedies which are astonishingly effective.

Everyone had demonstrations in plenty, during air raids, of the different way in which individuals reacted to the same cause of stress, but only the homoeopath could make full use of these in prescribing. No normal person would claim that an air raid was anything but a terrifying thing, even though most people were able to control their emotion and show no fear. I want to mention briefly one or two examples of how homoeopathy was used in the face of this stress when control gave way.

There were people who, in spite of great fear, were able to endure the first few raids. As each day passed the dread of the night made them increasingly terrified. They became more fidgety and unable to compose themselves, until they could bear it no longer and took flight to the country. If they were given Argentum Nit. 10M they were able to carry on again and they soon learned that a further dose would stop that terror of anticipation whenever it began to come back.

Others dreaded the nightly raids so much that one was constantly giving Phosphoric Acid 6c to prevent the diarrhoea of anticipation.

There were many who were seized with sudden panic and terror of death whom Aconite 10M calmed. I have a vivid picture of a woman during the first bad air raid looking more terrified than I have ever seen anyone. She was not injured but was shaking like a leaf and terrified of what was going to happen. She was convinced she would be killed. She did die, it was said, from fright, but I feel sure Aconite would have saved her.

There was the woman having hysterics – sobbing uncontrollably – who only stopped to take long sighing breaths. People tried to comfort her but it had no effect. She would not listen. Ignatia 6c helped her to control herself very quickly.

There was the unforgettable picture of the man in an incident who stood, stunned, apparently unaware of anything, with a fixed gaze like a sleep-walker, an automaton, whom Arnica 6c brought back to earth and activity at once.

There was a woman who was having coffee with two elderly relations when a flying bomb was heard and everyone scattered. The restaurant was hit and she spent two hours frantically trying to find or get news of her old people. Eventually she found them unharmed at home. For several months she suffered from dreams of anxiety and severe pain in the right shoulder. It was only when she explained that these symptoms all dated from that shock that Opium 10M was given and the pain immediately went.

I remember, too, a girl of sixteen whose parents had both been killed in a raid. Her aunt, who took her in, noticed a gradual swelling of her neck and an entire change in character. She had been a nice affectionate girl and had now become silent, irritable, difficult and resentful of any sympathy, and in three months had developed well-marked exophthalmos. She began to improve in a week after a dose of Natrum Mur. 10M and was quite well again in three months.

And finally, there were the numerous people who complained that their nerve had gone since the raids, who were frightened of being left alone, always better for company and consolation, and who were apt to burst into tears over any slight worry. They responded excellently to Pulsatilla 10M.

It is often said that it is impossible to run a busy general practice and prescribe entirely homoeopathically. After many years of experience as a general practitioner I know that it is possible. And now, when I go and stay in a village where I am fairly well known, I am able to prescribe on less than five minutes conversation in the street. I find that, 'Good morning, Mrs Smith, how are you?' is not taken as a salutation but as an opportunity to tell me how she is, in the hope of being given a box of pills. I am on holiday and cannot spare time to go into the case thoroughly, so prescribe a low potency remedy and have been astonished at the results. Here are some examples.

Mrs H. and her husband had been given notice to quit after being in the same cottage for thirty-three years. She developed acute depression and a congestive early morning headache and had had a backache for some time. Natrum Mur. 6c was given and within a week she was quite a different person.

Mrs K. was thinking of changing her job. She worked as a cook and loved cooking but thought that the heat and standing was giving her rheumatism – pains in her wrist one day, in her knees the next, and

24

all worse in bed at night. I gave her Pulsatilla 6c. She had no more pains after a very few days and there was no more talk of changing her job.

I was asking Mrs R. how her daughter was getting on. All right, she said, except that she was getting one stye after another. I knew her quite well – a fair-haired, good-tempered, bright, friendly girl. I was not surprised to hear a fortnight later that she has had no more styes since Pulsatilla 6c.

Mrs M. asked me one day if I would see her husband and cheer him up. He had had an operation and could not pick up and was worried about himself. He said he felt giddy and very scared several times a day, with sweating and nausea, ever since the operation. I gave him Arsenicum Album 10M followed by Arnica 6c and when I saw him in the street ten days later he looked a different man. He was delighted in the improvement he had made in a week.

Mrs C., a housemaid, reported that she had sprained her ankle and it was so painful that she would not be able to carry on. Arnica 6c and she was all right for work next day.

Mrs H. came hobbling up the hill and poured out the story of her very bad varicose veins and the cramps she had every night. I had given her some Cuprum Arsenicosum 3c and she asked me if she could have another supply as it had been so marvellous and the problem was now just returning.

One old lady in the village has much experience of prescribing for herself and her family. With her no constipation will resist a few doses in 6c of Hydrastis, Nux Vomica or Bryonia. Antihistamine for hay fever has been abandoned in favour of Sabadilla or Teucrium 6c with a real prospect of cure, and not just of relief for the time being. Learning from her I now prescribe, in cases of migraine, a single 10M of Natrum Mur. or some other indicated remedy, and give the patient Sanguinaria, Iris or Spigelia in low potency to take for any threatening attack.

I do not leave out the animals. When out to dinner once there was acute agitation about a horse which had been impaled on a railing two days before. It was off its food and very restless, and the vet was worried about the swelling, which was spreading up to the girth. I did not see the horse but as they were homoeopaths I suggested they should give Rhus Tox. if they could find any in the house. A 30c potency was produced and given, and by next morning the horse was entirey comfortable and the swelling gone. I did not have more than five minutes conversation on any of these occasions, but they were all satisfied with their improvement.

It was while doing this sort of thing on holiday that I began to wonder why we did not employ this low potency prescribing to interest doctors who might wish to know more about homoeopathy. We cannot expect to impress them with results with Aconite and Belladonna in inflammation as their predecessors might have been a hundred years ago, because they ask for nothing better than antibiotics. But there are many conditions for which they have nothing to offer and where they could try a remedy in a routine way, such as for teething, chilblains, shingles, rheumatism, tachycardia and extra-systoles, examination panic and many other complaints. A few trials with some of these would impress them before they went on to something needing a little more thought. Medicals already in practice with little time for study could do this, whereas if they are going to start high potency prescribing they must acquire a much fuller knowledge of the remedies.

Prescribing homoeopathically is rather like bird-watching. To begin with you study the flight, the size, the colour, the markings and all the rest and then have to go to some book. But, when you have been at it some time, one glance with scarcely a thought and you can name the bird. That does not come, though, without experience and study.

7
Some Illustrative Cases

Dr Compton Burnett went through what he called 'the laughing stage of ignorance', before he put the law of similars to the test. Eventually he decided to try Natrum Mur. 6c on himself. He expected no action but, to his amazement, developed a crack in the middle of his lower lip. He went on experimenting and was forced against his will to admit the existence of something in remedies which becomes operative in potency.

He described many interesting cases. One, a woman who was awaiting operation for cataract, having seen two eminent London ophthalmologists who had agreed on the diagnosis and treatment. Cures for cataract had also been claimed by homoeopaths. He smiled at his own temerity when he suggested trying to cure cataract with a homoeopathic remedy, but the lady was delighted and he consoled himself with the fact that at least he could do no harm in treating her whilst waiting for the operation. He saw her once a month and gave her various remedies in different potencies. Towards the end of twelve months, he heard some very loud talking one morning in the hall and the patient rushed in crying excitedly that she could see almost as well as ever. She had seen the parting in her hair and had rushed off to tell the doctor the incredible news! The opacities cleared and her eyesight remained excellent.

He became aware that varicose veins could also be affected by homoeopathic remedies and proceeded to put it to the test. He experimented on a lamplighter with an enormous dilated vein in his thigh – the result of an old sloughing bubo and contracting scar. After several months of Calc. Fluoride 6c it shrank to one-third of its size and became firm and strong in spite of the man's continuing his occupation, which meant carrying a light ladder and sliding down it scores of times a day. 'Considering the irremediable mechanical hindrances at its inlet,' he wrote, 'the result seemed to me so startling that I have ever since gone in very strongly for the medicinal treatment of varicosis under all circumstances, and the satisfaction one has in such medical treatment is truly great. Capable homoeopaths have herein followed in Hahnemann's wake for a good half century. Careless homoeopaths, more especially since surgery has advanced, decline the bother and trouble of finding the appropriate remedy.'

He eventually prepared a 30th potency of Podophyllum but hesitated to put it to the test. One day a child almost at death's door was brought in with a copious involuntary offensive diarrhoea. Here, he thought, would be a case to give this remedy. Next day he was sure the child would be dead and, not liking to enquire, he went past the house to see if crêpe was on the door. There was none so far, but he went out of his way later in the day to pass the door again. Instead of crêpe, a smiling grandmother stood in the doorway. 'The baby is all right this morning', she said, and he went home feeling better. He went on using Podophyllum 30c and found the results so different from anything he had ever seen that he determined to get other remedies in higher potencies.

I recall one of those cases that impress both patient and friends of the advantages of homoeopathy. This was a girl of nineteen who had come up to London for a dance. The friends with whom she was staying rang me next morning, reluctantly, as they disapproved of homoeopathy. Her temperature was 41°C at 9 a.m. I found her looking very ill, congested, with a thickly-coated tongue, severe headache, a bad cough and feeling very sick. She improved slightly after Bryonia 10M, and her temperature was lower in the evening. Next morning she was coming out in a rash and by evening she had the thickest measles rash I have ever seen. I gave her Sulphur 10M and she quickly improved and an early patch of congestion disappeared. Her father came by car at the end of a week and drove her back home and she went off to a different dance three days later. Everyone was impressed because they had other cases to compare her with. Four of her friends had developed measles on the same day from the same contact. They had all been extremely ill and they were all still in bed when she went off to the second dance. Two of them had developed pneumonia and had been in bed – one for four weeks, the other six weeks. This is the sort of case that makes even a homoeopathic family more convinced and enthusiastic than ever.

To the orthodox practitioner every case of shingles is the same, only varying in degree. To the homoeopath each patient reacts differently and is prescribed for on the basis of that reaction. The two following cases will serve as examples.

The first case, a surgeon, had not had any sleep for a week; his only ease from the pain was to lie in a hot bath twice each night. The pain became intolerable on lying down, analgesics were of no help, and he felt quite incapable of carrying out his long operating list in two days' time. He was given Rhus Tox. (poison ivy) in potency and to his amazement he slept for eight hours that night and operated with comfort two days later. A few years later an American woman was seen with a vesicular rash on her arm. 'If I had been at home,' she said, 'I would have thought I had been near a poison ivy bush – it gives you this kind of rash.' In its provings Rhus Tox. produced such vesicular rashes and very many other symptoms, all symptoms being better for heat, worse for resting and for beginning to move, and relieved by motion.

The second case was another doctor, a woman antagonistic to the word homoeopathy, who also developed shingles. The symptoms were described on the telephone – purplish rash and surroundings on the left chest, very sensitive, much worse for any heat, and better sitting on the edge of the bed with a cold mirror held against the rash. Quite a different picture. She was given Lachesis, made from the Surukuku snake poison, as provings from this substance produced a condition like the above condition. The first dose eased the pain. She became a keen homoeopath as a result.

I had looked after a man for years who had occasional gastric upsets. He generally cleared up quickly but this time I failed. I could get few symptoms: 'just exactly the same as last time Doctor' was about all I could get, but neither last time's remedy nor any other did any good. I took him to an orthodox physician because he and his family were very worried. Imagine my feelings when I heard him say, 'I do hope you will get to the bottom of this, Doctor, for it's affecting my business. I've always been able to make quick decisions easily and it's essential in my business, but now I can't make up my mind at all and its affecting the whole office'. He thought it was probably due to lack of nourishment. He had always lived on fish in previous attacks but he could not even digest that now. I had prescribed for him before the specialist had started to take the history! He clinched it when he was examining him. Looking at his hand he muttered, 'a little dry eczema but of no consequence' and I noted the palm dry and starting to crack. Graphites 10M cleared him quickly and the specialist is considered a genius in that family still.

Gold treatment and steroids by injection are used with some success in rheumatoid arthritis. Homoeopathy is capable of providing some interesting solutions. Some years ago I was asked by a doctor to see a woman of sixty-eight who was practically bedridden with arthritis. He had tried every modern treatment and had failed. She was a typical Pulsatilla patient and I gave it to her. I was not looked upon with a kindly eye when all it did was to produce an acute cholecystitis. She was admitted to hospital and operated upon. She had a chronically inflamed gall bladder with stones. Now, at eighty, she is generally well and active.

Other cases of rheumatism get better so slowly that it is almost imperceptible. A woman aged sixty-three when I first saw her was in constant pain, getting upstairs only with extreme difficulty and able to walk very little, even on the level. She had started rheumatism at sixteen, and after a perforated appendix at twenty-eight had got much worse. In spite of every kind of treatment the disease progressed. With continuous homoeopathic treatment she is in much less pain and often has spells without any and is able to walk about, even up and down stairs, fairly well.

Severe burns have lost their high mortality rate since the discoveries that saved the lives of thousands during the war. However, the homoeopath can help even here. A young woman was very severely burnt all down one side of her neck and body, and was admitted to hospital under an ex-R.A.F. surgeon who had had vast experience of burn cases. She was in the theatre for three hours and every modern method had been used. For four days she held her own but on the fifth she began to slip. The surgeon held out little hope and when an old friend of her father's asked his permission to allow her to see a homoeopath he acquiesced. I went along to the hospital, found her swathed in bandages, running a high temperature and too ill to speak. Maybe more on instinct than reason, I gave her Cantharis 10M every two hours. She immediately began to improve and had less pain and got on quite amazingly. The surgeon and house surgeon seemed unmoved but the Sister, who had been actually hostile on my first visit, was convinced that the powders had saved the patient's life.

I was asked to see a man of about fifty who had been off work for a year; in bed and running a temperature of about 38°C for months. Everything had been tried, even cortisone, and he had been told that he would never get up again. All joints were tender and swollen, his liver enlarged and tender and he had an old cardiac lesion. He came into hospital and for some weeks there was no improvement. He had no general or mental symptoms, as I often find in those long-standing cases. My interpretation was that the vital force had become a bit exhausted. Tuberculinum Bovinum 10M was the best I could do, and very little improvement followed. I then gave him Calc. Hypophos. 6c when he complained chiefly of his wrists and hands, Rhus Tox. 6c when he was restless and wanted a hot bottle, and Aurum 6c he sometimes found helpful.

The day came when I was able to get symptoms on which to prescribe a high potency. He had become very depressed, and from being very uncommunicative he now kept me talking a long time. He told me all about himself as he had never done before, and had always one more question to ask as I got up to go. He had lived in India and did not mind the heat, he said, but today he could not stand this hot room. Sister told me that he had been very restless and sorry for himself, always ringing the bell for something, which was unlike him. The weather had suddenly turned hot, and how grateful I was for it! I gave him Pulsatilla 10M and for the first time his temperature dropped and did not go above 37°C again. That was the beginning of his improvement and he steadily improved, being given a high potency when indicated and low potencies in between. I saw him first in the spring and in the autumn he went to India on business for his firm and felt very well.

We homoeopaths know from experience that most cases of Bell's palsy follow exposure to draughts, and that they clear quickly on Causticum. A maid of one of my patients sat in the back of the car on a long journey. It was a warm day but she felt the draught on her face and tried to protect it. Next day she had a Bell's palsy and my patient took her in haste to an eye specialist she knew. He was very gloomy and said she might never quite recover. So on the way home she was brought in to see me. She presented a typical case of Causticum and cleared within a week.

I want to mention one other group, which are the hopeless cases.

A man came in to see me one day to ask if I could see his wife in one of the big teaching hospitals, because she had been there for three months with a nephrosis. She had seen several urologists and they had pronounced that at most she now had only a week to live. He asked that if that was the case then might she see a homoeopath. So I went and met the specialists on the spot and was given all the necessary information about her. She had had a very intensive course of prednisone for twelve weeks. She was swollen everywhere. Her blood urea was 480. I gave her Eel Serum 10M and in forty-eight hours her blood urea was down to 140 and the registrar was delighted and thought she was going to live.

However, when I next went in he was very gloomy. She was semi-comatose, very bluish in appearance and while I was there came to suddenly and said, 'Where is my letter, who has taken it? I don't want my things removed', and sunk again into semi-consciousness. So I gave her Lachesis 10M and left a note for the specialist that it was one of the snake venoms, and that Lord Horder had said that the only people who knew anything about snake venoms were the homoeopaths. In twenty-four hours she was a different person and went out in three weeks, very well. No one acknowledged that the homoeopathic remedies had done anything, but when she had a slight relapse two years later I was sent for at once, and this time gave Eel Serum 12c with a good result.

In the second episode I was awakened in the middle of the night by an unknown doctor. A small boy with purpura had been sent home from a teaching hospital to die; nothing more could be done. The doctor could not sleep, he said, wondering if homoeopathy could help. He could not have anything to do with it for some reason, but would I go independently and see? I found the small boy covered with bruises and bleeding from every orifice and too weak to lift a new light toy from his bed to show me. I gave Crotalus Horridus 10M. By the end of the week he was readmitted to hospital for a blood transfusion. In spite of having been told that the child had had homoeopathic snake venom the specialist demonstrated the case as an instance of spontaneous cure, for which one could not account. I heard of the boy years later – by then a healthy adult in his thirties.

8

Homoeopathic Considerations Relating to Conventional Prescribing

I base these opinions on experience gained in a career in general and consultant practice, convinced of the truth of homoeopathy but trying to keep up with modern methods. We believe that before an organ is affected there has been some upset in the metabolism of the patient. Our aim is to restore the balance of the body knowing that the organ, if the structure has not been damaged beyond repair, will again take on its normal function. The allopath on the other hand attributes the general condition to the diseased organ, and most of his efforts are concentrated on getting that organ back to working order and hoping that the patient will then feel better.

The general trend of medicine today is in the realm of prophylaxis and prevention. We have ante-natal clinics, inoculation and pre-operative prophylactic treatment. Is there anything in the ante-natal· sphere that we can offer while accepting the use of vitamins? What about Phosphorus and Pulsatilla in the early vomiting of pregnancy and Caulophyllum as the time draws near?

Opinions differ more in the field of immunisation than in any other. Even we homoeopaths do not always see eye to eye on the subject. In these days when people fly from continent to continent at a moment's notice, it is not so much a matter of whether we can treat the disease with homoeopathy as whether the patient is likely to come in contact with infection. I vaccinate any patient against smallpox who asks me but, to ward against any permanent bad effects from it, I always give Aconite 6c for twenty-four hours when the reaction starts and prescribe afterwards on any general symptoms. I have never noticed any lasting bad effect from this method. I remember being very impressed as a medical student by Dr Tyler's description of how she and her mother were the only members of the family who escaped getting the disease in a smallpox epidemic. They together treated the entire family homoeopathically and they all recovered. None of them had been vaccinated. I believe she said the main remedy used was Variolinum.

Ethical problems can arise in the question of immunisation and treatment of diphtheria by homoeopathy, as well as in the treatment of other infectious diseases for which preventive measures are available. What is our attitude? I have seen two children in out-patients who had bad rheumatism of the knees, both attributed by their mothers to diphtheria inoculations, which cleared up rapidly on Diphtherinum 200c. Again I have seen two tragedies from the same thing. The mothers described in each case a sort of fit and drowsiness all day following the first injection. They were nervous about the next, but the doctor said it had nothing to do with the injection and gave the second. The same reaction happened again, only worse, and there was no further mental development from that day. One child died; the other is still alive. If we do not inoculate and have to treat the disease, can we do it?

It has been proved, as judged by the Schick test, that Diptherinum 200c gives immunity and that, in practice, it is effective in the case of contacts. A doctor who had been a Medical Officer of Health for many years started treating the diphtherias in hospital without serum when he became interested in homoeopathy, and was thrilled to find that the mortality rate decreased and the length of stay in hospital markedly diminished. In spite of these results, however, when the health authority heard of this unorthodox behaviour they compelled him to go back to serum.

A doctor, therefore, who wants to treat diphtheria purely homoeopathically must take his courage in both hands and run the gauntlet of public opinion. It is easier for those of us who have a purely homoeopathic practice, because our patients' ideas and ours are generally alike. If there is any doubt let us give the serum first, if we are going to give it at all. Most homoeopaths dislike immunisation and, so far, I have only been asked to do it three times. I watched carefully afterwards and prescribed for any reaction. What I generally do instead is to give Diphtherinum 200c to be taken in December, January and February of each year and I have found it satisfactory.

My own experience coincides with that of other homoeopaths in dealing with the treatment of diphtheria by homoeopathy. When I see a suspicious throat I give it the indicated remedy. If on the following day the throat is improving, all is well. If not, I take a swab and again give the indicated remedy. By the time the swab comes back positive it is the third day and the throat is generally clean. I know now by experience that the swab taken then or on the next day will be negative.

This often leads to strange predicaments. Many years ago, the mother of two small boys in the country rang me because they had bad throats. She had no Mercurius so I suggested Belladonna. Next day they were no better so I went to see them and found two dirty, suspicious throats. I would not be seeing them again so took swabs and gave Mercurius Cyanatus. Next day the report came – positive. They had no local doctor so I rang the community medical officer and asked him to deal with the matter. He was very irate on arrival to find two small boys, quite well, and with clean throats. He rang me to say I had made a mistake – they had not go diphtheria. I said if there was a mistake it was on the part of the laboratory and sent him the reports. Another case was a woman who was given Phytolacca and sent off on the third day to hospital. She got much amusement out of being the curio case. Every one came to look at her throat. It was positive on arrival, though clean, and negative soon afterwards.

Has the allopath anything to compare with the effect of a dose of Tuberculinum in the child with a TB diathesis, with its thin body and hairy back, its blue veins and blue sclerotics? Again, whooping cough injections have and still do give cause for concern. I have never used it but have seen its results. I have seen children losing appetite and weight after inoculation for several weeks but probably escaping whooping cough. If they developed whooping cough the cough has been as bad as ever, only the whoop was absent.

Has whooping cough any terrors for the homoeopathic doctor? I do not think so, with Drosera, Coccus Cacti and Carbo Veg. to hand. I remember treating a child in the country by telephone and the local doctor agreed to hold a watching brief. He had inoculated his own children, and in spite of this they had developed the disease and were well in the throes of it before my patient started. His children were still giving the family bad nights (though they had never whooped) after the homoeopathic family were at peace. In the end he asked for some Drosera for his children and has been interested in homoeopathy ever since.

Even with the knowledge of the risks of anti-measles inoculation, does the homoeopathic doctor feel that it is advisable to use that method rather than homoeopathy? To the allopath it can be a dread disease full of possible complications. To the homoeopath, on the other hand, measles causes no real anxiety when we have such infallible remedies in Bryonia, Rhus Tox. and Sulphur. The patient may be very ill but he responds well and quickly at every stage, and the parents generally remark how lucky the child has been to have such a light attack. What a thankless task is ours!

In the case of pre-operative prophylaxis, everything is done today before an operation both to build up the body reserves and kill off any lurking germs by giving antibiotics. Is this the surgeon's field alone or can the homoeopath offer something here? Arnica before as well as after an operation is as valuable as all the other means. What a happy day it would be for patients if we could be standing by with a dose of Arnica or Hypericum when a surgeon had knocked himself or caught his finger in the door. He would never forget the instant relief and might be induced to add Arnica to his pre-operative medicaments.

Homoeopathy is a blessing to the surgeon in the realm of fractures. Fractures treated by Calc. Phos. and Symphytum unite more quickly than those without.

Does the homoeopath send for the surgeon in a case of acute appendicitis? Yes, immediately. In my early days I had two cases which taught me a lesson. I prescribed for them and sent for a surgeon. All pain and sickness went, the pulse settled and the patient seemed well. How foolish I felt in having sent for a surgeon. He, however, on the history, operated that day and in both cases the appendix was just about to burst. Whether these cases were exceptions I do not know, for I have never put it to the test again. I wait till the surgeon has seen the patient before prescribing, unless he or she is in severe pain. In these two cases it seemed to mask the symptoms, although I have never found it do so in other acute abdominal conditions. It may be due to the anatomical character and blood supply of the appendix not being enough to effect recovery, even though the pain is eased.

The treatment of acute bacterial infection has been revolutionised by antibiotics. We homoeopaths know the use of these drugs in hampering germs but the homoeopath's aim has always been rather to raise the home defence. De we still stick to this in the light of the new drugs?

In an ordinary acute case, even the beginner in homoeopathy will feel quite at home in dealing with homoeopathic remedies only. Nature is playing her part and the patient is not in grave and immediate danger. The symptoms are clear – they have come on suddenly and the patient and friends are conscious of the changes that have happened. In a case of penumonia the patient will feel quite well within a few days, the lung will be resolving in an amazing way and the patient will never know she has had that dread disease, pneumonia.

There may be a different case, however, when either there is a virulent germ attacking or there is no reaction from the patient. One winter a man and his wife, both over seventy, went down the same day with pneumonia. There was little to prescribe on and I gave Baptisia on the dusky appearance. The next day they still had few homoeopathic symptoms but looked poisoned and ill. I therefore gave Lachesis but penicillin as well. One thing to guard against when giving penicillin is sitting back. When prescribing homoeopathically you know that the speedy recovery of the patient depends entirely on your prescribing, and if you have any homoeopathic conscience at all it keeps you on your tip-toes.

They both recovered slowly and I was disappointed. Had penicillin failed? Had my homoeopathic prescribing been poor? When describing the cases to an allopathic specialist who asked if I was seeing many cases of pneumonia, he said they would probably develop lung abscesses. He had seen six lung abscesses that week in just that type of case. I began to cheer up – neither of them had developed a lung abscess. I feel that in that type of case of virulent infection or poor reaction of the patient we do well to take advantage of an antibiotic, always provided that we do not relax for one minute our efforts to find the simillimum.

Cases of acute cystitis generally clear up quite quickly without any other medicine than homoeopathic. Post-operative cases seem to give more trouble. Antibiotics will have been given by the surgeon and the urine has cleared. The patient, however, often still complains of discomfort and frequency and only after something like Cantharis, Clematis or Terebinth is she comfortable again.

Allergy is another happy hunting ground of the scientist. They have many drugs and injections that make the life of the allergic patient more comfortable. Have they found a cure or are they doing the thing which they accuse us so often of doing – treating symptoms? I think so, only they are objective and not subjective ones. I think we have a great deal to offer in this sphere, not only of alleviating but of curing the patient of his allergic condition altogether.

Homoeopathy has not changed at all since Hahnemann founded it, and since it has not been affected by all the modern knowledge it is thought to be obsolete. Medicine, on the other hand, is advancing dramatically every year. But as I wander between Hahnemann's *Organon* and modern medical journals I conclude that homoeopathy started in advance and that orthodox medical knowledge has not yet caught it up.

Perhaps we do not realise to the full the greatness of our heritage. Homoeopathy, as formulated by Hahnemann, is the most scientific and the most successful system of medical treatment yet devised. Our responsibility for its pure and truthful presentation is great.

Constitutional Prescribing

9

Aluminium Oxide

As a student I once visited a laboratory in Harley Street, and the demonstrators showed us all sorts of experiments which were carried out. The only one I remember was when they cooked an egg for four minutes in an aluminium saucepan and traced aluminium inside the egg. I could not help being impressed with that. I thought that if in four minutes aluminium is inside the shell of the egg, what effect does it have on a patient? Many years ago there was a doctor at the London Homoeopathic Hospital who was very keen on aluminium poisoning, and who put all the young doctors off by attributing every possible disease to aluminium. He managed to get the Navy to ban cooking in aluminium at one time and the consequence was that the gastric and duodenal ulcers in the Navy went down fifty per cent. I do not think that everybody is sensitive to aluminium, but I am sure that there is a proportion of people who are.

Mentally Aluminium patients vary a lot. They may be contented, very much on the spot, competent, with intellectual powers alert, or else there is the type who is timid, not bright in the mornings and on top of their form later in the day. So the best time for Aluminium patients is usually later in the day. On the other hand they may be very contrary, take everything the wrong way and weep a lot. This second type gets easily confused – they take things in slowly and answer questions slowly. You feel that they are mentally rather slow and apt to be bored. Aluminium children are also peevish, whiny and rather obstinate.

The patient is usually pale, although the colour can vary. There is a greyish tint which I have always met in the cases that I have looked after. They describe it in the books as 'Skin as though white of an egg had dried on the face'. They have head symptoms, eye complaints, digestive complaints, and their extremities can be out of order. One or two examples will illustrate the sort of things that I have met.

The first Aluminium case I ever saw was a man well over seventy with a letter from his doctor to say that for some inexplicable reason he wished to try homoeopathy! He sent his X-rays and a report from a specialist which stated that he had an inoperable carcinoma of the gall bladder. The patient was very thin, drawn and lined and had the peculiar colour that I have always since associated with Aluminium. I took a lot of rather poor symptoms, nothing very definite. He complained of constant abdominal pain and a gripping sensation when he tried to eat, as if food stuck somewhere. He said he felt awful in the morning but that he might pick up a little later in the day. He thought he was probably hopeless, and if I would only keep him from too awful a death he would be grateful.

I asked if he had his food cooked in aluminium and he said that he did, but was sure that his wife would change if I thought it advisable. I talked to her and suggested she should change. So conscientious was she that she would not even have an aluminium spoon to stir anything. He had an aluminium beaker in which he put his teeth at night, and this was changed to something else. I gave him Sac. Lac. for a fortnight and at the end of that time he was a little better, which made me feel there might possibly be something in it, and I then gave him a 200c of Aluminium. I did not see him for two months and then he had put on half a stone. He was eating moderately well, but carefully, and had hardly any discomfort. He lived for another twelve years and finally died from an influenzal bronchitis. He has always stuck in my mind as the colour of aluminium and one of the true cases of aluminium poisoning.

The next case was a man of thirty-three. He worked for the BBC and was getting on well. He said he had constant indigestion and that he was fortunate because his work was always an evening stint and that this was the best time of day for him. He felt much better in the evenings, although he would have fits of apprehension and worry that everything would go wrong. When he had had a bad day he would go to work thinking, 'I shall never get through tonight', but he did. He said the indigestion was such that when eating he got quite painful constriction of his oesophagus and had difficulty in swallowing, as if there was an obstruction. Otherwise he had vague indigestion.

Then he suddenly broke off his history and said, 'You know, I have a little boy of seven and he has a lot of the same symptoms. At the weekend my wife was away and I saw much more of him than usual. In two of the meals he clutched his stomach and said what a pain he had in the middle of his food. He was really very unwell for about half an hour and then when it had gone off he was all right again'. He said the child had told him his stomach ache was much worse if he took potatoes. This was interesting because it was the first time I had ever met that symptom. He also used to eat strange things like charcoal and cinders and all kinds of funny things rather like the Calc. Carb. child. He was very constipated and so was the father. The boy had no desire for his bowels to act and often passed a lot of small ball-like faeces only. He seldom had a really good action. The patient said he had the greatest difficulty over his bowels too, and seemed unable to strain or expel the stool even when it was quite soft. He also had frequent headache, more like a pressure in the forehead, as a rule sometimes very severe on the top of the head. I think this is where your Aluminium headache is if you have one. It is more often on the vertex. His whole head often irritated him if he had a headache, and he would sit pressing his hand on top of his head to ease it off a bit.

I had great difficulty with his wife because when she came back on Monday she had a new lot of aluminium saucepans and was very unwilling to get rid of them. Finally her sister lent her three stainless steel ones and I made her buy a different kettle. I saw the wife some months later and was rather pleased when she said, 'My family's health is entirely different. They are all so much better, I can't believe it. You don't think it would really be the aluminium, do you?' I said I was sure it was and that I thought they were all sensitive to aluminium. It is likely to happen in one family rather than in individuals. They have not used aluminium for the last twenty years, not even to stir anything, and have been quite well.

The third case was a man who had not been at all well, with a great many abdominal symptoms. He had had four biopsies of his liver and all sorts of other tests. He had had X-rays which had not shown anything definite, although various specialists thought he had a carcinoma of the stomach and his doctor had been very serious about it. He was a nervous person and his wife had managed to ask the doctor not to tell him what he thought, but only tell her. The doctor had told her that he gave the patient another year and that he thought he had probably got a stomach cancer.

At this point I was called in. He lived in a flat on the ground floor in one of London's squares, and when I went into the room and saw him in the half light he looked absolutely greyish. He told me he had a very great deal of trouble and that he did not think I would be able to do anything about it.

I went to see his general practitioner, who was a very nice man, who told me what had been done. He said, 'You can feel how tender and how thickened he is over his upper abdomen' and I said, 'I quite agree

41

with you, he is very thick there but I doubt whether it is malignant. You have not found anything in all your X-rays and biopsies and therefore I am hoping that it is not actually malignant. I agree with you that it will be if we leave it, but I don't think that it is at present. I think he is aluminium sensitive.'

The first thing I did was to take him off aluminium utensils and I left him without any other medicine except Sac. Lac. for a month. I then gave him a 30c, 200c and 1M of Aluminium, night, morning and night, and Sac. Lac. to follow. Four years later I examined him again and he told me he could not be better. He still had a slight thickening in the epigastrium, but less than it was, and said he could eat anything.

10

Arsenicum Album

There is one aspect of Arsenicum Album which is a point of great likeness to Lycopodium, and it will be helpful to mention it first. Both remedies show a very definite miserly tendency, but each from a different cause.

The Lycopodium patient is always supposed to be a bit miserly and to take care of his money, in case he does not have enough to live on afterwards. I had a boy of eighteen who put away any money he got and saved it up. His mother said to him 'I wish you would spend your money sometimes', but he replied, 'What would happen to you if father died and there was nobody to look after you?' I also remember another patient with this same peculiar Lycopodium symptom, in hospital with a broken nose and a broken jaw and various other symptoms. One day I went into all his history because of his indigestion. Later he came to see me as a patient at my house and said, 'I did not know you thought I was a miser'. I said, 'I did not know you thought you were either'. 'Well', he replied, 'Lycopodium is a miserly person. And I think you are quite right. I love sweets and chocolates, and if I have some chocolate to eat, I don't eat it if the last bit is there. I wait till I get some more to take its place.' I thought that was a good description of miserliness.

The Arsenicum miserliness is different, although it is sometimes easy to mix them up and one needs to be warned. The Arsenicum patient may have a fear of failure or losing money, and then they can be over-careful. Much more often it is that they are really covetous of someone else's possessions. They admire beautiful things and have a good understanding of them, and would like to possess them. I had one old lady in my practice who used to have to defend herself from a friend's daughter who would come to see her and ask for this or that particular object. The old lady got out of giving away a lot of beautiful ceramics and other things by saying that they were in the family trust. In reality it was that this girl longed to have them. Sometimes, if you are considering Arsenic you may not think of that particular

43

symptom. They can be afraid of failure, afraid of losing money and really covetous, but it is desire for possession much more than a dread of poverty.

In appearance the typical chronic Arsenicum is the person who is quick, alive, restless, who comes quickly into the room, sits down and begins her history. I have seen many Arsenicum patients who have started giving their history before they had given their name – it is quite characteristic of them. They have a story to tell and they are so anxious to tell it. They are intelligent and rather finely made. They are pale and thin, and I always think when I look at a chronic Arsenicum that they have much too much energy ever to have time or to put on any fat.

They are nervous and fuss about all sorts of things. They fuss about their health, imagine all kinds of diseases, and quite often go from one doctor to the other. They fuss about their family and they are never happy unless they have some specialist they are going to, some X-rays or blood tests they are going to have done.

They love to have more than one iron in the fire. I once looked after a patient for several years, but never knew whether I was her doctor or not. She would say, 'Last week I went to see Dr So-and-so'. I would ask, 'Well, what did he say about you?', and would be told. She was also an awful fusser, and made her husband's life a misery. Her husband really was a permanent patient of mine. He smoked, certainly too much, but she made him cut down. Finally, to please her, he cut down to twenty a day. Well, if he got down to twenty why could he not cut down to ten? – she gave him no peace at all. As I did not then think it was doing any harm, I was not going to enter into the fuss of having the poor man cut out his cigarettes, particularly as he once said to me, 'I could not stand my wife's fussing unless I smoked a bit'. I did so sympathise.

They also like their families to go to other doctors. The woman I am speaking of had no children but had lots of nieces and nephews to whom she was very good. They came to see her and she would tell them to go and see either me, if I was her doctor at that time, or some other doctor.'You must get other advice. I feel quite worried about this'. Off they would have to go to yet another doctor and had a most miserable time. She was extremely unpleasant if they did not go. I would say, if she pays for it it did not really matter.' 'Oh,' they would reply, 'She does not pay for it,' – and this is the point – 'she expects us to go because she has advised it'.

They are very fastidious. If you go into a house of an Arsenicum patient it is very orderly, surprisingly so sometimes. I always remember a typical chronic Arsenicum patient who had hundreds of books in different parts of her room. She used to collect books – she was a great reader and used to like to read first copies of this and that and the other. They were all piled neatly along the back of the sofa, or else they were all one on top of the other on a table. If they were the same subject they were all put together. I was amazed at how neatly they were piled, when I thought a room could not even look tidy with that number of books. It did look orderly – but not comfortable – you could not sit on anything because there would be books on it. The pictures were all straight. I have even known an Arsenicum patient straighten a picture in my room on coming in – they nearly always glance round the room – and sit down after that. They also always like to be prepared for things. If their grandson is coming for the weekend they like to know when he is coming, what time he will arrive, whether anyone is coming with him, and they like to have time to prepare everything.

The chronic Arsenic patient will call himself a fussy person. They are oversensitive to all sorts of things, particularly to touch, smell, light and cold. The chronic Arsenicum does not like the dark. I remember a patient who had had a great deal of trouble, and lived in one end of a large house all by herself. There certainly were other people in the house but they were a long way away. She might just as well have lived alone, because nobody was in reach or within call. One day I said, 'If you feel like that why don't you have a night light?', and the next time I saw her she said that the night light had made all the difference to her life. 'I really find it such a comfort that I could not tell you'.

I often find that they really do like the comfort of some light, otherwise they hear a noise, or think they hear one. They think there are burglars and get thoroughly worked up and nervous. They have a very vivid imagination anyhow, so that it does not take much for them to think that something awful is going to happen. They are also very sensitive to tobacco, especially if they are not well. I always remember that when I went up to the women's ward with Dr Borland he always had a cigarette between the ground floor and the second floor. But he used not to light a cigarette if there was an Arsenicum or Sepia patient in the ward because he knew that they would be upset by the smell.

They are rather upset by food. Nine people out of ten can take radishes and be perfectly alright. The tenth, your Arsenicum patient, will be upset by them if they are not completely fresh. They are upset sometimes by other fresh vegetables and very juicy fruits, or sometimes by any fruit at all. They do get quite a lot of diarrhoea from a food upset – Arsenicum is the second great diarrhoea remedy. (Phosphoric Acid is the first.)

They have a fine skin and very fine hair, and tend to sweat. Alternatively, and equally commonly, they have a rough skin which gets scaly, coarse and unhealthy and tends to crack with no sweat. On exertion they get hot and flushed with an acute congestive headache. So, with the 'skin' of an Arsenicum you cannot definitely say that the remedy has one particular kind of skin. Sometimes you are surprised at how rough the skin is of a patient who is otherwise so neat and who may have, say, silver pins in her hair. I always remember a patient who had nearly two dozen silver pins to pin back every little strand of hair that stuck out. She must have had twenty showing, but everything was neatly done. They are also bad sleepers and wake at any noise. They are apt to wake between 1 and 2 a.m. They feel nervous and restless at that time and find it extremely difficult to get off to sleep again. They make tea, move about, have something to eat, and then perhaps they try and sleep again and finally do so.

Arsenicum children are definite entities. They are nervous and precocious and develop very quickly. They are very likely to be pushed at school and often by their families too, and are disturbed by awful night terrors. This terror of the dark and being alone really worries them. As a rule they are very fine-skinned, not like the Arsenicum adult. They flush up easily, are restless, and never sit still. They have a burning skin, never an itching rough skin, but rather inclined to burn.

I had a good instance of this in a schoolboy of twelve. He was very clever and getting to the top of his primary school, but I felt a little worried about him, thinking that he was being pushed too hard. He finished at that school with excellent results and went on to his next school, which had the highest academic standards. I was even more worried about him now, because I thought he would certainly be pushed, and if he was pushed it would ruin him. I asked his father whether I might write to the headmaster and just beg him not to push him too hard, to which he readily agreed. The headmaster wrote a nice letter back to say he would do his best, and that he had told the boy's housemaster that he was not to be pushed.

However, the housemaster pushed him as hard as he could. The boy did all the things he was meant to do and came out brilliantly with a scholarship to Cambridge. When he got to Cambridge he wrote me a letter to say, 'I feel absolutely awful and can't get down to any work. I can't sleep and what shall I do?'

I had a friend at Cambridge at that time, and asked him to call on this boy. I explained the situation and said that I had put him on a homoeopathic sleeping medicine. The friend went round to see him and had the greatest difficulty in the world in keeping him from going off his head and having an absolute breakdown. Without him he would never have got on.

Every now and then, once every five weeks perhaps, a 10M of Arsenicum just pulled him together and he was able to do the next spell of work. Then I would have another desperate letter or half a letter, just a few words, to say please send me some more medicine, whereupon I sent him some more Arsenicum. He recovered completely, was able to work, and is now a professor in another university. He was an absolutely typical Arsenicum, and that was the only remedy he ever had.

You may need acute Arsenicum at any time. A doctor who had just started to practise homoeopathy rang me up and said he was in great trouble. 'I have a youngish man with me and his wife is here too. He is absolutely off his head. He has not sat down since he got here, he wanders about the room all the time and has been threatening to throw himself out of the window. He can't possibly keep still and he seems to be in a very bad way. Can you tell me what to give him?' I asked what remedy he wanted to give him, and he said Arsenicum. 'Well,' I said, 'give him a 10M. Give it every few minutes and then, when it has worked a little, send him home.'

The next morning he rang up to say that it had worked nothing short of miraculously. 'Within an hour he was sitting down having some tea which I had made for them both, and was perfectly alright. The next morning he went back to work, although I must say I insisted upon their having a holiday'. There is no quicker-acting remedy in the world than Arsenicum.

The other great characteristic of Arsenicum is that it has a burning pain which is better for heat. The other drug that has a burning pain better for heat is Lycopodium. This is its other likeness to Arsenicum. The only contradiction in the whole Arsenicum make-up is that if they get a congested headache you sometimes get them sitting as nearly as they can in the fire, but with their heads out of the window or in some cool spot. They like cold to their heads, even though the rest of them is icy cold.

11

Calcarea Arsenicosa

Calc. Arsenate was proved by Hering in 1848 and many clinical proofs of its efficacy were recorded by various people and put into Clarke's dictionary. It is a good remedy for epilepsy – there is no doubt that these strange Calcarea salts are good for epileptic people. Calc. Arsenate patients nearly always complain of a rush of blood before a fit. They have headaches which begin in the forehead and go to the back of the head, and this sometimes occurs before they have the fit. The last patient to whom I gave this to said that when he exerted himself mentally he felt much better, but that he felt absolutely worn out when he stopped.

They cannot bear changing their diet. If there is anything new in their diet they say, 'Oh no, I think I am susceptible to this kind of thing'. Either they take very little, or else they take it and think they feel ill after it. They also get pain in the eye. It is nearly always in the right eye and quite often recurs weekly, and this periodicity is sometimes very useful. It is usually on the opposite side to the one that they lie on. Calc. Arsenate is a chilly remedy and the patient is worse in cold weather.

They have a rather irritable heart and get extrasystoles. They get them much worse with any mental or emotional strain, anything that upsets them or makes them angry, and are also rather depressed and pathetic-looking. With their extrasystoles they are apt to get violent palpitation which comes and goes, especially if they are agitated. This same patient said that he was so tired in his lower limbs that when he got up from a chair he felt that he could not walk properly, and he was really quite lame when he walked. I asked if he had rheumatism but he said he did not. I said, 'You came in almost lame'. 'Oh, but that is because I had been sitting about and had not moved.'

The queer thing about this remedy, which is where it can sometimes be very useful, is that it can help an alcoholic to get off his alcohol. (He has to want to get off it before you can help him.) This is one of the remedies as well as Nux Vomica and a number of others that may come in, according to the history. I remember giving it to a patient who told me he had lost his wife and that he drank three-quarters of a bottle of whisky in the evening. 'Well,' I said, 'if you would like to stop, I can probably help you with a homoeopathic remedy and make it easier for you.' He did well on some Calc. Arsenate and I heard later that he had become very abstemious in drinking. I would give it in a 6c or 12c potency for three weeks and then stop to see how the patient was.

12

Calcarea Carbonica

On the whole I would say that the Calc. Carb. patient is soft, fat and flabby; as Dr Borland used to say, a rather useless person. Personally, I do not think that this is quite correct. They can be very nice people, live full and useful lives and do much good. In adulthood they have a rather large head. What you notice is a rather scraggy neck which gives the impression that they are much fatter than they really are. You think of Calc. Carb. as a child's remedy and do not give it to adults nearly as often as it is needed.

The patients are mentally and physically slow. They have a slow deliberate walk, they are cold, damp (never icy-cold) and have damp hands and heads, and sometimes damp feet. They are flabby and have a boneless kind of handgrip. If you ask them questions they grow exasperating because there is a long pause while they take in the question. You feel irritated because they do not start to give the answer. Once you have given them Calc. Carb. and they have responded to it you cannot believe that they are the same person.

Everything is in a minor key. It is one of the remedies which I think is not used nearly enough for depression. When they are giving you their history they often rather go to pieces, or if you look at them you see tears dripping down their faces, quite silently. They never burst into tears as any other patient may, or show that they are crying, but the tears just drip down silently.

If you can get down to their story they give the same difficulties over and over again. During their history they will probably repeat some particular difficulty four or five times. Their families will tell you that they can almost hit them over their head by the time they have heard the same story half a dozen times; it is very difficult for the people who live with them.

If they are ill they are sure they are going to die and become quite spineless, and again they sicken their friends by saying this and seemingly making no effort. They often fear the dark and have an acute anxiety at night. One of their great fears is that they are going

50

insane. They feel mentally below average, which also worries them, and have confused memories. If you ask them what they have been reading or doing they cannot tell you. They are utterly confused and in rather a poor way.

They have a fairly good appetite, possibly not as good as you would expect from their fat and rather large appearance. The one thing I have always found is that the Calc. Carb. patient must have his breakfast. If they have to go out before breakfast, even if it is a Calc. Carb. doctor who has to go out on an emergency visit, they feel frightful and have a headache in a very short time. If one such doctor whom I know had to go out before breakfast she was useless for the day. Otherwise they can get very distended. They can get hard and uncomfortable tummies and dislike their clothes tight round them and have to undo them, and they complain about this. Sometimes Dr Tyler used to say that with their weak stomachs they got very rudderless at times and I think that this is true. They love eggs and they will eat them at any time. If they get ravenous and have eggs they can get sour vomiting, which they will also often get after a milky dish.

In spite of their complaints, sometimes making a nuisance of themselves to their families with all their troubles, they are very sensitive patients. If they are gone for or even just ticked off, or if as children they are told they are no good in any way, it upsets them very much because it makes them think they cannot keep up with the others. I always remember a little girl of ten being brought to see me. She was behind everybody in the form. Sweaty, with a damp head and damp, limp hands. She had a teacher who used to tell her, 'You can do so much better if only you would try'. The point is that she could not do better – she really tried her best but was simply slow. She was put into a games team and was turned out in about a fortnight because she could not keep up. She used to arrive home every day in tears, utterly miserable. She had eczema round her neck and a poor skin altogether and sweated profusely at night. She talked to herself at night about all her complaints and all her difficulties, and her sister was disturbed by them and refused to sleep in the same room.

She was something like twenty-first in her form. I gave her a 10M of Calc. Carb. and asked her mother to let me know how she was in a month. About eleven months later her mother wrote to say she would very much like me to see her again. When she came in I would not have known her as the same child.

She had jumped a class and was second in her form, playing games and doing everything, except that in the last month she had gone back a bit. She was worried and said, 'You know, Mummy. I am not as well as I was and I think I ought to be taken to see Dr Blackie again'. She is now twenty-four, has an extremely good job and speaks four languages. Every now and then I get a note from her to say, 'I want four of your special powders, please'. I send her a 10M of Calc. Carb. and that just puts her right. If you looked at her today you would still think of her as a Calc. Carb. with her rather large impressionable face.

The Calc. Carb. depressions are an important subject. The patient can come in, sit absolutely silent, not speak, not take an interest in anything. They are heavy and dull in appearance, have a great disinclination to work, and are despondent and dissatisfied and melancholic. The difference between them is that you can, by your personality, get the Calc. Carb. patient out of his depression, whereas you can never, never lift an Aurum. This is the distinguishing point between them.

The Calc. Carb. patient is worried and down, and they worry about the most unimportant and trivial things. Even the most cheerful Calc. Carb. child is a great worrier. They worry about whether anyone has been left in charge of the dog up the road because its owners have gone away; is anyone feeding it, etc. Is the child up the road very ill or is she going to get better? – there will be something or somebody that they are worrying about. They worry if they see an act of injustice or think there is an act of injustice, and this is the sort of thing they will talk about at night; they won't go to sleep because of it.

They never have the sense of unworthiness that Aurum has. They may be beholden, but they do not think that they are to blame. In the books they describe them as just sitting and bending pins. I do not understand about sitting and bending pins, for I have never seen a patient sitting and doing it. The Calc. Carb. patient has very little stuffing, especially in this depressed state. You are struck by their inability to pull themselves together or to do anything. If we do not give them their remedy they may sink back and become weary of life, but they never commit suicide, whereas an Aurum can be suicidal and even make a mess of a suicide. It is more that Calc. Carb. patients have become weary of life and think they are a failure. There is not the acute melancholy of the Aurum patient and they are a much less violent personality than the Aurum.

They have one great fear, which is very constant in the adults, that they are going insane. I always remember a patient coming up to my surgery on a Wednesday morning. I was rather horrified because she had been coming for six months. She came from a distance, had a long train and bus journey and took about two hours to get to me. I was worried to see her sitting there again. I thought she should be cured and wondered why she was not. So I went into the waiting room and said, 'Look, you live such a long way away, I am going to see you next'. She sprang to her feet very pleased and shook hands with me – and for the first time I felt her damp, limp, cold, absolutely boneless hand.

She had always been blamed by her family and her friends. They got sick of her because she went over things again and again, and because she had a terrible fear of going insane. She was living with a wonderful friend and was miserable because she felt she did not give her anything or keep up with her or add anything to her life. She went on for some time, and I thought to myself, 'Now what have I been doing all this time to miss a case like this?' Everything fitted, her appearance and her complaints, so I gave her a 10M of Calc. Carb. and did not see her again for two and a half years. And then she came to see me and said, 'I am not really that bad. I have been wonderfully better. I just thought the last week or two I was going back a little, so I've come again'. She added, 'You know, I have lost all my fear. I don't worry my friend any more with the stupid questions that used to sicken her'. She is quite well now.

Calc. Carb. children are slow and fat and obstinate, and they are slow walking because their legs are weak and will not bear them when they are young. They are very slow teething. One of the things you are nearly always told about is that they sometimes get very emaciated legs but are fat and flabby elsewhere. Dr Tyler used to say that they had fat without fitness, sweating without heat, bones without strength, and tissues of plus quantity and minus quality.

Calc. Carb. is very good for hair, teeth and bones. We had an actor in the practice whose dentist advised him to have all his teeth out, because he had the most awfully sore gums and the dentist thought they were not healthy. I said, 'Oh, you can't have all your teeth out like that. Don't do it'. 'Well', he replied, 'I need them terribly. I don't want to have them out'. So I gave him some Calc. Carb., and in two and a half years the gums had improved to such an extent that the dentist was amazed. It helps pain in teeth. It is good in the early difficulties with teething, and also helps the second teeth to come through well.

It is a very useful remedy for little children who have rather fine, rather miserable hair with no real life in it. A dose of Calc. Carb. bucks it up very quickly. In the days when we saw a lot of rickets, it used to be one of the great rickets remedies. It is still very helpful in children who walk slowly or who do not get on, and it helps their bones enormously.

It is also one of two remedies that are good for the patient who gets a lot of exostoses. I had a patient who used to get them down his shins and occasionally in all sorts of odd places. He was an artist and found it very aggravating. First of all I gave him Calc. Carb. which helped him considerably, and he thought he was much better. He then got a spur under his foot, which was lucky for me – I gave him Hekla Lava and it cured them all. After all, the sheep under Mount Hekla get exostoses from feeding below the mountain. Therefore when we meet it in patients we give Hekla Lava in potency.

Calc. Carb. is also good for several odd things. For example, children who get a lot of glands with every cold or slight throat. One of the things you can make a shot at is polypi – somebody who is developing polypi in his nose, or polypi in the ear, or a cervical polyp. It is good for rheumatism. It is the chronic of Rhus Tox, and often when you have got so far with this, you can follow on with a few doses of Calc. Carb.

Calc. Carb. patients are bad at going to sleep. They say they cannot go to sleep because they have so much to think of, and their thoughts worry them. If they are small children they usually scream in the night from their dreams. If they are older they just find it difficult to go to sleep because they cannot manage to stop thinking. They get eczema and eruptions, especially infantile eczema, with the other Calc. Carb. symptoms of sweating and perhaps caring for milk, perhaps also of being very chilly.

They get colds in the eyes. It is interesting to notice how often the old books claim that cataracts can be cured by Calc. Carb. I am quite sure of that, when they are getting dim vision. I had two cases where the eye specialist and I were quite sure that both were beginning a cataract, and both reported that he said he could not find it. I have had that experience through the years.

It clears things – it is good for discharges in the ear, for old, stubborn catarrh which may be offensive. It is good for the patient who gets too tired and suddenly chucks his hand in, gives up everything and says he cannot work any more. It is good for this if you get it in time – usually you do not.

As a rule they have menses which are too early, too profuse and too prolonged, and often there is a murky leucorrhoea. They are worse before and after the menses, and their leuchorrhoea has a lot of itching and burning. They can have quite increased sexual desire; they can also have impotence – this is one of the things that Calc. Carb. men sometimes complain of.

In spite of a soft motion, and really no difficulty about their bowels, they do get haemorrhoids and sometimes bleeding, but more swelling and pain. The Calc. Carb. patient would describe to you, 'My bowels are really quite alright probably, but I get an action which is at first hard, then liquid and often containing undigested food.' On the other hand, Calc. Carb. patients are much happier and much more comfortable when they are constipated. Sometimes children are given a slight aperient so that they should have their bowels open every day, and if they are Calc. Carb. they are made quite ill by it.

A mother will bring her child with an Autumn cough, and say that if it is not treated it will continue for the rest of the winter. The cough is loose as a rule, accompanied by a blocked nose and catarrh. They get a sort of painless hoarseness and are scarcely able to speak in the mornings. They get a tickling, dry cough at times and a night cough. If they get any expectoration it is usually sweetish.

They also get very short of breath on walking up hill, and with that they can have palpitation and rather an anxiety.

They get a certain amount of weakness and bruised sensation in the long bones and also in the small of the back. It is quite common to have a Calc. Carb. adult who complains of backache. It is always worse when they have to move about, and even when they are sitting or standing their back feels rather beaten and their legs are apt to go to sleep. All Calc. Carbs. are apt to get numbness in the arm lain on, with a general weakness and fatigue and lack of power on walking and going upstairs. They also take cold very easily – I think they are one of the first who gets a cold in the autumn.

Another instructive case was a charming boy of fourteen with osteochrondritis. I saw him first in the country and he came in on crutches. He had severe pain on the insides of both heels, did not even like them touched, and his legs were rather chilly to feel and soaking wet. Sweat just trickled down and his shirt was very wet from his axillary sweat. He told me that he was a worrier, that his father had had a heart attack, that his mother an operation on her back, and that he had felt quite desperate with worry.

He had had to leave his school and have a tutor to help at home. He had seen six orthopaedic surgeons. Four of them had suggested cordotomy but the other two were very strongly against it, and the parents decided to hang on and see what happened. Then the boy got such pain that they thought the operation should be done. They arranged for him to go into a nursing home but brought him to see me four days before the operation was fixed.

I felt that this operation was unjustified so I tried to see the surgeon, but he was away. I then rang the Matron of the home and explained that I wanted to stop the operation and could she help me. She could not have been more thankful, because she was horrified by this suggestion and thought it was all wrong, so it was put off. I gave him Calc. Carb. 10M and arranged to see him each week. No crutches after the second time. Now he is well and does everything. He passed his examinations and has learnt the trumpet and piano, and works extremely hard. He rides and swims and dances and does everything, and looks like making something of his life.

13

Calcarea Fluorica

Calc. Fluoride is an invaluable single salt, and is used chiefly in dispersing bony growths. I always remember a boy of fourteen coming in to see me. He complained of a lot of pain round his elbow and pain in the top part of his arm. He found that at school he could not play tennis and that it was very hard to join in any games. He had seen the school doctor who was genuinely most interested in him but thought that he had strained it in some way. He had it X-rayed and there was nothing very special, so he encouraged him to play games. However, it was a sarcoma beginning in his arm, and he was taken into one of the teaching hospitals in London under a very good bone man who was there at the time.

This man met me one day while I was seeing the boy, and I said, 'Would you allow me to give him something homoeopathic?' 'Well', he said, 'why not? After all, I am not giving him any special medicine. I am watching to see if we can do an operation to save him, because this is growing fast.' I gave him Calc. Fluor. 30 three times a day. He improved so much that the orthopaedic man thought that he would be able to save him from having an operation. He was not in the end. The point is he had had two terms absolutely wasted, without any treatment, which I always felt had taken away his chance of getting well.

The same orthopaedic man took in another patient of mine later and rang up to say, 'You are coming round with your homoeopathic medicine, aren't you, because I thoroughly approved of what they did and I should like you to treat this patient too'. I was allowed to treat that patient too and he did quite well. If I thought the improvement was stopping I would either go up or down in potency, probably up. I might give 10M and sit back for a week and see what happened, but I would not stay on the same potency for too long.

I think sometimes that Calc. Fluor. can remove bony spurs on the heel of the patient almost as well as Hekla Lava. I would give Hekla Lava in the first place.

I have a very interesting patient who grew all kinds of queer nodules on her hands and then began to get them behind her ears. I gave her Calc. Fluor. 10M and saw her again in a fortnight and could not find a trace of them – they had all gone. I did not see her for months afterwards until she came back because she had one little nodule behind her ear and asked if I would give her the same remedy again. So I repeated it and every trace of it disappeared.

This remedy is also useful for eyes, particularly where cataract opacities of any kind are beginning.Usually the eyes ache and are worse on pressing or closing.

The other thing that these patients have is deficient enamel on the teeth. It sometimes gives you the hint that this is going to be Calc. Fluor.They occasionally have a bony growth in the nose, like a septum which has grown out more one side than the other and is increasing in size and blocking the nose, usually also with a thick yellow catarrh. They are worse for rest, they like to move about gently and always say it makes them better. They are better for warmth – they like warm drinks, warm food, warmth of any kind, fomentations and all the things you associate with warmth. They are also better for rubbing.

14

Calcarea Hypophosphorosa

I use Calc. Hypophos. every day. It has all kinds of characteristics, strangely enough, which you sometimes do not remember and do not think of. Fullness is one of its characteristics and can be anywhere. There is a sense of great oppression and fullness round the heart, feeling of fullness in the chest, often with breathlessness. If you can teach these patients to breathe properly I am sure that they respond very much better. Sometimes they have this awful full feeling and are so breathless that they cannot get up from a chair.

I use it mostly for rheumatism in the hands, fingers, thumb and wrists. In treating rheumatism I always try and get the constitutional remedy and then give a high potency. I am certain that the right thing to do, if you are going to cure the rheumatism, is to give six doses of a very high potency. The patient feels she is progressing daily, and is pleased with her improvement, but comes in and says, 'Oh my hands, they are so bad. This knuckle is enlarging. I have got awful pain down in the bottom of my thumb'. She tells you all about her hand pains and her wrist pains. That is where I find a 6c of Calc. Hypophos. quite invaluable.

It is one of the low potencies that I put in quite often when treating a rheumatoid. First give the constitutional in high potency, which is essential, and then follow with low potencies as they are needed. If a patient had trouble in one knee, rather than in her hands, I might give Pulsatilla, or low Ruta. There are different remedies for different parts. If they are doing well on their high potency 10M, and come in with a very sore right shoulder which will not get better, I would think of Sanguinaria. One must think of the low potencies to help on one area, or one particular part, which is so painful that they do not remember how much better they are. This sometimes makes you think that you are not on the right remedy when in fact you are. It is always wise to wait and see whether the high potency is really doing it before you change.

A patient with rheumatism can sometimes be associated with these queer feelings of fullness. I had one who came in and was terribly breathless, sat down and puffed and blew. I was inclined to take notice only of the puffing and blowing until she suddenly pointed out her hands. She was on a 10M of Pulsatilla and I thought she was going to do well on it. I felt that Calc. Hypophos. would possibly help her other odd symptoms as well while the Pulsatilla was going on working, and I am sure this was right.

Having had rheumatoid arthritis myself and being completely cured of it, I speak from personal experience. Sometimes you think that you are not so well and you want to change your high potency. Fortunately, somebody else usually gives it to you, which is much more sensible. Do not treat yourself if you have complex pathology. If you are prescribing on subjective symptoms you may not change the potency correctly, and in that way interfere with cure. In my own case I never had any low potencies. I had only four doses of a high potency which went on improving me for seven months, and did not have a repeat during that time. But it is essential, when you have got your high potency, that you know the low potency remedy that may come in.

15

Calcarea Iodata

Calc. Iodide is another invaluable Calcarea and one time was used very much more than it is now. It was one of the great eye remedies used by the homoeopaths at the end of the last century and it has many eye symptoms. It has conjunctivitis, acute lacrimation, any inflammation of the eyes, burning pain in the eyes, a pain that is worse if you touch the eye – if by any chance you press against it, it is always worse. There is nearly always redness of the lids. And, very occasionally, you get exophthalmos.

With their eye symptoms these patients often get a lot of coryza, which can be any colour and not necessarily thick or thin. Yet they always complain of dryness of the nose. A patient might say, 'My nose runs, but strangely enough, when it has finished running I always feel that it is much too dry, and it gets a little sore inside when it is dry like that.' They will often have no appetite at all for some days at a time. As a rule they pass very little water and often have a lot of digestive symptoms, such as fullness, sour eructations, and a sort of pulsation in the stomach which is very common and which they will nearly always mention.

They also have some glandular enlargement. They sometimes get nodules in the breast, which are painful when they move their arms and very tender to touch.

It used to be a frequent remedy for phthisis. I remember Dr Wheeler, who was very keen on treating this if he could, having four patients on the balcony of King Edward ward, all with acute T.B. I recall him saying, 'You know how fond I am of Calc. Iodide for these patients. But you can't give it to this patient – she is not hot enough. She has the chilliness of the Calc. Carb. although she does not look like it entirely. She does not have the scraggy look of a Calc. Iod. patient who is losing weight rapidly and who has an enormous appetite, which is one of its characteristics. You must think of something else. There is a Calc. Carb. element here that you cannot miss'. He used to give Calc. Iodide, never more than a 6c, and with good results.

61

It sometimes has a wonderful effect in convulsions. I always remember a man who got frequent blackouts. When he got blackouts, and I was once there when he did, he would shake and quiver and jerk and do the most extraordinary things. He then used to be quite unconscious for a while after. Calc. Iodide was the first remedy that helped him.

Whatever the symptoms, the Calc. Iodide patient is usually better for open air. Although they have a great tendency to take cold they cannot bear to be in too stuffy or too hot a room. This again was one of the points that Dr Wheeler used to take into account, although they are also better for open air. Many symptoms are aggravated or come on before food, and are better after food. Here again your Calc. Iodide is better for breakfast – but also better after each meal, which Calc. Carb. is not. Again like the Iodine, alone among the Calcareas, they lose weight very rapidly at times and become weak.

They feel they cannot go for walks or take any other exercise, and they are trembly and twitchy and not at all well. If the man with the blackouts went into a hot room he was quite apt to faint away, sitting in a chair. His feet and hands and face were always very cold. These patients are anxious, worrying people. Like Calc. Silicate patients, they too get rather angry over nothing. Otherwise I think of Calc. Iodide as dull and rather despairing.

16

Calcarea Lactica

I only use Calc. Lactate for one thing. I use it for the snuffly baby who really snuffles and you do not know why. They clear up very quickly on this remedy.

17

Calcarea Phosphorica

Calc. Phos. is an important Calcarea, with its own very particular symptoms. On the whole, I think that Calc. Phos. patients are more dark than fair. They often have long lashes and rather dark blue eyes, and when you see them at first you think of Tuberculinum Bovinum. Their skin is not fine but it is fairly active, usually pale, almost sallow and sometimes rather like a suet pudding! In general make-up the Calc. Phos. is above average weight and height. There is usually a history of growing very quickly and of wearing themselves out by putting on height so fast. They are long-legged rather than long-backed, which is a useful point to remember. They have damp hands and feet, and another very interesting thing, which I have tested out many times, is that they have damp clammy faces.

Calc. Phos. is mentally tired and they give all sorts of signs of it. They have weak memories and an inability to concentrate, and at times a great indisposition to work. They have poor school reports and are often brought to the doctor because they are not working well and have got exams ahead, and what can one do about them?

When they are tired their reaction is one of irritability. In fact, they are so irritable that you almost sometimes feel like giving them a dose of Chamomilla. They are fretful and peevish, and even if they do not show it you can feel it. They are full of fears and dreads in the evening. If they are anxious they complain of an anxiety in the pit of the stomach and they can quite easily get diarrhoea. The diarrhoea is always particularly bad if they have had a shock, or are very anxious about something, or if their exams are coming up and they have not done enough work and are rather worried.

They really do have queer symptoms – one that I have seen dozens of times is an aggravation from talking. The Calc. Phos. patient is exhausted by people quarrelling and by having to talk to people who entertain them, and they are very bad about staying as guests in another person's house. They are apt to go out of the room and disappear, and do not help the family when there are lots of people who would like to meet them. The Calc. Phos. child will probably not undertake her share at all.

They are restless and do not want to stay anywhere for any time. I remember a typical Calc. Phos. patient with her long legs – she had grown very quickly – coming in to see me. She would come in and sit down; her mother would sit here and she would sit there and in about two minutes she was up. First of all she would look at all my flowers, then she would look at something else that she had not seen before. Then she would go round the mantlepiece and look at all the things there. There was nothing in the room she had not examined and she never sat down. I used to say, 'Caroline, come and sit over here now and let me hear about you', and she would still walk round all the time.

Calc. Phos., adolescents are real grumblers and very discontented with their surroundings. They grumble about the school they go to. If they have been sent to one school, another school would have made them so much happier. They grumble at the friends they have got, the people they see, and they often blame their parents for not having done something better or different. When they are fifteen or sixteen they get a real mood of discontent which goes on all the time. It is quite possible that they will even take to drugs, although if you give them Calc. Phos. in time they do not.

Calc. Phos. children of twelve, thirteen and fourteen are very apt to get headaches. The headaches are brought on by intense application or by exposure to cold, especially a cold wind. They are much better from bathing the head in cold water. They can be made worse by driving in a car which is a bit jolty and they are much worse for pressure, so they cannot wear a tight hat.

They are worse for both physical and mental effort and they are worse at night. The last patient I had with this typical history was a boy of fifteen. I went to touch his head, and a colder, clammier head you could not have found, just as I expected. They have them when they come home from school, particularly if they have had to concentrate hard. Occasionally they feel as if there is a vice at the back of the head. This is a peculiar symptom and very rare.

They get a lot of chronic catarrh. They are apt to get coryza in a cold room but this stops when they get warm enough.

Their teeth have always been late in coming, and in adolescence they are very sensitive. They will quite often have been a Calc. Carb. baby or little child and then they come into a Calc. Phos. stage, and they may end up as Phosphorus. This is quite a common thing.

64

They like salt very much but prefer to have it as salt bacon or salt meat or some other salty thing, rather than the salt itself. They get an easily disordered stomach and sometimes find that milk, or very cold drinks, which they are apt to take on a hot day, or ice cream, will upset them. Fruit can also upset the stomach. As a rule, if they are upset by any of these things, they get a certain amount of pain and diarrhoea.

They sometimes get very painful periods. Through the years I have found that this starts for many of them when they caught cold during their first period. It may then go on for a bit, but usually Calc. Phos. will stop it.

The lower limbs are always rather cold – it is the cold feet of these patients that get rheumatic, and they are better for warmth and rest. They have a bit of the Calc. Carb. make-up – the weakness, the worse for cold, worse for movement, the sweating and the ability to push themselves to excess. They do not give up their jobs in the same way as Calc. Carb.

18
Calcarea Silicica

This is a deep-acting remedy and I am quite sure that it is not used enough. Calc. Silicate patients are often pale and anaemic and are apt to get bad catarrh with a thick greenish-yellow discharge. They are chilly, and very sensitive to alcohol. After half a glass of alcohol they can feel their heads swimming as if they could not walk straight. They have no special hour of feeling at their worst. One symptom that distinguishes them from Calc. Carb. is that they are rather apt to feel worse after breakfast.

Another thing about them is that they are weak. They will go out and fall down one step and slightly twist their ankles. It will be a major problem for a few days because they do not stand pain well and they are not at all well afterwards. (The other two remedies that strain their ankles easily and feel excessive pain are Arsenicum and China.) Most Calc. Silicate symptoms are worse for motion.

One patient of mine had all sorts of Calc. Silicate symptoms – the after-breakfast aggravation, the great chilliness and weakness generally. She had had to carry a heavy suitcase and had pain in the muscles of her arm. This pain went on for ten days, until I gave her Calc. Silicate. I had first given her Ruta and thought it was a ridiculously undue result from such a small thing. I gave her Calc. Silicate and it cleared up in twenty-four hours.

They complain of numbness a lot, and as a rule the numbness is on the side lain on. I had a new patient to whom I almost gave Calc. Silicate, but finally did not. She had this exaggerated pain after a sprain caused by carrying a heavy weight, but she did not quite fit – she was a little too restless. While she sat and explained her symptoms she undid and did up a button, and then undid and did up her bag, and was never for one instance quite still, so I gave her Arsenicum Album in the end instead.

They often describe their pain as burning, and can get excitable and angry. On the whole they are much too weak and too indifferent to get really angry. If they do, they are much worse for the anger.

They are always tired and they worry over everything. They particularly worry when they are going to go to sleep at night, because they often have vivid dreams which disturb them. One very good case was a girl of twenty-seven who came to see me. When she came into the consulting room I put her down as being thirty-five, just to show how much older she looked than she really was. She walked in with a total lack of vitality, as if she could hardly get to the chair. She said she never felt completely quite well, and that she had a miserable life because she was always dead beat. She was apt to get pains in her legs which were always going numb.

She gave one curious symptom. She said, 'I don't really sweat, but I can get what I call moist. But if I go into a cool room or into a draught of air or out into the open air, it stops at once. If I do that I feel thoroughly mussy and a bit sort of swimmy in the head afterwards. The great characteristic was that her sweat, which was never very profuse, but definitely there, would stop instantly. Her feet tended to sweat at times but it was just the same; they would dry up at once if she went into a different room.

She came to see me not only because she never felt well, but also because she recently had an ulcer in her leg following a blow. She could not get rid of it and it made her feel run down and miserable. When I looked at her leg there was quite a large ulcer with a greenish-yellow plug of discharge in it, thick and horrible. That was the first thing which made me think of Calc. Silicate. She also had a tendency to eruptions, and the day I saw her there was a patch of ezcema. It began at the lip and went out onto her cheek, and she could not help scratching it. 'I don't mean to, but I sit and find myself scratching away at this bit, and afterwards it is likely to bleed and can be very irritable. It is much worse for scratching, and rather inclined to look burning and red.'

She also said that she was extremely constipated and that she had to strain very much to pass the stool. If she did get her bowels open every day she felt much better, but that it was almost never the case. She was rather stiff in the back and hated it being pressed. She also had a lot of cracks in her hands and fingers, rather reminding one of Slica.

There is a strong element of Silica in Calc. Silicate, and this comes up every now and then. You think the patient has got to be Silica as they describe their slightly damp feet, or whatever it is, and their slight sweat everywhere. And then there are the cracks in their hands, and you think immediately of Silica again, but they do not really fit into Silica.

67

19

Calcarea Sulphurica

Calc. Sulph. is a mixture of Calc. Carb. and Sulphur. It is like them both and has symptoms of them both. It is likely to be in patients who are apt to get boils, abscesses or suppuration of any kind, and just at that point it is rather like Pyrogen. But Calc. Sulph. heals up from below. It is the best of all the acne remedies, unless there are strong indications for something else. The lesions are slow to heal and the patient is very sensitive to cold air and draughts and takes cold easily. But in some complaints they feel the heat, as in their headaches, croup, choking and pains and for that reason are really a mixture of Calc. Carb. and Sulphur.

They get complaints from over-lifting and over-straining and pulsating pains in their chests, or pains in their limbs. These complaints are all worse on standing, and from walking fast and getting overheated. Sometimes they are worse from the warmth of the bed.

On the whole they are irritable. They are easily angered and have a great anxiety about their health, their future, and what is going to happen to them. They are full of imagination when trying to go to sleep, and if ill are quite apt to feel that they will not recover, especially in hot weather. I think on the whole that they are discontented people. If it is just an acne they are merely troublesome. I do not think that acne patients have this general discontentedness. In these circumstances I would give only the Calc. Sulph. and then as a 6c. I would not expect it to be their constitutional remedy. I possibly should give them a 10M of Sulphur or whatever it was, or even a 10M of Calc. Carb., and wait a bit and then follow up with Calc. Sulph. 6c, because I think it is an easier thing to do. I would give them Calc. Sulph. 10M if they are discontented at all times and have rather weak memories, cannot make up their minds, cannot remember, cannot add up correctly, and never get anything quite right.

They have rather poor bodies generally, which is why they are always complaining of something. They like to sit and meditate over all their misfortunes but lose the thread of what they are going to say, and with all this you nearly always find that they have very cold feet. They have heat everywhere else – they do not want too many bed-clothes on, and cannot bear too many clothes at all, and on the whole they are better in the open air.

They have all kinds of eruptions – not only acne – on the scalp, crusty eczema, pimples and the hair can fall out.

A young man came to see me with the most awful acne. His father was ashamed of the sight of him and had sent him to a skin specialist, who put him on to deep X-ray treatment and hormones. I had cured one of his friends so he came to see me on his own, and I gave him some Calc. Sulph. A month later I got a letter from the specialist to say, 'So-and-so tells me that he has been to see you and I would very much like to know what you gave him, because his skin is much better'. So I wrote and told him what I had given him.

The joke was that the skin specialist was enraged to think that homoeopathy had done it. He got on to the father who then forbade his son to see me again. So the next thing I had was a letter from the young man to say, 'If I call at your house would you mind putting me out a box of pills? I can't come and see you because I have been forbidden to do so by my father and the skin specialist, and as my father is paying I do not feel I can come and see you.' He wrote later to say that he had been better for the last year and to ask if I would mind putting out another box for him to collect.

They get quite a lot of periodical headaches, often in the morning and afternoon which are always better in the open air. They have crusts, often round their nose, and they sneeze a lot; that again is better in the open air. They get cracked lips and a lot of flushing of the face. Otherwise they are rather pale and sickly, often looking like a mixture of Calcarea and Sulphur.

Sometimes you get swollen glands with Calc. Sulph., just as you do with all the Calcareas. The patients get glands in the groins, glands round the neck and glands under the arm. They have ulcers and vesicles in the mouth, and skin complaints characterised by burning, itching and often a degree of suppuration.

20

Cuprum Metallicum

I use this remedy several times a week and find it most valuable. It is principally a convulsive remedy, characterized by violence – spasms, cramp, diarrhoea and coughs. I have always found it useful to remember those four aspects in its complaints. In appearance Cuprum patients are pale and rather distressed-looking, or they are bluish and in extreme distress. They often present with a lot of jerkings, spasms and twitchings, which you can see very easily. Their mentals vary. When feeling awful they chat incoherently and it is difficult to stop them. If extremely ill, they tend to become delirious, and cannot remember anything about themselves.

A curious thing about Cuprum patients is that they are bored stiff if they are idle, even though they are disinclined to work. Therefore, they are always doing something. If they are not tossing about in bed they are up and down or moving about, but never content to do nothing. They are fretful and are apt either to burst into tears or else to be very amusing and show off with a sort of buffoonery. They often have vertigo, and tell you that they will fall forward or that the head feels as if it is falling forward, and that they are better for motion and are better for lying down. They have all sorts of frights, nothing particularly definite.

It is interesting to note that copper has been known and used for generations. A hundred years ago there were hardly any people in the East End of London who did not have copper insoles as a protection against getting epidemic diarrhoea or possibly cholera or any other illness that might be about. Most of them, particularly Jews, had copper insoles. At another time they had copper discs over parts of their back if they had acute backache. The third thing is the copper bracelet. I do not approve of them at all. However, the ones who tell you that these are useful and have done them good will often have quite a number of symptoms that fit in with Cuprum.

The Cuprum patient nearly always complains of a metallic taste in the mouth. There is only one other patient who complains consistently of a metallic taste and that is Rhus Tox. They nearly all have relief from cold water. If you can get a Cuprum patient with a really awful cough to risk taking a few sips of cold water it helps enormously. They have a lot of eye symptoms, dimness of vision, rolling up of the eyes, itching of the eyes.

They have constriction of the throat, too, as well as a variety of abdominal symptoms, colic, violent vomiting and acute pain. They eat fast, which makes their pains worse as a rule. They prefer cold food and have a great thirst for cold water. They are greedy patients and have not got a true appetite. They come down to a meal and think they will finish it as quickly as possible, and gobble it down. They can also get nausea and severe vomiting at times, always relieved by drinking cold water. They can get cramp with their abdominal colic with gushing, sudden stools, also better from cold water. Cramp and colic are common and the abdomen, if they are getting colic, is very tender to touch.

Respiratory symptoms are common. They get a spasmodic cough, which can be an awful nuisance with suppressed respirations and violent dyspnoea, and you can hear it at a distance. I always remember standing in a room and hearing the patient above coughing this spasmodic cough. It made me think, even downstairs, that he was going to need Cuprum when I got up to him.

The following four cases show the type for which Cuprum is useful. The first was a man whom I looked after for years. He had been gassed in the first world war, and had only half a left lung but a fairly normal right lung. He had a great tendency to get bronchitis. If he had bronchitis he would get pneumonia by the next day if you had not been to him in time. If I got to him in time with Bryonia I usually stopped it. He then went on as a rule to Natrum Sulph. and three or four times he cleared up well and effectively, and I was very pleased.

One night I had just got home when I was called urgently to come round at once. I arrived to find him having the most terrifying and violent attack of coughing that I have ever seen in my life. He was sitting in a chair and the attack of coughing was so violent that he toppled out of his chair and lay on the ground with his hands contracted, his thumbs drawn in, looking absolutely awful and apparently quite unconscious. He lived in a hotel in London and I sent for the porter. We took the mattress off his bed and put it on the floor because we could not have easily lifted him into bed.

I then found that in my pocket, by a bit of great luck, I had a 30c of Cuprum. I pulled down his lip and put a few granules on his tongue. I stayed for an hour and every quarter of an hour I put another dose on his tongue. Then I thought he was a little better. He was still intermittently unconscious and did not know where he was. I held a cup to his lips and he thankfully drank down some cold water which obviously relieved him. At the end of an hour I went away. It was by that time half past nine at night and I said that I would come round very early in the morning to see how he was.

When I went round in the morning the only person who had had an absolutely perfect night was the patient! His wife had been up all night. The porter, who was very fond of him and had known him for some years, had come up three times in the night from his room. He completely recovered, but never for the rest of his life – and he lived another twelve years – did he go about without his Cuprum.

I then had a man who used to go every year to his regimental dinner. This was one of his great functions and weeks beforehand he would say to me, 'I hope I shall be all right to go. Two great friends of mine are there and I am very anxious to go.' Then he said, 'The last two occasions I choked in the middle of dinner and had to go out. Can you stop it?' I said, 'Of course I can stop it. No doubt about it!' I gave him some Cuprum 30c which he put in his snuff box and carried in his waistcoat pocket. He got to the dinner and when he thought he was going to choke and became scared stiff about it, he took one of his pills and never thought any more about it again for the whole of the evening. He too carried Cuprum for the rest of his life. It stopped his tendency to choke, his throat to contract and the awful spasm of coughing to follow.

One of my patients, about eighty years old, sent for me at five o'clock one morning because he had the most awful cramp from his ankle to his knee. His whole leg was in a state of complete spasm. There was no question that it was just a cramp which would go off. It was agonizingly painful, and he was in very great distress. I gave him Cuprum straight away, because there was obvious violence of contraction, and ten minutes later it had all gone off. The contraction had lasted for an hour before I arrived. Again, this patient carried the remedy for the rest of his life.

Another interesting case was that of a woman who used to get the most queer symptom. Her upper eyelids would both contract and close so that she could not see a thing. She had to prop them up in order to see. Then, if she let them go, they would contract again. It was a most embarrassing situation for her because she did not know when it would come. I sent her to an eye specialist and to various people to see what it could be. They all said it was an acute contraction of her upper eyelids and that it was obviously troublesome to her. The condition cleared up with Cuprum.

The fourth case is a young woman singer who lives under great strain. She got terrified when she was about to sing, because her leg would go rigid and she was not sure if she would be able to walk across the platform. It was not painful, strangely enough – just an acute spasm. I expected it to be painful from the look of her and the description she gave, but she said it was not, just that it was terrifying. She has carried Cuprum for the last four months. She rang up one day to say, 'I have got a very important concert three nights running this week, do you think I could take a dose of your medicine even if I feel the cramp or not?' I said, 'Certainly, take it beforehand, take it as a preventitive', which she did and so far has met with success.

21

Ferrum Metallicum

The outstanding characteristic of the Ferrum patient is that they are always clear-skinned, as a rule with an unstable circulation. They are liable to become pale, or else flush up on any emotional excitement or exertion, or on a stimulus of any kind, either food or drink. The typical patient has a fair skin and a fair amount of colour, particularly round the cheek bones, accompanied by pale mucus membranes. They are definitely anaemic, very easily tired, and without exception will tell you that if they attempt to hurry they get out of breath and are often faint and giddy. Faintness and giddiness is one of the things that runs right through them all.

The next constant thing is that they are chilly – they feel the cold intensely and usually have very cold extremities, and associated with their cold extremities they get troublesome cramp in their feet. This tends to come on either when they are sitting still or after over-exertion. Another thing they will tell you is that they are perfectly all right going about in the house, but that immediately they go out of doors and have to go a little faster or a little further, they get exhausted at once.

Mentally the Ferrum condition is a state of despondency and they weep easily. In that state they tend to become confused, and if you ask what is worrying them they usually cannot give you a clear explanation. Mostly they are irritable, and one thing which irritates them more quickly than anything else is noise. I know one typical Ferrum patient who becomes nearly distraught with rage if the maids in the house are brushing up and making a clattering – she has almost gone out and pushed one of them down the stairs. All you have to do is drum your fingers on the table and in no time they sit up and say 'For heaven's sake stop that'.

They are also sensitive to pain. I remember one man who had to have some typhoid inoculations. I stuck a needle into his arm and he fainted at once. He said he always had a fearful time at the dentist's.

They strike you as gentle, pleasant people, a little under the weather, a little depressed, with rather a minor key outlook on life; and yet they will not tolerate any opposition – this often gives you a useful lead.

Ferrum and Pulsatilla patients are rather alike in appearance and temperament, but you will not get the intense opposition from Pulsatilla that you do from Ferrum, and their temperature reactions are different. Another point I have noticed in Ferrum patients is that they often suffer from bad constipation. They are always worried by it and their depression is much more marked when they are constipated.

A 10M dose *may* do it, but a 6c certainly will. In small chilly boys with that variable colour in the face, and awfully little to go on in the way of indications, and the fact that he has not a definite liking for eggs and has a definite enuresis, you will almost certainly clear him on Ferrum. In adults a certain amount of incontinence also may be cleared up.

Another point in Ferrum is that they cannot deal with dry wine, and yet are perfectly all right with sweet wine. They get a stomach upset (without vomiting) and diarrhoea after dry wine.

If you ever have to treat a chronic diarrhoea and get the statement that it comes on while the patient is actually eating – not after the meal – the only remedy I know that has it is Ferrum, I have seen it clear up a very obstinate case of nine months standing. The urging occurs immediately they put anything into their mouths. I have also seen it clear up summer diarrhoea of babies, where they got diarrhoea immediately you started to feed them.

22
Graphites

Graphites patients are difficult to distinguish from Calc. Carb. patients – they can look very much alike. The only difference, in my view, is that Graphites have a slightly mauvish look. I gave Graphites to a patient for the most frightful rash on her face. She came in wearing a veil, and her face really was terrible with all sorts of symptoms, cracked and oozing yellowish stuff, but behind it all there was this mauvish look. She was incredibly better after a 10M of Graphites – one of the greatest of all skin remedies. It cleared up entirely and she never had it again.

Graphites patients are heavier-looking and more heavy-featured than the Calcareas, although they look awfully like them sometimes. You often sit in front of a patient and think she must need some Calc. Carb. when in fact she really needs Graphites. Both Calc. Carb. and Graphites tend to have pale mucous membranes, and they both have pale lips and hands. Only one of them has bluish extremities – the Calc. Carb. – you never find bluish extremities in a Graphites, which is a very useful distinguishing point.

Another distinguishing point is that a Calc. Carb. is generally nervous when seeing the doctor. You occasionally see a Calc. Carb. child of eight, nine or ten, with dilated pupils when they come to see the doctor, because they really are so nervous. They are not going to show it otherwise. You do not get this in Graphites, but you do get another queer symptom which I have seen dozens of times, and that is a little droop of the upper eyelids, as if they would not hold up, especially if they are nervous or if they have decided to have another opinion. They look as if they have been awake for several nights and are really overtired. Graphites also get a tendency to styes whereas Calc. Carb. do not. The styes are on the lower lid (which is useful to remember: Pulsatilla – upper lid, Graphites – lower lid).

Graphites patients very often have another symptom, which is that their eyelashes are stuck together when they wake in the morning. They get a sort of gluey discharge from their eyes in the night. I always remember a child of about eleven being brought to my outpatients, and I tried to get a history out of the mother. I asked dozens of questions and got nothing at all from her. Finally I said, 'Does this child always have these stuck-together lashes?' And all the mother said was, 'Didn't you wash your face properly this morning?', which was not what I wanted to know. There were no symptoms to go on, absolutely nothing, except that she was rather chilly, and I gave her some Graphites.

The next time the little girl came she was with her father. He said, 'I have come up this time because I want to thank you, and ask whether your medicine might also have helped her with another problem'. He explained that she had always been a particularly indecisive child. If they asked her to go to a picnic, well, she might like to go. She would probably ask to come at the last moment, but would have all sorts of reasons which she must think out first. Or perhaps she had to arrange a bookcase in her room. She would not know what books she was going to put into it. Whether she took the one that belonged to her round the house, or whether she borrowed some of theirs – she would not be able to make up her mind. He said that this time she was entirely different and that this had made all the difference to their lives.

The patient whose awful skin rash I describe above also had the same problem – the indecision of Graphites. She had a famous father who wrote books, and when he died she was left with the whole of his library to look through and to put into bookcases. All the bookcases were there. She changed them round every day until her family were more or less demented. Her two sons called on me to ask what they should do and I gave her then, although it was five or six years since I had treated her previously, another 10M of Graphites to see if it would help, which it greatly did.

Graphites patients also have a degree of depression. They get a sense of foreboding and a feeling that there is some kind of trouble ahead. It goes with their indecision, and they really are very depressed. They seldom weep – they just tell you about it – and rather badly, as a rule.

Graphites is one of the great skin medicines, and it is not the soft moist skin of Calc. Carb. at all. It is much rougher. If you feel the Graphites skin when they are quite well, even when the patient has been cured by the remedy, you still find that the skin is rather rough – rather dry and harsh-feeling.

Graphites and Calc. Carb. both have a feeling of a rush of blood up to the head, although there is a difference. In Graphites it feels as if the blood flows up from the feet, and they can have quite severe nose bleeding. In Calc. Carb. it starts in the abdomen and surges up the neck – not into the head.

Graphites patients do not necessarily get on with Calc. Carb. patients, because they are very critical and can be quite bad-tempered. They are both fond of music, but the Graphites patient gets a peculiar sensitiveness to music, and can weep from music where they will not weep from anything else. Calc. Carb. are often very musical but are not affected in this manner.

Graphites patients have their own particular type of skin complaint, and it can be anywhere. The skin cracks – awful cracks down the fingers – and oozes a honey-like sort of stuff, slightly sticky. They often have one thing which is a good hint. They nearly always have a rash and a skin complaint at the back of the ears, also with cracks and oozing. This is sometimes at the side of the nose and sometimes all round the hair, although it can be more or less all over the place. If I was uncertain as to what to give and found a lot of rash behind the ears, and cracks, I would be inclined to give Graphites if it fitted at all, because I have found it so good in skins.

Graphites patients are disturbed by their constipation (in contrast to Calc. Carb.) They get blown out with a lot of vague pains and are much better if they have their bowels opened regularly. They also sweat. Their sweat is sometimes offensive – any discharge the Graphites gets can be offensive. They complain of it and do not like it at all.

Graphites has another queer symptom. In certain complaints, if the patient has rheumatism in the spine or anything like that, Graphites is better lying on the back, covered up to the neck, in a draught. They are chilly patients, but they do feel better if they are in a draught, so long as they are covered up warmly enough. There is also extreme photophobia in sunlight. They can also have one peculiar symptom, which you will meet perhaps once in a year and which could not be more strange, rare and peculiar. They feel as if there is a cobweb over their face. They try to move it and cannot – this awful sensation of a cobweb stretched over their face.

The remedy is also valuable for all the digestive things. They get a lot of stomach pains and are nearly always better for eating. They are also better immediately they have eaten. They sometimes get ulcers and keep food by them in the night, which eases off the pain and makes them feel quite comfortable. They get all sorts of queer food aversions. Nearly all Graphites patients have a marked aversion to fish. Sometimes, if they are not well and have a lot of stomach symptoms, they get an aversion to meat, to salt and to sweets. Their pains are practically always better for warm milk. That is why they go to bed with a biscuit and a thermos of warm milk, so that they will not have to drink it cold, if possible. If they drink it cold it helps a little, but if it is warm it helps a great deal more and they will tell you it gives them a great deal of comfort. They also get a lot of flatulence, which is better for belching. The Graphites patient can get incarcerated wind, which can be painful, sometimes also with extreme tenderness.

Occasionally in their skin complaints they get itching all over the body. Occasionally they get very swollen glands in the neck, which are quite painless. You do not know why somebody's glands are coming up and you are sure it is not glandular fever, and you are sure it is none of the other things, and it may be helpful to remember this.

23

Kali Bichromicum

There are certain points of similarity running through all of the Kali
salts, but their differences are very definite. The only way to compare
them is to take the remedies one after the other, take the outstanding
characteristics of each one, and mention the similarities of the others
as we go through.

I always visualize the Kali Bich. patient as a definitely fair, fat,
somewhat sluggish individual, either male or female, with an air of
general puffiness. Their faces are puffy, and they give the impression
of having an unhealthy skin, the majority having a definite tendency to
acne. The next thing you notice is that their eyes are muddy – they
may have the definite yellowish tinge of the conjunctivae, and there
may also be a blepharitis; altogether they give you the impression of
being definitely weak-eyed. That, I think, is the way they strike you at
first. The next impression you get is when you begin to talk to them.
Suppose you take a man. He will be rather above the average height,
and looks strong and muscular, but begin to talk to him and you find
that he is unduly easily tired out, and when he is tired he wants to
stretch out in a chair and do nothing.

As to what they come complaining of, I find that they fall into three
definite classes. The common Kali Bich. patient is the typical catarrhal
dyspeptic. You get a certain number of Kali Bich. patients in whom
the catarrh is further down and who tend to get bronchitis and attacks
of asthma. Then there is a third group.These are not so fat and not so
heavy, they have more colour in their cheeks and have darker hair.
They are the people who come along with definite rheumatism.

There is one other condition in which you may need Kali Bich., but
where the patient does not correspond in appearance to the typical
picture, and that is the migraine patient. A certain number of
migraines will not respond to any other remedy.

There are apparent contradictions in temperature reactions. Most
patients tend to be definitely worse in summer, to get rheumatism in

hot weather, and at the same time skin irritation and acne tend to develop. Actual respiratory conditions such as bronchitis and asthma tend to be worse in spring and autumn. Yet you will find that when they are actually ill they often complain of feeling the cold. They are definitely worse from damp cold weather and when they are seedy they do become shivery.

They have one or two definite time reactions during the twenty-four hours. In all the Kali salts you get a definite early morning aggravation, varying in time but round about 2 a.m. to 5 a.m. In Kali Bich. it tends to be earlier. Kali Bich. is definitely more seedy on waking in the morning, and respiratory troubles in particular are worse. That is not the early aggravation, but a separate and definite aggravation at the ordinary time of waking up. Another characteristic of Kali Bich. worth remembering is that they have a definite aggravation after food – they feel more uncomfortable, heavier and have less energy.

One useful point is that they tend to have definite alternations of symptoms. Their rheumatism will clear up and be followed by digestive troubles or diarrhoea, or you may have migraine clearing up and being followed by eye trouble. In rheumatism first a knee may be affected, and when it clears a shoulder becomes affected, when that is better the trouble shifts to an ankle, then the other knee, and so on.

Let us consider the various types of illness they complain about. The typical catarrhal dyspeptic complains of catarrh, tending to be very troublesome in cold and damp weather. They get the kind of cold in which their nose and nasal sinuses are choked up with stringy yellow mucus. The mucus may be white if the complaint is chronic – the more chronic it is the more the mucus tends to be white, the more acute it is the more the mucus tends to be yellow. There may be involvement of any of the accessory sinuses, but in all of them you get a typical Kali Bich. boring pain, as if a blunt plug was being forced into the affected area. The most common area to be involved with a pain of this character is the frontal sinus, often severe general headache, and you may get similar pains over the maxillary antra or just over the eyes, depending on which of the sinuses are picked out.

In between their attacks the appearance of the throat is very suggestive. There is very marked deep congestion of the whole of the back of the throat, often with strings of mucus hanging down from the posterior nares, an oedematous appearance of the tonsils, uvula, and soft palate. It is a typical throat and you cannot miss it if you have seen it once.

Following the catarrhal condition further down you get it extending into the lungs. The kind of condition you get there is a definite capillary bronchitis and with that there is a very troublesome cough. One point that often leads you to Kali Bich. is their marked tendency to choke. With the bronchial irritation they choke on solids – they can swallow liquids, but solids make them cough even to vomiting. In the morning they cough and bring up abundant, stringy, difficult muco-pus. They often feel better out in the open air as far as the respiratory condition is concerned, provided the air is not too cold and damp. They tell you the most comfortable thing is to get into bed and get as warm as they can. They often complain of a sensation of coldness in the chest. One of the commonest complaints is a pain in the chest going from the sternum right through to the back.

Now take catarrh going down to the stomach instead of to the lungs. You get a typical acute gastritis, or gastric ulcer. The patient complains of loss of appetite and attacks of nausea and vomiting coming on quite suddenly. They have a lot of flatulence and a distressing sense of weight in the stomach after food.

Their food likes and dislikes are very marked. They have a marked dislike of meat, a bad taste in their mouths, and water tastes particularly unpleasant. Usually they develop a dislike of fats during their attacks. They often crave for sour things and have a marked longing for beer – the chronic beer drinker is fairly typical of Kali Bich. They have a definite aggravation from beer – it makes them sick and often sets up acute vomiting and diarrhoea. As regards the vomit, they may vomit pretty well anything, but an important point is that practically all the material is sour. It is a watery, yellow, stringy vomit. Occasionally they vomit up a meal, and after the stomach is empty start bringing up a quantity of glairy white mucus, although this is not as common as yellow glairy material.

In gastric ulcer you may get blood – fresh or stale blood – but gastric ulcer is not so common as acute gastritis. The patients tend to get a certain amount of hepatic congestion, a feeling of weight, and a feeling of heaviness in the right sub-costal region. Associated with that there is often a certain amount of diarrhoea, with clay-coloured, bileless stools.

Kali Bich. is peculiarly liable to develop catarrh of the bladder accompanied by the passage of urine in which there are strings of yellowish white mucus. Where this condition is present, a strong indication for Kali Bich. is a peculiar pain in the region of the coccyx coming on during micturition.

The commonest cases in which I have used Kali Bich. are acute rheumatism, and they all tend to sweat. The principal indication is the wandering nature of the pains. One joint gets inflamed and tender, then clears up, and another starts. The next point is that the pains tend to come and go quite suddenly. The patient is lying comfortably and suddenly gets an acute pain that does not last long.

Although the rheumatism comes in summer it is definitely better from heat and worse from cold; it is aggravated by motion and relieved by rest. You get a certain amount of sciatica in Kali Bich. which is definitely relieved by motion, although pains in other structures of the body are aggravated by it. The sciatica occurs in hot weather and is better from applied heat, but not to the same extent as the rheumatism. It is also better from flexing the leg and is particularly sensitive to weather changes.

You get a number of patients suffering from migraine. The type that calls for Kali Bich. is where you get a warning by visual disturbances that the headache is coming on. The vision is blurred, dim, or hazy. This comes on suddenly some time before the headache, usually clears before the pain develops, but may continue throughout the headache. These migraine headaches are definitely one-sided, sometimes right, sometimes left, and the pain is particularly violent. Often it is situated in a small area in one or other temporal region, and it is definitely relieved by pressure over the area. It is helped by warmth and hot applications. These headaches often tend to be periodical in their recurrence. They are aggravated by stooping or by violent motion. They often develop during the night and are particularly bad on waking in the morning. Often the headaches are accompanied by violent sickness in which the patient brings up this typical, white, stringy, glairy mucus in the vomit. That is the typical migraine headache, and it is quite different from the catarrhal headache which begins at the root of the nose and extends up into the head.

24

Kali Bromatum

There are a few conditions in which Kali Brom. is particularly useful. The majority of Kali patients tend to be fat and Kali Brom. is usually fat and fair, definitely lethargic in type, rather depressed, heavy-looking and dull. Although there is this apparent dullness there is a certain amount of local restlessness. They have fidgety hands and feet and there may be a tendency to twitch. They often complain of being sleepy and that they fall asleep in their chair if they sit down. They also often complain of a tendency for their hands and feet or legs to go numb. Associated with this numbness the legs tend to become uncomfortable and get a trembling feeling. These symptoms make them fear that they may be going out of their minds.

One type of patient I always found difficult to fit before I came across Kali Brom. was the child who is not getting on well at school. He or she is dull and apparently lacking in brains, rather like Pulsatilla, but with too coarse a skin for Pulsatilla. The first thing that put me on to Kali Brom. was that they all tend to get acne. If you get acne severely in a child and no other definite indications it will clear up on Kali Brom. every time. It is the same with acne during menstruation in a woman, if there are no other indications. Occasionally you get a girl of that type who gets very long periods and that too is a strong indication for Kali Brom.

Kali Brom. is a hot-blooded patient worse from heat, worse in summer and in hot rooms. The kind of aggravation you get in a hot room is that the patient has a general feeling of chilliness. They are better in cold weather, and like all the other Kali salts tend to have an early morning aggravation, round about 2 a.m.

There are three pathological conditions in which I always consider that Kali Brom. may be indicated. The first is when choreic symptoms have developed after a shock or fright. The next is the semi-convulsive condition that you get in Bright's disease – the patient seems heavy and sleepy with a besotted appearance and threatened convulsions, and there Kali Brom. will often help you out. Third, if you have a bad case of infantile diarrhoea, and the child is beginning to develop signs of meningeal irritation, then Kali Brom. is strongly indicated.

A number of epileptic cases respond to Kali Brom. In the male the epilepsy is not always associated with over-excitement, and without that over-excitement I have never found Kali Brom. of any help whatsoever in the male. In women you always have a definite relationship between the period and the onset of the fits. They occur either during or near the period, and without that relationship I have never seen any good result from using Kali Brom. In both the male and female there tends to be an aggravation at the new moon. In all of these epileptics who require Kali Brom., the fit is followed by a severe headache. One other epileptic indication is an aura before the onset of the fit. It is a sensation of swelling – sometimes they feel as if their whole body was swelling.

25

Kali Carbonicum

The first impression you get of Kali Carb. is that the patients are soft.
That is not the impression you get in Kent – the Kali Carb. he gives is
the irritable, highly-strung, nervous type, but this is not the kind I have
met. I visualise them as not taut at all, but pale, soft, flabby
people – any exertion tires them, and when tired they always get
backache. They always tend to be fat and very often have flat feet. I
visualise a rather fat, rather dark, slightly sallow, back-aching woman
coming into the room. They all say they are very tired and when their
back aches they are simply compelled to lie down. Their mental
picture is very much the same sort of thing; the slightest effort of
thought or excitement tires them and they get into a state of mental
confusion. The ordinary description they give is that they get up in the
morning knowing that they have got a fair amount of work to do.
They start on something and immediately it dawns on them that there
is something else they ought to be doing, so they leave the first job and
dash off to do the second, and have no sooner started it than they leave
it for a third, and so they get into a thorough muddle and end up by
completing nothing at all.

They tell you that they are constantly misplacing things. A man will
say that he can never find his notes in his office – that he puts them
away carefully enough but cannot remember where he has put them.
They also get the fear that they are going out of their minds. With this
inability to get things done they get harried, they make mistakes in
their speech, miss words out, put wrong ones in, and forget to finish
their sentences. They get annoyed with themselves and scared. They
get annoyed with circumstances and they become jealous and suspicious of those who are working with them. When they are in this state
they are very difficult to get on with and often show a strange
vindictiveness. Another thing they will tell you is that they get worn
out with the slightest physical or mental effort, and that if they have
any excitement they are quite exhausted and have to go to bed; it takes
them two or three days to get over it. You get a good deal of fear in

Kali Carb. patients – fear of poverty, fear of the future and fear of death.

With this fear they get a marked hoarding instinct. Kali Carb. is essentially possessive. They tend to hang on to everything – they hang on to life and are afraid of dying, even though their life may appear hardly worth living. They hang on to their husbands, even when they appear to loathe them. They hang on to their children, even when their children appear to be nothing but a worry to them and when they treat them none too well. They hang on to their money and may be positively miserly – though this is often the result of their fear of poverty.

Another thing that very often crops up is a feeling of failure. They become timid and cannot stand up for themselves, and if anyone accuses them of a mistake, especially a mistake they have not made, they simply lie down under it. Another important point about Kali Carb. patients is a dislike of being touched – they simply cannot bear it.

The kind of thing they usually complain of is the feeling of breaking down. They have a general catarrhal condition, are very susceptible to colds and usually have some digestive disturbance.

As far as general reactions are concerned, Kali Carb. are chilly patients, in fact as cold as any remedy we have in the pharmacopoiea. They are not only sensitive to draughts but to any cold air. The next thing about them is that their complaints are aggravated by any exertion, mental or physical and they are very susceptible to damp. An apparent contradiction to this aggravation from cold and amelioration from warmth is that they do get an aggravation from warm drinks. What really happens is that they get warmed up by the hot drink and then immediately get chilled down again, and the aggravation is due to this chilling down and not to the warm drink. Usually their complaints are all worse after eating – they are generally more uncomfortable and more aggravated after meals. Kali Carb. always feel particularly seedy and lacking in energy when it is time to get up.

The character of the pains is general in Kali Carb. Wherever they have a pain it is of the same type, whether in the arms, the back, the chest or the joints and whether due to respiratory, digestive or rheumatic troubles. The pains are always sharp and cutting and are constantly flitting about from place to place. Next, they are almost always relieved by heat, are sensitive to cold and mostly aggravated by pressure. Occasionally the pain comes on during rest and is slightly better for gentle motion, but is definitely made worse if the patient moves fast.

I remember an old lady with a typical trigeminal neuralgia who was about the best example of Kali Carb. I have ever seen. She was not only sensitive to draughts, but also so acutely conscious of any movement of air that if you waved a handerkerchief in front of her all the branches of her trigeminal nerve were literally mapped out in pain. The slighest movement of any sort brought on the pain – eating, talking, laughing or smiling. She was so sensitive to touch that she simply could not bear to wash her face, and she was the typical worn-out, tired-out, backachey middle-aged woman. This is very like the description of Mag. Phos. – they both have the great sensitiveness to cold, but Mag. Phos. is relieved by pressure, whereas Kali Carb. is aggravated by pressure.

Kali Carb. is as catarrhal as any remedy we have. The patients are always catching cold and get a certain amount of nasal discharge when overheated, either by exertion or by being in a hot room and going out and getting chilled afterwards. They also tend to develop a violent headache from the same cause. It is usually a temporal headache, either on one or both sides, and is so acute that it gives rise to nausea.

The nasal catarrh quickly tends to spread down into the throat. They have very typical dry, painful, hot tonsils with a large quantity of white or sometimes yellow tenacious mucus hanging about the throat. There is early enlargement of the tonsillar glands, which are painful and tender and markedly sensitive to cold; this is a valuable diagnostic point. If the condition is not checked immediately the patient quickly tends to get an early bronchitis with a paroxysmal, dry, hacking cough. There is not much mucus and what there is is mostly swallowed rather than expectorated. The cough is so violent that it is liable to go on to vomiting, and with that there is the typical Kali Carb. violent stabbing pain in the chest.

In pneumonia you hardly ever want Kali Carb. in the early stage – it is after consolidation that it comes in at all. The things that may put you on to it are the time aggravation in the early morning, the character of the pain, the character of the sputum, the character of the cough and the fact that they get definite relief from sitting propped up, leaning forward. They have an aggravation from lying on the affected side, and as a rule it is the right lower lobe that is affected. There is often marked dyspnoea. They can only sip fluids, as they cannot hold their breath long enough to take a decent drink, and they cannot take anything solid as it starts them coughing and the cough goes on until they are sick. They always tend to get a pallid, slightly cyanotic, puffy look about the face.

The great danger in Kali Carb. pneumonias is a failing heart. You get very early and very dangerous symptoms of a toxic affection of the cardiac muscle.

The remedy most likely to be confused with it is Hepar Sulph. This has the same respiratory trouble, the same cough, the same sensitiveness to cold air, the same involvement of cervical glands, but it does not have the 2 a.m. to 4 a.m. time aggravation. Its time aggravation is much later, 7, 8, or 9 a.m., and it does not have the same puffy face – it is always much thinner, more drawn, more anxious-looking.

Kali Carb. patients always complain of a tendency to digestive difficulties, and a constant complaint is the tendency to flatulence – they get absolutely blown out after food. They have the greatest difficulty in getting rid of this distension, which involves the whole abdomen and is not merely a gastric one. They also have a feeling of emptiness in the abdomen – they feel hungry and want something to eat, but are no better after eating as it is not a real hunger at all.

They all tend to get dental trouble. You hardly ever see them with a sound set of teeth. They usually have inflamed gums, an unhealthy offensive mouth, and a pale and flabby tongue. You may get the usual Kali tongue, thickly coated at the root, but more commonly it is pale and swollen-looking.

Another frequent symptom is a sensation of internal coldness in the abdomen, and in respiratory troubles you will find a similar feeling of coldness in the chest. These patients often strongly object to being examined because of being so acutely sensitive to cold.

Kali Carb. patients are liable to get colic. It may be intestinal or it may be hepatic, often it is just a feeling of fullness and tenderness over the liver. It may even go on to biliary attacks, but you are more likely to get a threatening rather than the development of actual gallstones.

Practically all of them are constipated, and they have a marked tendency to the development of very painful piles. These come down as large masses and tend to thrombose, and occasionally you get them bleeding, but the special thing is their painfulness and hyperaesthesia – the patient simply yells if you touch them.

Most Kali Carb. patients are thirsty and have a definite desire for sour things. In acute illness they have a desire for sweets – it may be for chocolates or sweets, or it may be an actual craving for sugar. As a rule there is a definite aversion to meat, and although it is not in the textbooks I find that most of these patients tend to eat an excessive quantity of starch.

One other point constant to every Kali salt – and I think Kali

Carb. has it more marked than any other with the exception of Kali Phos. – is that they are all aggravated after sexual intercourse. It leaves them absolutely played out. In Kali Carb. there tends to be an unusual degree of excitement and yet there is this prostration afterwards. In Kali Phos. there is not the same degree of excitability, but the prostration is even worse.

There is a marked haemorrhagic tendency in Kali Carb. – the periods may be too frequent and they are always too profuse. There is often a history of periods which become so bad that the patient is never free from an oozing of blood, at times there is almost flooding and then it slackens down again into this state of oozing, but never really stops. The pathological condition you are most likely to find is a polyp or fibroid.

It is repeated in all the textbooks that Kali Carb. is a dangerous remedy. Kent warns against its use in acute gout, but the few cases I have seen have never called for Kali Carb. It is a remedy that can safely be used in rheumatoid arthritis. I have seen many patients in whom there were definite indications for Kali Carb. and they got Kali Carb. straight away in high potencies and got well on it. In pneumonia I have given it many times and have never had dangerous results. It is, however, dangerous in T.B., as it may promote miliary spread. You have to be very careful what potency you use as these patients do not stand the reaction well. I have also given it many times in stomach conditions and have never seen any bad results. I would not give Kali Carb. for gallstone colic in a Kali Carb. patient, just as I should avoid giving Lycopodium for hepatic colic in a Lycopodium patient. If you give the patient's own constitutional drug you do tend to get a marked aggravation. If Kali Carb. was indicated in a Kali Carb. patient with colic, and no other indication could be found, I would give it, but I would give it low. As a rule, if you get Kali Carb. patients with gallstone colic you can very nearly match it with Aconite. You can relieve the symptoms with this and then follow up with Kali Carb. later when the pain has disappeared.

26
Kali Iodatum

First there is the acute group in which one gets indications for Kali Iod. Secondly there are the rheumatic conditions in which you get indications, and associated with these there are the heart affections. The typical chronic Kali Iod. patient tends to be pale and delicate-looking with a definitely unstable vasomotor system. They flush up very easily. They are usually fair-skinned and very often fair-haired. The acute type you mostly find is fatter than you would have expected them to be, more flushed, deeper red, than the chronic type, heavier-featured, rather cyanotic and heavy-lipped.

There are certain constant features all through the type of patient who calls for Kali Iod. The first thing about them is that they are hot-blooded and definitely better in the open air.

Next, and constant to both, is that they are depressed patients, very easily discouraged, and very often taking a definite disgust to life. They are bad-tempered and irritable, and if annoyed tend to be abusive. They are also restless, which becomes more marked if at all agitated, and if any attempt is made to control them they are liable to burst into tears. If they are trying to make you understand anything and find themselves incapable of putting it into words, they get so agitated that in despair they burst into tears because they are so worried about themselves.

There are certain definite times when their conditions tend to get worse. They have the ordinary Kali aggravation early in the morning from 2 a.m. to 5 a.m. as well as an aggravation on waking up in the morning. The kind of aggravation they tend to get then is a headache, dry throat, and general depression. They are susceptible to damp weather. They are upset by cold food and get a marked aggravation from cold milk. They tend to get urticaria which is usually worse at the seaside; some also get asthma which also tends to be worse at the seaside. Kali Iod. patients are definitely hungry people, usually they are thirsty too, and they all tend to get flatulence.

Kali Iod. is a very useful remedy in rheumatism and also in sciatica, and here there is one characteristic feature. There is a point of tenderness over the sciatic nerve and a diffuse area of tenderness much wider than the nerve. It is the same in the rheumatic condition; you get the tender joint, but also a diffuse tenderness both above and below the joint. The next thing is a definite heat aggravation both in rheumatism and in sciatica – the patient wants the affected part uncovered or wants cold applications. There is a definite amelioration from movement, particularly so the more they keep up the motion. It may be painful to begin with but the pain steadily improves as they keep moving. As regards the sciatica, they are definitely worse from lying on the affected side, worse sitting, worse standing but better when moving about.

There are valuable indications in eye and nose conditions. Of all the inflammatory eye conditions, I think that acute conjunctivitis, particularly of intense violence with blepharospasm, is the most usual in Kali Iod. You always get the typical flushed face, marked oedema of the eyelids, all the outside of the eyelid is red, the face round about is red, and the redness and swelling spreads up on to the forehead so that it looks swollen and puffy too. There is intense photophobia, marked headache and the conjunctivae are red and oedematous. The discharge is a thick greenish-yellow discharge, and when you do open the eyes they simply pour tears. The patient complains of a burning pain and in practically all cases there is an early tendency to ulceration of the cornea. This condition, when associated with aggravation from warmth and love of cold, almost always clears up on Kali Iod.

There is another condition, and that is acute inflammation of the accessory nasal sinuses. What draws your attention is the puffiness of the forehead spreading down into the eyes. Associated with that you get an acrid watery coryza with burning in the eyes and intense lacrimation, a tendency for the nose to become sore and raw and for the upper lip to become swollen. With these nasal conditions you get mouth disturbances, commonly small ulcers situated on the tip of the tongue. One confirmatory symptom is an intense pain at the root of the tongue on trying to put the tongue out. That picture always calls for Kali Iod. It does not matter whether it is conjunctivitis, cavernous sinus, antrum, or ethmoid disease, provided there is the heat aggravation it will clear up on Kali Iod.

There is just one additional clinical tip. If you get a hot-blooded patient with singing in the ears and no other indication, give them Kali Iod. If you get the same thing in a cold-blooded patient, very often a dose of China clears them.

27

Kali Phosphoricum

There is a definite difference between Kali Phos. and the other Kali salts. In the others there is a tendency to excess fat deposit, whereas in Kali Phos. you do not have that. The average patient is a thin person with a typical pale, waxy skin. Most of the ones I have seen have been dark and they have all been obviously tired out. It is a curious state – a mixture of extreme nervous and physical exhaustion. They usually walk with a slight stoop, their movements are uncertain and there is a tendency to stagger. Sometimes this is due to giddiness but more often it is due to actual weakness of the limbs. They are despondent and anxious, and almost always of the neuraesthenic type. Their irritability comes in spasms, for instance when someone annoys them. It is the irritability of weakness and exasperation and a conscious inability to cope with things. They usually get into a state of exhaustion with tremor and fears, and feel that they would like to scream. They want someone to hold on to them, either to save their reason or to help them to keep control.

They are always shy and are particularly nervous of going away from home. This is said to be homesickness but I think it is more a fear of strange surroundings. They are not only shy of strangers but definitely suspicious of them. Another thing you will find in Kali Phos., and which has been brought out in the provers, is a fear of open spaces. This is a symptom that is often difficult to place in the materia medica. In spite of their nervous and physical weakness they often become restless. They are also easily startled and peculiarly sensitive to noise. And yet, in spite of their apparent weakness and fear and exhaustion, a curious obstinacy runs through them. It is especially noticeable if you are trying to get them to do anything to benefit their health – you find them remarkably obstinate and difficult to handle. With their extreme lassitude you find a definite dislike for life, they loathe it, although they have a fear of death and are never the sort of people who commit suicide.

You often get this state after a long illness or chronic debilitating

93

disease. They are always pale and obviously ill, but under stress or excitement you get a tendency to flush – a hectic flush over the malar region. They are also troubled with flushing after meals and an associated tendency to sweat, particularly about the head and face. I mention this because it is often difficult to differentiate between Kali Phos. and Phosphorus – both have a tendency to flush and get hot – and yet otherwise there are no end of differences. With the weariness of Kali Phos. you get a peculiar pain at the seventh cervical vertebra, involving the whole of the dorsal area of the spine. This is one of the most common complaints, and it comes on whenever they are tired. This pain in the back is definitely worse if the patient is lying down or sitting, a little better if they move about gently, and there is a feeling of weakness about the back generally.

These people are peculiarly sensitive to cold. In fact, most of their modalities are aggravation reactions – they have very few ameliorations at all. Warm weather makes them worse, they are aggravated by food, they are usually worse in the morning on getting up, always worse from exertion, and occasionally slightly better from moving about gently. They are always hypersensitive to noise. As a rule there is a premenstrual aggravation, with definite relief when the period starts. They are more distressed, more apprehensive and more weary in the early hours of the morning. They are particularly sensitive to touch, and any emotional excitement normally leaves them trembling, for instance, bad or startling news. They are aggravated by the stress of talking to people, especially to several people at once, and yet they have a definite fear of solitude. They have a fear of crowds, and in a crowd become tremulous and frightened.

In other words, it is the typical picture of what the patient calls 'general nervous prostration'. The main complaint is a feeling of general weakness, associated with various pains and disturbances in their arms and legs, and you may even get definite nerve degeneration. I have seen typical disseminated sclerosis markedly helped by Kali Phos. All these patients with numbness, tremor and pain are aggravated by exertion, whereas gentle movement seems to keep their circulation going and they feel better for it.

Practically all suffer from digestive disturbances, and certain points are characteristic. As far as their appetite is concerned there is an apparent contradiction. They often have a feeling of hunger – more a feeling of emptiness – which tends to disappear at once on taking food, whereupon they feel full immediately, as if the whole abdomen were swollen out. Even if they take only a small meal they have bad flatulence, and yet, within a few minutes of stopping eating, they again have the feeling of emptiness. You get the characteristic nervous dyspeptic who is always nibbling. Practically all of them have a dislike for bread, so most resort to sweet biscuits or to sweets such as chocolates.

One useful diagnostic point is that they tend to get an acute gnawing hungry pain when they wake in the morning, at about 5 a.m., and usually you find they have a box of biscuits by their bed in order to relieve it. They suffer a lot from flatulence which they find very difficult to move – a sort of obstructed flatulence which gives rise to colic. You often get longer periods between the taking of food and beginning of discomfort, and between that and the definite hunger pains, but as a rule you do not find actual duodenal ulcer nor the immediate relief from food you get in duodenal ulcer. Another point about the digestive disturbances is that these patients have a definitely unhealthy mouth, with inflamed and tender gums which tend to bleed easily. If their teeth are not very well looked after they decay and they get definite troubles, for instance, the tongue becomes flabby and has a suggestive mustard-coloured coating.

They often have a craving for ice cold water, which is a peculiarity as they complain of a feeling of coldness in the abdomen. They have a great liking for sweet things, as well as sour things, and sometimes have a craving for vinegar. If I ever get a tired-out woman with backache and a liking for vinegar, the first two remedies I think of are Sepia and Kali Phos. Both are chilly, both tired and excitable, both pale, both rather better for motion. In Kali Phos. the pain is mainly in the dorsal region, in Sepia in the sacral. Kali Phos. is rather worse lying down, while Sepia is better. Kali Phos. tends to be pale, Sepia to be sallow, and the rings round the eyes are brown in Sepia and black in Kali Phos. Like all the Kali salts, Kali Phos. patients have an aversion to bread and meat.

Practically all these nervous, debilitated patients suffer from headaches. Another type of patient with headache in which you get a definite indication is the student who has been doing intensive study. They get the kind of headache that comes on during the night, is very acute on waking up, often slightly better on getting up and moving about, and gets bad again towards night. It is generally worse from cold and aggravated by noise – it is about the most sensitive remedy to noise of any we have. It is an intense headache which seems to involve the scalp, and even the hair, and the whole head becomes tender to touch. It is helped by eating a little food and comes on again when the patient gets hungry – rather like the digestive symptoms. It is helped by wrapping up the head and keeping it warm, and is much aggravated by any excitement or mental effort.

Associated with the general tremulous weakness you get marked palpitation. On physical examination you find a poorly-acting heart and low blood pressure, and occasionally you get a patient with true anginal attacks. In these attacks, after the acute radiating pain has subsided, a sensation of numbness is left.

Practically all get urinary disturbance, usually a typical bladder catarrh. In an elderly patient, tired-out and debilitated and with a tendency to incontinence, Kali Phos. will often clear up the symptoms and re-establish sphincter control. They get a marked burning pain on micturition, starting with the flow of urine, continuing after the flow is finished, and usually situated in the bladder, not in the urethra. If you consider the sugar-loving, tremulous, worn-out, hungry, emaciated, debilitated patient, you will see that you quite frequently get Kali Phos. indicated in the diabetic.

There is a definite menstrual aggravation and as a rule a scanty menstrual flow. If these patients do get leucorrhoea it tends to be excoriating and highly coloured. You frequently get this with acute ovarian pain.

There are two other useful points concerning Kali Phos. Apart from the tendency to sweat on the face and head after meals or from excitement, the sweat glands are generally inactive and these patients do not perspire easily. Their sleep tends to be disturbed and they get violent dreams and nightmares.

It is an immensely useful remedy. I have seen quite a number of people whose appearance suggested the presence of a carcinoma which has not been found, and who have cleared up on Kali Phos.

28

Kali Sulphuricum

To my mind Kali Sulph. is always a cross between Sulphur and Pulsatilla. The typical appearance is one of heaviness and sluggishness. They are usually highly coloured, rather fat, definitely slow in their movements, and tend to have a coarse skin. They always complain of feeling tired, which I think is often laziness more than physical exhaustion. They have a definite aversion to work, either physical or mental, and are usually very sorry for themselves.

They are rather depressed, often lack confidence, and may actually be timid. A feeling that their brains will not work is often associated with their depression. In spite of their timidity they are often impatient and liable to be changeable, lively one moment and depressed the next. You do all you can to cheer them up, and they respond and buck up, but the next minute they lapse again. They tend to become anxious about themselves, think they are very ill, especially in the evening and during the night, and take a gloomy view of life when waking up in the morning. They become snappy if you attempt to jolly them out of their serious view of their illness, and they are always obstinate.

With their mental confusion they complain of giddiness. Their heads feel full and their faces hot. Another characteristic is skin irritation – they are always troubled by itchy skins, all over the body, and this itchiness is a useful peg to hang most of their symptoms on.

They are always catarrhal. The catarrh may be anywhere but is usually in the upper respiratory tract. The typical cases in respiratory conditions are flushed. With the chest catarrh they get an enormous secretion of mucus, the whole chest bubbles and tends to be worse on the right side of the chest. They get catarrhal conjunctivitis in which the eyelids are gummed up and itchy, with yellowish crusts on the margins. The discharge is yellow – it is the same with all the body discharges, they tend to be irritating and to itch.

There is an intense irritation of the nose, and often some degree of ulceration, always aggravated in a hot room and in hot weather. It is the same throughout in Kali Sulph. – for instance, it is one of the most indicated drugs in chronic otitis media. Patients also tend to get haemorrhoids and here again you get the intense itching.

Everything is aggravated indoors. Warmth in general aggravates them, and they are always better in the open air. They tend to be worse in the evening, and worse from exertion, which makes them over-hot and they perspire and catch cold. They tend to stagnate when at rest, so they are better when moving about gently. They are worse on waking up in the morning, when they are often quite besotted and usually have a headache, and they are worse after food. One peculiarity you would not expect to find in such a sluggish patient is the intense aggravation they have from noise. They tend to catch cold after a bath, and it does not matter whether it is a hot or a cold one.

They are always liable to headaches. The kind they get is the full congestive headache with an intense feeling of heat and heaviness in the head. As a rule these start over the eyes, are worse there and in the forehead, and then tend to spread over the whole head, being more marked on the right side. Unlike most congestive headaches they are better from pressure and better lying down.

The next thing is a cough which is aggravated by eating and helped by cold drinks and cold air. The patient has a feeling of irritation low down in the trachea, great difficulty in bringing up sputum, and brings up this typical yellowish discharge. Their mouths are also typical. They have a slimy appearance with a yellowish coating, the patient always complains of an unpleasant insipid taste, and specially complains of water tasting badly. If you can imagine a slightly sour drink which instead of being clean and refreshing has gone flat, I think that conveys the idea. You may find in addition that they have the ordinary desires – for sweet things, sour things and cold food.

You may also require Kali Sulph. in acute rheumatism. The kind of patient is the one with the typical appearance – general aggravation from heat, amelioration of pains from moving about and being in the air. Associated is the dry skin, usually scaly in character and itching, and there may be urticaria. The pains wander about, start in one joint, go to another, leave that one and go to a third. With their rheumatic pains they often complain of very cold hands and feet – which immediately eliminates Sulphur.

In connection with their sleep, particularly in febrile conditions, they have appalling dreams of ghosts, death, robbers, murder and so on, all with violent struggling, and they wake up terrified out of their lives. In that way, and in many other respects, Kali Sulph. is not at all unlike a hot-blooded Rhus Tox.

29

Lachesis

I treated a patient once who has always struck me as the very essence of Lachesis. She was a middle-aged woman with reddish-brown hair and a high colour. The particular point about her colour was her venous engorgement – little veins standing out on her cheeks, little veins standing out on her nose, and a definite bluish appearance of her nose and ears. Her eyes were bright and clear and very much alert. What impressed me first was not so much the intent attention to what I was saying, but that she was looking all round the room to see that she was not missing anything that was happening. The next thing that struck me was that her hands were also rather congested – red, a little puffy, and tremulous. The next point was that she was very restless.

I then began to talk to her, and there you get an experience which is absolutely typical to Lachesis. They talk, and it is awfully difficult to keep them to the point. It is not that they keep things from you, but that they do not pay attention to what you ask. Often they have not got the drift of your question and something else appeals to them, and they start off on what they want to say, not on what you ask them. They are at no loss for words – these always stream out of them. She was perfectly frank in telling her tale and her symptoms were well given.

I began to ask about her life and conditions, and the outstanding thing was the jealousy she had of those members of the family who were well. Her husband was a strong, healthy man who went to his business every day and played golf at the weekend, and she was jealous that he was fit, whereas she had to stay in bed. Her daughter was married and had four healthy children, and this old lady was jealous that they were healthy, whereas her own daughters had always been seedy and a worry to her when they were children. I went and saw her one morning, and after I had finished, she turned round and said, 'Oh, would you not like a little tea? It is just tea time'. They are always mixing up the time of day, which is also very suggestive of Lachesis.

Another characteristic was an obvious self-consciousness and a weird conceit, which interested me because it was mixed up with another typical Lachesis symptom – a narrow religious outlook. She belonged to some small sect, but was perfectly certain that it was the only sect on earth, and her whole day was spent trying to make everyone she met join it. Yet she kept telling me the amount of money she gave to keep it going, and the self-gratification she got was evident. The next moment she was saying that she was a very poor member of the sect and was no use to them; and in the next breath, if only she had good health like her husband she would be able to do so much more.

One other thing she trotted out was that all the people she helped had done her down. Her husband told me that for two years she developed the most appalling suspicion, even of people she had known for years. He said that life was awfully difficult. 'I don't want to offend my wife because she isn't well at present, and one of the things she dislikes is that I should take any alcohol. I am not narrowly religious, but she wants me to keep to her standards. I go out to golf and I do want a drink occasionally, and almost the first question I get asked when I come in is, "Have you had a drink?" She is always wanting to know where I have been and whether I have done anything contrary to her own religious beliefs.'

Another woman I know has the Lachesis suspicion even more markedly. She lives in a small village in the country and is always in trouble because of her suspicion of her neighbours, looking for offence and slights and suspicious that people are doing her down.

This is only one side of the Lachesis picture. There is another, which I have only met in connection with the chronic alcoholic. In this case you get a more congested appearance. There is the same tendency to the venous stasis, dilated veins on the face, nose, and so on, but you do not get the brightness or the same mental sharpness – the edge of things is a little blunted. You get the same tendency to wander, to half finish one subject and drift off to the next one. You get the same tremor, perhaps even more noticeably, and rather more irritability, even though the ordinary Lachesis patient has quite a useful temper. These alcoholics do seem to develop the worst side of the remedy – they are also more malicious in their statements about other people.

Another point about a Lachesis alcoholic is that they get a marked aggravation from food. They are more drowsy, more heavy, more muddled, liable to get a congested face, and awfully difficult to treat. I remember one such patient who had to be given his medicine without his knowledge, as he would not take it. He was very suspicious and thought he was going to be poisoned – pretty constant in the Lachesis alcoholic. Another common reaction in the alcoholic is that they are very conscious that they themselves have been responsible for the state they are in. They are very melancholic about it, and are hopeless about your being able to do anything for them.

All Lachesis patients have the typical Lachesis sleep aggravation, and are all sensitive to heat. With a congested patient like that they are intolerant of any tightness round them – tight collars, tight belts, or anything of that sort. If they have any cardiac embarrassment they get very short of breath and want to push all the blankets down and open the windows.

I have seen a pale Lachesis patient, but never one without pigmentation.

30

Comparison of the Natrum Salts

Natrum Muriaticum

Far and away the commonest is Natrum Muriaticum. The best thing to do is to start with this one and then take up a comparison with the others.

I think the ordinary textbook description of Natrum Mur. is misleading. They tell you that Natrum Mur. patients have a pale, waxy skin; in most cases it is nothing of the kind. They do tend to have an oily skin, but you do not get the waxy pallor which Kent stresses. You are much more likely to get a patient with a fair amount of colour and, very often, a tendency to flush. When you are talking to them, or if they are embarrassed, they tend to get a high, irregular colour. The circulation is unstable, they quickly become embarrassed, the pulse runs up very quickly, and it is then you get the oily look. The modern woman does not come into your room with a greasy nose, but before you have done with them they tend to be greasy across the forehead. They tend to get small vesicles at the corners of their lips and along the margin of the hair along the ears. The margin of the hair is a help sometimes; usually you do not see the ears nowadays.

The extreme emaciation of Natrum Mur. is also stressed in the textbooks but, certainly in the industrialised countries, it is the exception to see extreme emaciation. They are often thin about the neck but they need not be thin otherwise. As far as colouring is concerned, I do not think there is much to choose whether they are dark or fair. One pretty constant thing is a certain amount of yellowness of the skin. You do not notice it when they are flushed, but you do notice it when the flush begins to disappear.

You notice that the patient is slightly embarrassed, a little self-conscious. They have usually screwed themselves up to come and see you; yet they do not want you to see they are finding it a strain. They often come in with an appearance of self assurance – almost of opposition – they are not the most friendly of patients who ever come into your room! They definitely seem to be on their guard. They will answer your questions, usually briefly, often abruptly, and tend not to give anything away at the beginning of the interview. After you have got their confidence they often pour it out.

Natrum Arsenicosum

The Natrum Ars. patient has nothing like the same degree of flushing as the Natrum Mur. The patient is pale, with a much bluer pallor than the yellow sallowness of Natrum Mur. You often notice blue rings round the eyes and the lips tend to be pale, and instead of the eruptions of Natrum Mur. they tend to get dry, cracked lips. The next thing is that they are more nervous and less resentful. Their hands and fingers are restless and when you are talking to them there is often a slight twitch of their shoulder, arm, or the muscles of their face. A certain amount of perspiration develops, but you do not get the same greasy sort of look. When they come in they are obviously tired: Natrum Mur. plants the feet firmly down on the floor, Natrum Ars. comes in rather shyly. Natrum Ars. is alone among the Sodium salts in being prostrated by sexual intercourse.

Natrum Carbonicum

There is a general Sodium similarity with all these patients and I am concerned to stress the differences. Here you have, instead of the taut Natrum Mur. a much more fleshy person. The impression you get is of a pale, doughy, indefinite sort of outline to their features. They tend to be more plump than the Natrum Mur. patient and they may be fat. Most Natrum Carb. patients have a certain puffiness about their ankles. You may get Natrum Mur. patients quite neat and trim but you hardly ever get a Natrum Carb. patient who does not have rather thick ankles. When you talk to them they tend to flush up, somewhat like Natrum Mur., but it is a much more blotchy redness.

There is not the same degree of definiteness in their character. They are tired, and sort of waddle across the floor rather than stamp across it as the Natrum Mur. does; sitting in the chair they tend to slouch, whereas the Natrum Mur. sits up and looks you in the eye. One thing that will clinch the matter if you are in doubt about it being Natrum Carb. is this: if you have a big book on your desk and let it drop with a bang on the floor, they will fairly damn you. If you do not get that reaction to a sudden noise it is not Natrum Carb.

They always get acutely irritable. If you fidget with papers on your desk they get more and more worked up and finally say, 'I do wish you would stop doing that'. Natrum Mur. patients also dislike it, but not to the same extent. They may look at you in resentment but they will not spit out at you when they cannot stand it any longer.

All the Sodium salts have the thunder aggravation, but Natrum Carb. has it more markedly than any of the others.

The time for the Natrum Carb. general aggravation is about 5 a.m., and that is particularly the case in its stomach conditions. They often wake feeling horribly hungry, with definite gastric pain, and their only relief is by getting up and eating something. They are definitely ameliorated by heat, provided they do not overdo it. They have a second aggravation at 5 p.m., but that is a general aggravation, not particularly a stomach one.

Natrum Phosphoricum

The Natrum Phos. patient is the thinnest of all the Sodium salts. I have never seen one who was not definitely underweight. They are often tall and scraggy. They are almost always pale but flush up under stress, and it is usually a hectic flush—a bright spot on the cheek, usually on both cheeks.

The skin of the Natrum Phos. patient does not have the same degree of oiliness as the Natrum Mur., but it tends that way. Most of the Natrum Phos. patients I have seen have been over middle life, and most of them have struck me as having let themselves down. They are not so trim and tidy as you would expect from their general outlook and from the way they talk; they have rather lost their keenness. When you are trying to get their story they find it an effort to remember details of what is troubling them. They are quite ready to help you, but either they cannot remember or, for some other reason, they cannot get it out. Another thing is that they are hopeless about their condition. They do not think you are going to do them much good and have usually come to see you under some compulsion—someone has been badgering them.

Natrum Sulphuricum

Natrum Sulph. is a definite entity. Practically all are fattish and rather undersized. They usually are high-coloured and may be florid, but with an underlying yellowness. In acute conditions they are the kind of people who very often develop a stagnant liver and may get jaundice. They tend to get skin eruptions, much like Natrum Mur., and they do have a slightly greasy skin.

The main impression you get is that they are rather discontented and bad-tempered people – although you do get some who do not show any bad temper but just the signs of depression and hopelessness. I think they are as near as one ever meets to what used to be looked on as the typical livery subject – the sort of outlook that popularly used to be considered as an indication for a dose of salts.

You will occasionally get a Natrum Sulph. patient who is not typically like that, and here you get the high colour and the greasy face, but not the excessive fatness. They all have fat necks and tend to be plump. The only cases I have seen of this type are people with definite exophthalmos plus thyroid. If they get on to emaciation they have probably moved away from Natrum Sulph.

That is more or less how these different salts strike me when seeing patients when they first come in. When you begin to question them, certain distinctions in their mentalities become apparent as you go into their case more fully.

MENTALITIES

All the Sodiums are, without exception, hypersensitive – sensitive to noise, surroundings, music, thunder and to people.

There is a lack of balance in them all and the Natrum Mur. patient very often runs to extremes. They may either be over-conscientious or they may lose all interest in what they ought to be doing. They may either be over-affectionate or they may have no interest in the people round about. They may either be afraid of all sorts of things, or else they may get into the state when, as they say, they are damned if they will be afraid of anything. The same patient may spring about from one state to the other. One day they will tackle anything; the next day they have lost all self-confidence.

The Natrum Mur. patient is stated to have an absolute intolerance of consolation. In fact they crave for consolation from the right people, and if they get it will often knock them off their legs altogether. If you happen to strike the right note with a Natrum Mur. patient they strike you as entirely different people. They crave for understanding and appreciation but hate what we used to call 'plastering'. They dislike being touched, and if they have pain it is generally aggravated by touching.

They are always rather keyed up and restless. They move their feet or fidget with their bag. They constantly complain that whenever they attempt to relax, or as they are falling off to sleep, they are liable to get sudden muscular jerks. If one takes that as a starting point and compares it with Natrum Ars. mentalities, Natrum Mur. are much more nervous and frightened, and get all sorts of fears – of disease, of impending evil, of something going to happen.

They are also usually over-conscientious and this is one of the points where the typical Sodium make-up comes out – they do things though it is a fearful effort to do them. If they undertake anything and meet with opposition they fly into a fury, and anger simply exhausts them. After being angry they get into a state of trembling; their hands and feet tremble. Any mental effort is very trying for them. They always have the sense that they are being hurried and that they are doing it against time – which always brings on a fearful sense of mental and physical weariness. These patients will tell you that after anything of that sort they simply must go and lie down.

If you take Natrum Carb. mentalities, they correspond more nearly to Natrum Mur. than any of the other Sodium salts. But the hypersensitiveness, particularly to noise, music, thunder and people, is even more marked in Natrum Carb. The reaction you get to any of these is either irritability or even palpitation. Music upsets Natrum Mur. emotionally; they weep from it. The common Natrum Carb. reaction is the same, although occasionally you get a patient who cannot stand a full orchestra whereas they can stand music that is not loud.

There is a degree of difference in their reaction to sympathy and social relations. Natrum Mur. want to be looked up to and thought well of. Natrum Carb. feel their friends do not understand them, and it is this feeling of being cut off that often starts their dislike and criticism of their relatives. Of the two, Natrum Carb. is much more sensitive to atmosphere from people than Natrum Mur. and they take marked dislikes for certain people for absolutely no reason, particularly for strangers. Natrum Mur., on the other hand, is more likely to take a sudden passion for somebody.

As I have already remarked, the Natrum Phos. mentality is one of being tired and discouraged and a little discontented. That is their ordinary state but they do, under interference, become irritable and often very impatient of friendly advice – not of criticism as some of the Sodium salts. In spite of this weariness they will delay seeking medical advice, often due to a fear of illness. As a rule they are restless and fidgety in spite of their weariness, and will tell you that it feels as if their nerves were all in a fret. Any effort of concentration produces this state of nerves. In the Natrum Phos. patient you get the critical side that comes out in most Sodiums, but it is liable to be a criticism of somebody who is not there rather than the sudden unpleasant reaction of the other Sodium salts to somebody who is present. They usually have a grievance of some kind.

Natrum Sulph. patients are practically always depressed, and the depression may go on to definite thoughts of suicide. In this depressed state they have a dislike of people; they do not want to talk to them or see them. They resent your questions and are rather suspicious of what you are getting at. That is the main outline and yet, underneath this sullen exterior, there is always a sort of apprehension and it is not quite the same as in the other Sodium salts. Their discomfort and their anxiety appear to be more marked if there are people about, and they have a definite fear of crowds. They often have a shunning of people – I am never quite sure whether it is a fear or a dislike. They have a fear of evil. What form it is going to take they do not know; it is just a fear of something hostile to them.

TEMPERATURE REACTIONS

The next thing you get out of Sodium patients is their temperature reactions, and these offer definite help in distinguishing between them. Natrum Mur. is very much like its mentality – typically a hot-blooded patient. They are intolerant of heat in general and you have to establish exactly how it affects them. They are intolerant of any stuffiness rather than warmth. A stuffy room crowded with people definitely upsets them, though they are also sensitive to cold and draughts. The easiest way to remember is that they get a greasy face under stress, and immediately they are greasy on the surface they become uncomfortable.

Consider in contrast the Natrum Ars. patient. They are chilly; they like as much warmth as they can possibly get, but they have a slight mental amelioration in the open air. If they have had an emotional upset, they are again better in the open air. They are always worse in winter and very sensitive to damp – damp cold upsets them intensely. They are aggravated by exertion, either mental or physical, and usually worse after food.

Natrum Mur. tends to get an aggravation of all symptoms round about mid-morning – 10.30 a.m. to 11.30 a.m. – and they may get a sun aggravation, worse at noon and tailing off at sunset. Natrum Ars. has a definite aggravation on waking up and another round about midnight.

The Natrum Carb. is a chilly patient. They are much aggravated by cold and are better for heat, with one exception – they cannot stand a hot sun on their head; it will always produce a headache.

Natrum Phos. patients are more chilly than any of the others, possibly with the exception of Natrum Ars., and more sensitive to draughts than any of the others. They are sensitive to cold, miserable in winter and much aggravated by any change in the weather. They are aggravated by damp and are often upset after a bath. It is usually their chest conditions that are upset by it – cough and cold. They get a good deal of digestive trouble as well, and that is also worse after a bath.

Natrum Sulph. is a hot-blooded remedy, much aggravated in warm weather and extremely sensitive to lack of air, a warm room, a stuffy room or to a room full of people. They are sensitive to damp, wet weather – hot muggy days lay them out entirely. One peculiar thing is that in spite of their aggravation from heat they are most susceptible to night air, particularly if there is a little mist about. It is a common asthmatic remedy – people who get wheezy at night commonly call for Natrum Sulph. They tend to a spring aggravation in most of their complaints. I suppose it is due to the softer, damper weather of spring. They are better when moving about and tend to be worse when keeping still. Natrum Sulph. can be at its worst in the morning when waking. They are singularly unpleasant before breakfast; after it they are bearable, but before it are best left alone. They often tell you they feel more cheerful after they have had an action of the bowels.

FOOD REACTIONS

Certain constant factors recur in Sodium salts. One outstanding feature is their aggravation from milk – they all have it, some more than others. The one in which it is most marked is Natrum Carb. They all have an aggravation from rich foods, particularly fatty foods. Another constant thing is an aggravation from starch, although it is much less marked in Natrum Carb.

In addition to these generalities, certain of them have aggravations peculiar to themselves. For instance, Natrum Ars. has an absolute intolerance for fruit, Natrum Mur. does not. The other three – Natrum Carb., Natrum Phos. and Natrum Sulph. all do. After Natrum Ars. the second strongest aggravation is in Natrum Sulph.

There is a marked aggravation in Natrum Phos. from sour things. It has the fruit aggravation but it needs to be definitely acid fruit. Natrum Ars. and Natrum Phos. have aggravation from alcohol.

108

Natrum Carb. has an aggravation from sweets. Natrum Sulph. has an aggravation from vegetables of all kinds, particularly green ones and Natrum Sulph. also has an aggravation from coffee.

Sodium patients display certain contradictions between their desires for food and their aggravations. In spite of having a definite bread and starch aggravation, many of them have a definite desire for bread. This is marked in Natrum Mur., less so in the others, but is present in Natrum Carb. as well as in Natrum Ars.

Most Sodiums have an aggravation from alcohol, yet they all have a definite desire for beer and sour drinks. They all have an aggravation from milk yet, occasionally, a Natrum Mur. patient has a definite desire for it.

Sometimes you get contradictory indications – a desire and an aversion for the same item of food. You do not get the desire and the aversion in the same patient, but rather in different patients requiring the same remedy. For instance, a Natrum Mur. patient may have a definite desire for sweets or may have a definite aversion to sweets. You find some Natrum Mur. patients with a definite desire for meat though the majority of them have a definite aversion to it. You find a certain number of Natrum Mur. patients with a definite craving for salt and a certain number with a definite aversion to salt. Some may have a definite desire for wine or beer, and others will have a definite aversion to it – this is more marked for wine than for beer. One relatively unrecorded peculiarity is that Natrum Mur. has a definite desire for soup.

Another constant feature is that they all tend to be thirsty and practically all have a desire for cold drinks, athough a certain number of them have an aggravation from cold food. Natrum Ars. and Natrum Phos. have an aggravation from cold food even though they have a desire for it. Natrum Ars. has more desire for sweets than most of the others, with the exception of Natrum Carb., which most constantly has this desire. You find it moderately marked in Natrum Mur., a little in Natrum Ars.

Natrum Ars. patients often have a craving for bread and almost always a desire for juicy things. They have a definite aversion to fat. Natrum Carb. have practically all the desires of Natrum Mur., particularly for sweet things, and they have a desire for all sorts of stodgy, heavy, starchy, farinaceous foods. Usually they dislike coffee and fat and have a definite loathing for milk.

There are one or two peculiarities about Natrum Phos. They often have a desire for eggs, which you do not find in the other Sodium salts, as well as a desire for fish – particularly fried fish – and for all sorts of highly-seasoned food. You do sometimes come across an exception in Natrum Sulph. in connection with the loathing for milk. They rather like boiled milk, and often have a definite craving for ice cream. I think there are no exceptions to Sodium aversions, but one or two points come out in Natrum Mur. which are not constant to the others. For instance, Natrum Mur. has a definite aversion to tobacco. I think the aversion to salt can be more common in Natrum Mur. than in the other Sodiums. The aversion to coffee is common to both Natrum Carb. and Natrum Mur.

DISCHARGES

There are various distinguishing points in the character of discharges in these five remedies. The typical discharge in Natrum Mur. is white, very much like white of egg, and you may get it coming from any mucous surface. It is frequently less transparent than the ordinary unboiled white of egg but the general impression is that it is white. Associated with the discharge, the patient will always tell you that the affected mucous membrane feels dry. They get pharyngitis and you find this discharge all over the back of the throat, and yet the patient feels it is dry – so dry that they have difficulty in speaking, even though there is all this glairy material hanging about. You do not get the same complaint of dryness in the other Sodium salts (with the exception of Natrum Ars.). They may have a burning sensation but they do not complain of it being dry. The typical Natrum Ars. discharge is usually yellow in colour; rather watery, rather sticky and definitely yellow. It is practically always offensive.

Quite commonly you get an offensive discharge in Natrum Carb. and you may get it in Natrum Sulph. but Natrum Ars. is the most offensive. Natrum Carb. patients tend to have two types of discharge. It can be white in colour, but not so thin, tending to be lumpy and come away in pieces, and usually more ropey and stringy than Natrum Mur. The other type is a rather thick, yellow, offensive discharge.

The Natrum Phos. discharge again tends to be yellow, but it is much more pussy than any of the others. It varies between a creamy colour and a definite yellow, and the feature that distinguishes it from the others is that it is an acrid and excoriating discharge, and often has a peculiar sourish smell. The discharges in Natrum Sulph. are usually thicker, and instead of being yellow are yellowish-green, definitely pussy and usually fairly profuse.

TONGUE

The tongues in the five Sodiums are fairly suggestive. The Natrum Mur. patient complains of the whole mouth feeling dry, and the tongue is either one of two things. It is either shiny red or has a general shiny, red appearance broken up by patches of white exudate. That is the typical Natrum Mur. 'mapped' tongue. In the Natrum Ars. the tongue and mouth generally are rather flabby and toneless. The thing that draws your attention is the quantity of viscid mucus hanging about the mouth. The tongue is always a little like the typical Mercury tongue – large, flabby and pale but without the typical discharge you get in the Mercury mouth. In Natrum Carb. the tongue is characteristically sensitive, slightly inflamed, with a tendency to the development of small blisters along the margins. It may be moderately coated, but it usually has a bright red tip which is also sensitive to touch.

The Natrum Phos. tongue is typically a coated one and tends to be yellow at the base. It may not be definitely yellow – it may be white – but it always has a thick coating.

The Natrum Sulph. tongue tends to be dirty. It is thickly coated, and the coating varies from a light colour to brown. There is always a good deal of mucus. Occasionally you get blisters, but the blisters are on the cheek or on the inside of the lips rather than on the tongue itself.

The typical Natrum Mur. taste is salty. The Natrum Ars. taste is bitter. In Natrum Carb. the patient complains much more of a burning sensitiveness of the mouth than of the actual taste, though if they have a stomach upset there is a degree of acidity. In Natrum Phos. the patient complains of a sourness in the mouth. Natrum Sulph. commonly complains of loss of taste and a feeling of disgust at the sliminess of the tongue.

DIGESTIVE TRACT

The Natrum Mur. stomach tends to be sluggish and acid. The patient will always tell you that they feel uncomfortable after meals and that it feels as if their food takes an awfully long time to digest. During that period they often have a feeling of acidity and a burning feeling in the stomach. The great bulk of them also suffer from obstinate constipation although you will occasionally have to prescribe Natrum Mur. for chronic, persistent diarrhoea, particularly in a patient with a red, shiny tongue. All the digestive disturbances in Natrum Mur. tend to be aggravated by eating. If they are suffering from an acid stomach they are liable to become extremely thirsty, and it is with stomach complaints more than anything else that Natrum Mur. get thirsty. If they have a thirst they have a desire for cold drinks, and these often relieve the stomach disturbances for a time. In abdominal disturbances you get flatulence as well as intolerance of any pressure. Both Natrum Mur. and Natrum Carb. tend to get a feeling of hunger. Kent says Natrum Mur. get hunger feelings at 11 a.m. He also says Natrum Carb. get it at 10 a.m. to 11 a.m. I think Natrum Mur. tends to be later – 11 a.m. to 12 noon. However, I think the typical Natrum Carb. period is not 11 a.m. but earlier, round about 5 a.m., with a secondary one at 11 a.m.

In Natrum Ars. you are more liable to get an acute digestive upset with burning pain, usually in the stomach, and vomiting, either an acute gastritis or a gastric ulcer. One peculiarity in Natrum Ars. is that they get a feeling of emptiness without a feeling of hunger, particularly in stomach conditions. If they do take food it immediately produces a sensation of nausea. The next thing is that with most of their gastric pain they develop thirst and want very frequent small drinks; even when that pain is not present they are hypersensitive to hot drinks, which always produce a burning sensation in the epigastrium. There is a sense of sourness in the stomach in Natrum Ars. rather than a sense of acidity, and they are much more liable to get attacks of diarrhoea. These are usually painful, accompanied by tenesmus. They often get diarrhoea after food that is taken in the evening, and the attack is often precipitated by catching cold. The stool is that it is usually a very bright yellow.

The outstanding characteristic of the Natrum Carb. digestive system is flatulence. All Natrum Carb. patients get a certain amount of flatulence and they all tend to have a lot of loud, noisy eructations. Very often the patient suffers from troublesome waterbrash heartburn, and most of the abdominal symptoms are definitely relieved by eating. They want food every two hours and get a special hunger period in the early morning and late in the evening. If they have an acute gastric upset and you put them on milk they will be sick and become as sour as can be, and if you persist, they will almost certainly get acute diarrhoea.

Most Natrum Carb. patients are thirsty and desire cold fluids, although not too cold. Apart from their acute diarrhoea Natrum Carb. are constipated – just about as constipated as any remedy in the materia medica – and when you consider the type of food they like to eat you are not surprised at their flatulence and constipation.

Natrum Phos. have one or two odd points about them. They have the Sodium hunger but the circumstances are peculiar. They get a feeling of emptiness, and it is aggravated after meals. Another time they get this aggravation is after they have had their bowels moved, and that emptiness is not relieved by eating. Apart from that, you do find fullness after meals, and eructations which are definitely more sour than any of the other Sodium salts.

There is a good deal of general abdominal irritation in Natrum Phos., a pretty marked tendency to diarrhoea, and of a kind which is a help to diagnosis. It is usually a greenish watery diarrhoea accompanied by flatus. There is always marked urging before and a feeling of weakness in the rectum with possible incontinence of faeces.

Natrum Sulph. are the typical sluggish liver patients that feel as if they have a spoiled stomach. It is uncomfortable, full, and often tender, with a sense of fullness and weight under the right costal margin. There is a certain amount of dragging sensation in the liver; it feels heavy and congested, and if the patient lies on the left side the liver feels as if it drags over the abdomen. Associated with that there is a good deal of nausea, that develops after breakfast. It is not there first thing in the morning, but immediately they take food it develops and, with it, they get a horrible slimy taste in their mouths.

Further down the digestive tract they get a tendency to a congested, stagnant colon, and you may get an obstinate sluggish action in the region of the caecum. They often complain of a feeling of weight there, and on examination you find it tender and full. They also tend to get a chronic appendix. The whole caecal region is thickened and the appendix will be aggravated by lying on the right side. They may have jaundice.

Often, with their torpid colon, they get urging to stool. It feels as if they were going to have an action but all that happens is that they pass a quantity of flatus. The aggravation time is 4 p.m. to 8 p.m. for abdominal conditions, particularly for appendix and cholecystitis.

Another point concerning the lower abdomen is that they tend to get morning diarrhoea, in which they are not unlike Sulphur. Remember that Sulphur diarrhoea comes on before the patient gets out of bed, whereas Natrum Sulph. diarrhoea does not come on until after the patient gets up.

Natrum Sulph. patients are also liable to develop piles. If they do, these are usually congestive and bleeding, but not very painful.

31
Plumbum Metallicum

Plumbum patients are as a rule pale, and what I call a sort of dingy hue. They have not got a good fresh, bright complexion at all. They often have yellow sclerotics or are rather sallow, and nearly always have an expression of anxiety. Sometimes they have very dilated pupils. Mentally they can be active and intelligent and absorbed by their work, but more frequently they are indolent and disinclined to work, and rather melancholy and slow of perception. They are slow in answering, give names and words wrong, and are generally rather apathetic. They are restless sleepers and get into a state about not sleeping. When acutely ill, particularly with severe colic, they can have paroxysms of screaming because their pain is so frightfully acute. They do not know where they are or where they are going. They often talk to themselves. They think they are going to be poisoned by somebody.

I have had many Plumbum patients and have never seen a violent one yet, although this is the description in the books. The Plumbum patient also has an inclination to cheat and deceive. I remember a girl telling me about her brother, to whom I gave this remedy with very good effect: 'He always cheats at games. We are such an honest family, but he always cheats and then pretends he has had some reason for doing this, that, or the other. It astonishes the rest of us'.

I had a patient who came to see me looking very drawn, pale and anxious. Her main complaint was dimness of vision and an inclination to get an inflammation of her nose, which made her look conspicuous and worried her a lot. It was very red and sore-looking when she came and I was not surprised that she was worried about it. She then told me her difficulties. She said that her husband, son and daughter all had some difficulties, and that they all did the wrong thing by her. She grumbled away and I felt very sorry for her by the time she had finished. I gave her Natrum Mur. because I thought it would help her to live under such a strain. I then saw her once a month for the next six months but she did not alter. Natrum Mur. had not touched her, and somehow I felt that this woman needed help badly.

I took her history again. I said, 'I am going to treat you as though I have never seen you in my life before and you are to tell me everything as if you have never seen me'. The first thing she mentioned was her intense, distressing thirst. She had not mentioned that at all the first time! Also, that she had a very sweetish taste. She had vomiting and retching with tightness and pressure in the abdomen; pain in the groins and a pain down the legs. She told me all sorts of things which she had never mentioned previously. She had bouts of constipation. She also passed, as I think all the metals are apt to, very small balls of faeces. (They are all constipated remedies.) She sometimes had difficulty in passing water, and she had some vaginismus. I then repertorised her and it was very interesting. I took twelve symptoms that she had given, and in every one Plumbum came through in lowest type. It did not once come through in black type. I gave her some Plumbum 10M and in a month she was an absolutely different person.

A woman I knew quite well socially, but had never seen as a patient, suddenly lost her speech. She was taken to see various doctors who all thought she had some cerebral trouble. She asked if I would see her, and when she came she was quite unable to talk. She could not articulate properly, and on the history I gave her a 10M of Opium thinking she had possibly had some cerebral accident, with no effect at all. A week later I tried to get more details from the husband. He told me of her excessive thirst, which he said was an entirely new symptom, and that she had had a tightness in the throat for some time and her voice had been nasal for some weeks, and that she had complained of a numbness in her arms and legs sometimes, particularly in the thighs. She also had a feeling of a tight band feeling round one thigh. On this I looked up Plumbum and gave her a 12c for a fortnight and she got steadily well. I met her later and she said that she had never had any difficulty speaking again.

Shortly after this I was extremely interested to have a patient who came in because of constant pains in the limbs. She could not sleep well and could never get comfortable. She had a very dull colour and looked poor and anxious. The chief symptom was that she had a feeling that there were tight bands tied round her legs. When I asked her what she did for recreation, whether she was fond of music or whether she looked at the television, she said, 'Well, you know, I play bridge'. I said, 'Oh, do you? And are you good at bridge?' 'Yes, I am good at it. My family always say I cheat'. I thought this a gift and gave her Plumbum.

Another patient may complain of a cough. I had a patient with expectoration which quickly became purulent. Within two days it was short and dry-sounding, almost like a nervous cough. It was such a silly cough to bring up so much phlegm, but there was blood with it. He complained of tightness and distress and a feeling of oppression, felt very ill indeed and was constantly sighing. I asked a physician in one of the teaching hospitals if he was meeting this kind of cough, and he said, 'Oh, yes, and I will tell you what will happen. There is an epidemic of it. They start with rather a stupid cough. Their sputum is rather as you describe and you will find that they usually get a lung abscess'. I gave my patient Plumbum 30c on his chest symptoms, his sudden and excessive thirst, his apathy and lack of all other mental symptoms except sleeplessness. He did not get a lung abscess and was soon quite well. He was getting quite elderly and his wife said he had never had such a thirst before.

32
Pulsatilla Nigricans

Pulsatilla is one of the most commonly needed remedies. It is made from the meadow anemone, the wind flower. It blooms in the spring and the patient who needs it is like an April day.

The best picture of the remedy as a whole is perhaps shown in the teenage girl. She is fair-skinned and usually well covered. She is pleasant and affectionate and must have fuss and attention. The patient is sometimes described as taking everything but giving nothing. I do not altogether agree with that as some of the finest characters I have known have been typical Pulsatilla patients when not well. However, I remember a very nice family of six who had a sister in her teens who was extremely pretty, and I noticed that the brothers and sisters all waited on her. In my long experience I find the Pulsatilla patient is, as a rule, sweet-natured, yielding and very loving.

Under stress, whether mental, physical or the result of an infection, this patient becomes like the April day – everything about her is changeable. She will be smiling and apparently very happy and then in tears the next moment. These tears are perhaps the most characteristic thing about Pulsatilla. She is easily depressed, particularly in the evening, and hates to be alone. If someone comes in cross and irritable with her she will burst into tears, but a little attention and the feeling that you want to help will dry these tears quickly.

The Pulsatilla patient feels the heat, she wilts in a hot summer and can never sit in the sun; even a baby left in the sun gets very upset and miserable. The patient gets upset in a hot airless room and is better moving about gently in the open air. The tongue is moist but feels dry to the patient and she is usually thirstless. She hates fat or fatty foods, which upset her and cause nausea, vertigo and often a headache. The headache is worse on stooping or pressure and is relieved from cool air and gentle movement. She may sleep in a characteristic position on the back, with the arms above the head. She is often slow in getting to sleep, and if she has anything on her mind will go over it again and again, but once asleep she can be difficult to wake in the morning. She can complain of pains everywhere, but like her general personality they are changeable, going from one place to another. There is a history of the pain coming on suddenly and going off gradually; also that one joint, particularly the knee, is often swollen and painful and distressing. The joint is worse from bandaging, which produces heat and pressure which she never likes, and again the pains are often better for moving about gently.

In the cold this patient's nose runs and in a warm room becomes very stuffed-up. Any discharge is usually thick and yellow but not excoriating, even in a leucorrhoea, for which Pulsatilla can be good. The remedy is useful for menstrual troubles in this type of patient and can be excellent for hot flushes and morning sickness.

It is also a great stye remedy. I always remember the porter who took me up to the fourth floor when visiting a patient in a hotel in Eastbourne. The porter had one of the worst styes I had seen. By the time we reached the floor I had extracted a bottle of Pulsatilla from my case and asked if I might give him a very safe powder which would relieve him quickly. I did not mention this to my patient, because she was a most difficult person, and was very surprised to get a letter from her three days later asking me to send some more of those powders. The porter's stye had discharged within two hours and he felt so much better. Now the waiter and another porter both needed them as they too had styes, so I sent each of them three Pulsatilla 10M powders to be taken night, morning and the following night.

I do not want to give the impression that Pulsatilla is a remedy only for women or girls. I have had male patients whom it suited perfectly, and I have given it to men very often.

33

The Sea Remedies

The sea remedies are very useful, all of them in between the picture of Sepia and Natrum Mur.

Medusa

Medusa is a cross between Sepia and Natrum Mur. Everything is slighter. The patients have slightly greasy hair and skin, never as marked as the very greasy hair of the Natrum Mur. They are rather sallow, but not as sallow as Natrum Mur. They have the brownish appearance of the skin and the face of Sepia, but to a lesser degree. They often have very dark rings under their eyes and yellowish, slightly brownish faces. It is not as marked as in the Sepia, except that they are very tired-looking, as a rule.

Now there are two types of Sepia. There is the rather bright Sepia who goes off the deep end on the slightest provocation and is exceedingly irritable. There is the other Sepia who is rather stupid. They are tired out and they are stupid, but Medusa is neither of those. It comes between all of them. It is useful because when you are listening to the patient's history and looking at them you think that they must need Natrum Mur., or that they must need Sepia – and they do not.

You know the walk of the Natrum Mur. You can go along the road behind them; you know perfectly well if you have walked behind them for a minute that they must need Natrum Mur – the deliberate walk of 'him who means to get somewhere'. That characteristic always comes into your Natrum Mur., and it is not nearly so marked in the Medusa cases. Nor is their handshake quite so deliberate as that of the Natrum Mur. You think that it cannot quite be a Natrum Mur., but what could it be? – and probably they need Medusa. Nor do they flush up and go pale and greasy like the Natrum Mur.

Through the years I have found it a very useful remedy, particularly in the adolescent who finds his life rather difficult. The following three cases are absolutely typical.

119

One day a young women of about twenty-three was sent to me by her boss, who rang up about her and said she was not doing at all well. 'She is such a clever girl. There is nothing she can't do in her work, but she just feels tired out and can't tackle it, and will you please see if you think there is anything wrong with her?' I saw her for three weeks running and then he rang up again and said, 'I suppose you could not take her into hospital and get some tests done and really see if there is anything wrong with her, because she is invaluable when she is in her good form and useless when she feels she can't tackle her work'.

So I took her into hospital, and as I had a very ill patient in the ward at the time, I used to call each day to see her. Each time she stopped me to say, 'Doctor, there is something else I did not tell you'. That is quite typical of Medusa patients. They never give their history in one go. They always think of something else that they consider has a great effect on them, and they catch you and tell you about it if they can. She gave the history that she could be working well and then suddenly feel that she could work for an hour and no longer. This was most exasperating for the man she worked for, who wanted her to do a heavy day.

I did every kind of test on her and found absolutely nothing physically wrong. She gave me an interesting history of when she was at school. She said that when she had an exam ahead she had always done all the work, but that when it came to the exam itself she could not tackle it, and that was why she had rather failed in all the things she had done through life. She was lucky to have found such an understanding person to work for.

She was one of twins. She told me her twin sister had a good job and was doing extremely well, whereas she had had to come into hospital and was not doing at all well, and her work was too hard, and somehow or other she was always thwarted. She also rather resented those of her friends who were getting on well. She even resented her twin who was getting on so much better. Medusa patients do get full of resentment about all the other people of about their own age who are getting on well and really enjoying life, and here they are absolutely miserable. I remember the twin calling to see this girl. It was a very interesting thing that, although we could find nothing wrong with her, she got more and more untidy each day. Her twin came in and said, 'How frightful you look. Why don't you do your hair and make your face up a bit and look decent? How can the doctors endure to see you looking like that?' This made her furiously angry but from that moment she looked quite different when we went round.

120

When she did her hair and got her appearance very much better I said to her, 'Well, how nice you look'. 'Oh,' she said, 'my twin was in yesterday and said I looked absolutely frightful. That is part of my trouble. I sometimes get to the stage when I can no longer bother about my appearance or anything else. That was just another helpful point in her history and I gave her four doses of Medusa 200c. I have always used Medusa 200c. She soon became absolutely well. She went back to her job and was promoted.

A year later her boss rang me up to say, 'She is perfect. I could not do without her. She is my right hand, and I think it was having her in hospital and getting the medicine that obviously suited her. By the way, what was the medicine?' I did not know whether to say jellyfish or not. However, I said, 'It is a medicine called Medusa and it is made from the jellyfish', which entertained him a lot.

The Medusa patient can be very silent. They do not want to talk and they sometimes do not want to answer questions, in spite of the fact that they stop you in the ward to tell you the next thing. They nearly always have a full headache, rather like a Sepia headache, not like the much more severe headache of Natrum Mur.

They do not as a rule sleep well. This girl told me that she needed to have eight or nine hours sleep or she was no good. Sepia patients are also very much better for sleep.

Sepia are better for three things. Medusa are better for the same three things, to a lesser extent, these being sleep, movement and food. It is quite a useful thing to find a patient who says, 'Oh yes, I feel better for an hour after food. It quite definitely bucks me up'. Sepia are better if they go out for a walk, and if occasionally they go out to a dance they come in feeling absolutely grand. It is very helpful to have these three characteristics in Medusa to a lesser degree than in Sepia.

Occasionally you need Medusa in a younger patient than this girl. I had another typical case, a boy, whom I had looked after since he was seven, when he developed asthma. For two or three years homoeopathy kept down his acute attacks and he very seldom missed school, and he also stopped having his night attacks. This went on until he was about thirteen when he changed to another school near his home.

When he went to this new school he became more and more silent. The housemaster and his form master complained. They rang up his father and said that he was quite uninterested in his work and was doing badly. Although he never got acute attacks of asthma again he did get wheezy at times. He told me that he could not keep up, and when he was pushed at all he always got a headache.

He was a very intelligent boy in other ways, and I always remember interviewing his parents. His mother was the most difficult woman I had ever to interview about anything. His father was much more easy. I said, 'I don't think he should go to a normal school. He can't cope with it. He has had seven years of being delicate from his asthma, of being looked after morning, noon and night, and I don't think he can cope with an ordinary school at all. I think he is just going to take this attitude all the time and just be uninterested in his work, and I suggest that you send him to a coach'. At that moment I knew of a coach who took six boys and said he could take a seventh, and rather boldly I said all this, and in the end they sent him to the coach. Before he left I gave him a 200c of Medusa. That was at the end of the term and he was going to be six weeks at home before he started with the coach. He was a different boy. He became quite a famous painter, and kept Medusa ever since then, taking it if he felt he was headachy. Whenever he found he was getting a little uninterested in his work, or that it was a very great effort, or when he was doing a portrait and had to be very much on the spot for however long the sitter was there, he would take an occasional dose of Medusa.

There was one even younger patient, and this is the sort of thing that does not often happen, I am glad to say. He was a small boy in my practice who could not adjust to anything. If there was any change in the family or in the daily routine he reacted very badly. His father was offered a better job and the whole family moved suddenly to another place. He found himself at a different school, with different friends, doing all sorts of different things in entirely different surroundings, and it is difficult to describe how thwarted he was. He would not speak or answer and was very difficult, and said it was because everything had changed.

Medusa does not like a lot of changes and prefer to be able to go on in a pleasant routine. For a bit this boy, who was nine or ten did very badly. Then I sent him a dose of Medusa, although I had not given it to anyone as young as that, and rather regarded it more or less as an adolescent remedy. And from that time he became daily more and more amenable. He did very well.

Squid

Squid is another remedy that I find extremely useful. It is not synonymous with Sepia. It is often needed at the menopause in the most normal patient you can imagine. They are bright, quick, energetic women who find that their periods are perhaps getting more scanty or a bit irregular, and before their periods they are getting mastitis which they had not had for years. They start to find their work an effort, but they do not think that anyone else knows that they find it an effort.

The best case I ever had of this worked in an office and another patient of mine worked under her. She did not know that the latter was a patient of mine too. I happened to mention her one day to the second patient and she said, 'You know, there are times when we have to jump to it. It is only for a few days occasionally, but she absolutely drives us, and we all take very good care to have everything on the spot and that nothing is left undone'. She did not realise that she was menopausal and I did not tell her. This would happen just before a period, or perhaps on the first day of a period that was late and a bit irregular.

The Squid patient is one who is well and apparently absolutely normal but who is getting irregular and feels that her work, just that week, is an effort, and will be a bit impatient, hurrying everybody. They are not self-centred people like Sepia – they are really the least self-centred of all the sea remedies group. On the whole this group are not very interested in other people. The woman I have just described always had three or four nights of sleeplessness before a period, as well as mastitis. She was extremely chilly, and during this week that she was perhaps not quite herself she was more chilly than usual and complained of it bitterly. One thinks of Sepia, because if you meet her in her depression she is a bit depressed. The Squid patient does not have that certain degree of backache nor that certain degree of very marked irritability. I always use a thirtieth of Squid.

Sting Ray

Sting Ray is the only one of this group to be useful to both men and women. I have had several men patients who needed it and who have done well on it. They are sallow, usually dark, and they have rather heavy rings round their eyes. They look tired, are chilly, yet at the same time cannot stand a stuffy room. They are sensitive to all weather change, but as rule can stand real heat. Again, they tell you of their need of sleep, how many hours they need, how they must have it or else they are no good at all.

They get a slight headache as with Medusa, like a Sepia headache but even duller. It usually starts in the morning, strangely enough is usually better in the evening, and is made worse by noise or jarring, rather like Sepia although to a much lesser degree. One of these patients, the best case I had seen, was a dark, tall, rather tired-looking man who used to faint if he had to stand for long. He found it humiliating when he had fainted at two cocktail parties where he had had to stand for a long time. He asked if I would give him something to stop him doing that. He had a headache and said that when it came it lasted more or less all day but was always better in the evening. These patients also tend to be a bit sensitive to tobacco smoke and I think that this is why he had fainted.

In one year, just after using Sting Ray the first time, I had two soldiers who fainted continually, especially if they had to stand for an injection. Both of them had fainted half a dozen times each within the last so many weeks. They had had a lot of injections and had had to stand for rather long. One of them had taken part in the Queen's birthday parade and had fainted. He had been held up between two other soldiers who had held him on his feet until he came round again, but he felt frightful. Both these men did well on Sting Ray and neither of them ever fainted again.

I never inject a man standing up. Although I can inject any number of women standing up, I find I can get a man who faints, and feel that they are safer sitting down.

In women, you think the patient must be Sepia. They come in looking pale and drugged and very tired, with rather dark rings. You think they are going to be Sepia, but their chief complaint is of lower backache and gradually they tell you (and Sepia of course also tells you) that it always improves if they walk about. A Sepia backache goes if the patient walks about. The only difference is that with Sting Ray it does not come back, but in Sepia it always comes back when they sit.

This type of patient also gets quite a lot of palpitation, the men as well as the women. If the men have a tendency to faint, they think their palpitation has something to do with it. The woman gets palpitation quite a lot but forgets it again if she is walking. The history is typically that if she gets bad palpitation, and has to go out because she has a very busy morning, by the time she comes back from shopping it is gone, which surprises her very much but which is a good symptom.

They are rather tired-out patients, but in no way so despairing or such martyrs as Sepia. Sepia can be real martyrs if they go on getting tired out and have a lot to worry them, especially if they have to look after various members of the family and will not accept any help that is offered to them. Sting Ray patients are much less like this, but they do get rather hopeless.

34

Comparison of Lilium Tigrinum, Natrum Muriaticum and Sepia

It is a good thing to have a comparison of these remedies, which have certain conspicuous likenesses. Lilium Tigrinum is the least commonly needed of the three, but they are all very useful.

Lilium Tigrinum

Lilium Tig. is difficult to explain. You cannot say: 'This is what they look like . . .' because there is no fixed plan. They are rather compact people, firmly set up, fairly full-blooded, fat rather than thin, and fair rather than dark. Most of them have quite definite personalities with a sense of their own importance. They are not the soft and yielding type, nor are they unduly aggressive as the Natrum Mur. can be, and they are different from the resentful attitude of the Sepia, so you have here a quite separate personality for your Lilium Tig. One thing which is always present when they come to see you is that they sit there pushing their coat back, or something back, because they are too hot. They have a poor colour and as a rule rather blue lips. They are apt to be a bit cyanotic generally and full-lipped.

One helpful point of similarity between these three remedies is that they are all apt to be bad-tempered. They get all sorts of strange ideas into their heads, particularly that people have done something that they should not have done and are against them. If you try to explain, they deliberately take you up the wrong way, and if you persist in your explanation they get really angry.

Lilium Tig. have definite mental symptoms. They get a crazy feeling in their heads at times and do not quite know how to explain things, what to do and what to decide. They get depressed and low and sometimes very weepy, although I do not find the weepiness as common as they say in the books. They always feel – and this is characteristic of them – that they have something most important and urgent to do, which they are responsible for, which nobody else can do, and that they are the people who are left to do it. They are often quite indifferent towards their families but can be tormented about their own future, their salvation, about anything to do with their own lives. They are always hurried. They are all in a fidget; they do not have time to explain things, and are characteristically full of 'rush' – a sort of tormented rush that they have to get off their chests.

They feel the heat. If you have somebody who is very hot, and you are rather surprised as they are otherwise very like Sepia, do not forget Lilium Tig. It belongs to the same group and has a great many of the same characteristics, except that the patient is hot. They are snappy, exacting, and nothing pleases them. The following example of a Lilium Tig. patient gives such a perfect picture.

When I first saw this patient she was about forty-eight. She had an elderly mother and one older step-sister who was, fortunately, a schoolmistress in Gibraltar, so got away from her for a good part of the year, but what a life she gave her when she came home! This patient had been trained to be an actress and given every opportunity to learn acting. At last she was put into her first play and, with a great deal of help from leading actresses, was given a leading part.

She went to the First Night and was an absolute failure. She thought she had a wonderful career in front of her and suddenly found she had nothing at all. So, from that time she was determined to be the centre of the stage somehow. She went to bed and stayed in bed for the rest of her life. The only thing that ever got her up was an air raid. Her mother waited on her all the time, and so did her poor sister when she came home for holidays. She always felt that she was the pivot of the family, that they could do nothing without her, that they had to ask her advice over everything. She managed all their affairs. She also thought she had some fatal disease which the doctors had missed. I was always thinking out some way to convince her that she did not have anything, but it did not help much.

The family got rather worried about her – she could be so beastly to them – and suggested that I call in a psychiatrist. I did not want to do this much, although I did it, but he did not suggest anything helpful. So I then asked Dr Borland if he would see her. He visited her and was too sympathetic for words! She told him how she had had to have a psychiatrist in and how she felt humiliated about it. He was not at all surprised and said all the right things.

She told him of *all* her responsibilities, of *all* she had to do, and *all* she had to decide. As he went out he said to me, 'She's shouting for Lilium Tigrinum'.

126

So I gave her Lilium Tig., and am bound to say that whatever else it did not do – and it did not get her up – it did make her much nicer to her family and the people she had to deal with.

Natrum Muriaticum

Natrum Mur. is not so much a definite personality as a definite character. It has much more character than the Lilium Tig. As a rule they are square and well built, except in children. The children are very thin – you sometimes get a run of Natrum Mur. children who are all thin and scraggy. They have no particular colouring – they are sandy to dark, not as a rule black-haired. Their skin at rest is nearly always rather sallow, but there is one very misleading feature about this. If they are excited or pleased, or going to enjoy themselves very much, they can come in with such a bright flush that you think for a moment they must be a Phosphorus; In a few minutes you look up with surprise to find that they are quite sallow. The flush is from excitement only.

They have a definite walk – usually on their heels first – with definite movements. If they come to see you and you fetch them from the waiting room, they shake hands deliberately. If you do not fetch them from the waiting room and they just come in, they walk in very deliberately as if they have come to see you and the sooner it was over the better. 'Please get on with it' is their whole attitude. They sit down with a certain amount of strain, which is a funny thing because they look so deliberate. It is very common for the Natrum Mur. patient to put her parcels down with a little tremor. It is not a permanent tremor by any means but occurs just in putting down and picking up parcels, getting up from the table – a sign of the strain that they are undergoing in coming to see the doctor.

If they have a cold or if they are not well they are apt to have herpes round their lips, and they are also likely to have a crack in their lower lip, especially in the winter. In one winter I had a run of patients who had either a boil in their nose, very swollen one side and frightfully painful, or some kind of painful spot under their nose or on their chin.

The textbooks tell you that the Natrum Mur. patient does not have red lips. I do not think that is true – I think they practically always have red lips. They have a great aggravation from consolation when they are depressed. They quite like consolation if they are seedy or have a headache, whereupon they will break down and weep. If they are really ill they just want to be left alone. They do not get the same irritability and annoyance as Lilium Tig.

There is no doubt that Natrum Mur. has an unstable mentality.

That is one of its characteristics. They are actually very nice people. They can be absolutely up at the top and laughing or they can be down in the depths in two minutes, but they do not have a sense of humour that helps them to see the funny side of something. As you know them more you will find that they are really a mass of contradictions. They will pretend they do not want attention but grumble if they do not get it. As Dr Borland always said – they are very nice to know but not so nice to live with.

Natrum Mur. is also one of the most impatient of all the remedies. If they ask somebody to do something and it is not done quickly they are apt to go for that person thoroughly. They get a certain amount of palpitation and are very sensitive to sudden noise.

I remember a patient who was really the most perfect Natrum Mur. She had a large thyroid and had been advised to have an operation. Natrum Mur. just took down her thyroid and she never had any further trouble. She told me one day, 'You know, I can't bear noise'. I asked what effect it had on her. 'Well,' she said, 'last night I was reading a book and my sister dropped something behind me and I turned round and hit her over the head with the book!'

Another thing I have met many times is that they are very susceptible to music, although they are in no way musical. You can find them listening to the most drivelling and sentimental music you could possibly imagine, over which they are quite capable of weeping.

Another most useful point about Natrum Mur. is that it is the greatest of all the shock remedies. If you have nothing else to go on, give them Natrum Mur.

I had a girl in outpatients who got an enormous goitre after her parents and her brother were killed in an air raid. She was the only one alive in the house. She was taken in by an aunt who thought she was a useful girl of fourteen who could more or less look after her family. So the girl was left with half the work to do and treated very badly. The aunt brought her to the hospital because she began to swell in the neck. Her eyes became more prominent and she got a slight tremor. I put it all down to the shock she had had in losing her parents and her brother, but also followed on by the bad treatment she had received from her aunt. I gave her some Natrum Mur. which did her a tremendous lot of good. I got her away from the aunt and ultimately into nursing, where she did extremely well.

These patients will also remember anything that they thought was unfair from the time it happened for the rest of their life. They do not get away from it and are touchy and easily offended.

They are very changeable. They will have a great friend one week and the next week you find they are not on speaking terms with that person.

Sepia

Sepia tend to be fair with mouse-coloured hair, rather than dark, though I have in fact seen plenty of dark ones. When they are brought to see you they are often resentful of having to come to the doctor. They do not in the least want to see you. They say 'Good morning' without any politeness or any sort of smile. They can look so tired that they look stupid, in contrast to Natrum Mur. In Sepia it sometimes almost seems as though they cannot answer a straight question.

Sepia seems a fatter patient than you expect, more because they have fat faces than because they are fat in the body. They have rather well-filled, full faces, but are otherwise thin and tall, and they get a sallow colour that you do not get matched in any other remedy. The shadows under their eyes are halfway down their cheeks and very often, although not always, they have a saddle across the nose. When they do it extends across the nose to their cheek bones and up to the shadows under their eyes. They commonly have warty growths on their neck, sometimes also right up on to their face. As a rule they have pale lips and look physically absolutely done, as if they are too weary to do a job. They nearly all have long backs, and they look as if they could not possibly hold these backs up.

In their mentals they have a general resentment against their fate and feel that they have had a poor deal. If you try to console them they will often round on you and feel even more resentful than usual, and may get weepy. As a rule they do not weep unless you can break through all the defences they put up. The point about their getting weepy is that they feel much better and more cheerful afterwards.

They have quite as much sensitiveness to noise as the Natrum Mur. but their mentality is different. This is the really tired patient, mentally, physically and nervously, and definitely giving you the impression of being rather dull. They are dull sometimes in a sort of despairing state. At times they tell you they are simply not fit to go on and they just sit down and cannot take up the struggle. If you try to cheer them they change into an obstinate mood and feel that they are real martyrs. It is then very difficult to help them – they do not even want to be made well.

They are always afraid of something dreadful happening. If their husband is ill this is frightful. They are going to be destitute because he will not be able to work again, and here are the children to be looked after and they will have no money and what will they do? They do have a terrible fear of poverty. They tell you they have always been independent, that they have never asked for anyone's help and that they do not want to begin now. Yet if you have a patient living next to a Sepia you will soon be told how they would really like to help this woman, but since they get their heads snapped off every time they do not know how to do it.

These remedies are all sensitive to stuffy heat, particularly Natrum Mur. This usually gives them headaches. Equally they are all better for the cool, although draughts and extreme cold upset them. Of the three, Sepia complains the most about the cold. They all often have cold, clammy extremities.

All three of these remedies have bad headaches. The Lilium Tig. headache is always associated with a degree of mental strain. They get muddled and cannot think. They get a certain degree of ocular disturbance. If it is bad enough they are said to develop a squint. If their headaches are very bad they spread to the back of their neck, just to the top of their back. They nearly always also get some kind of abdominal discomfort with their headaches.

Natrum Mur. is one of our chief headache remedies and is a wonderful migraine remedy. It has a severe headache. Nearly always the patient wakes with it – a sort of dull head feeling almost as if it will burst. It can be a sick headache the whole morning. Very often they have certain ocular changes like zigzags in front of the eyes. They certainly cannot read and their eyes look heavy and dull, and sometimes the headache is so acute that they cannot even raise the eyelids.

I have seen patients with a severe migraine with these characteristics where Natrum Mur. has put them on their feet again. The headaches start in the morning and last into the second night, and may disappear by the following morning. If the headache persists, it is likely to be less severe thereafter. These headaches are associated with menstruation, usually before or afterwards, and not during the actual period.

Another curious headache that Natrum Mur. has is much more of a summer headache. It comes on between 10 a.m. and 11 a.m. and continues acutely until about 3 p.m. or 4 p.m., and then it fades away.

Sepia has an 'all over' headache. It tends to get worse till early evening, when the patient tends to be sick, and at that time it goes off. Usually it is better if they have applied heat. (Natrum Mur. is never better for applied heat.) Sepia is also better if you wrap up the head. Both are worse for light and for jarring noise, and worse in a very hot room.

All three tend to be hungry remedies. Lilium Tig. probably has the biggest appetite. They do not get any real satisfaction from eating and may remain hungry after a good meal. Natrum Mur. does not have the real hunger of Lilium Tig. It has much more an emptiness. They have a very definite salt craving. They like beer, fish, and occasionally milk. They do get an aversion to meat, coffee and to fat food, and they have a great aversion to sour wine because it thoroughly upsets them. The Lilium Tig. aversion to meat is really strong. Sepia patients have a definite desire for vinegar.

The one that has the most intolerance of tobacco is Sepia. Every now and then Natrum Mur. has a real dislike of tobacco and says it upsets their digestion. You must remember that they are all hypersensitive to the smell of food and to other definite smells. They like spicy pungent foods, sometimes craving stimulants such as wine.

Two other things are common to the three of them in different ways. The Lilium Tig. patient gets a certain fullness in the abdomen, especially as they are getting on in age or getting near the menopause. They feel that the whole of their inside is going to drop out. This is a very real complaint in Lilium Tig. They sometimes want support for the perineum in order to stop it dropping out, so great is this feeling. At the same time they are very sensitive in the epigastrium, so that you cannot give them a belt because they cannot stand the pressure, which makes them extremely difficult to deal with. They get a sensation of a lump in the lower abdomen. Sometimes they get an urgent desire for their bowels to act with this feeling of loading, but it is all controlled if they are kept very busy.

Natrum Mur. does not have this to anything like the same degree. They have irregular periods, and they have a general period aggravation either during or after menstruation. With this is an associated backache which is very bad in the morning but rather better when they get up and move about. It may be painful to touch. You will sometimes find the Natrum Mur. patient lying on the floor with a pillow in her back.

Sepia has almost as much drag as the Lilium Tig. but not nearly so widely spread. They do not feel that everything is going to fall out of their tummy – they feel that just the pelvic organs are going to fall out. They often have a retroverted uterus and a certain amount of prolapse, and a sensation of something bulging into the rectum. But it is rather different from the Lilium Tig. history. Lilium Tig. feels that there is a large lump there and the whole of it is going to fall out. Sepia feels that something bulges into the rectum and that it is going to fall out for that reason. Sepia always feels as if it were rather full down there, though there is never any urging to stool and no tenesmus; but they do get acute dysmenorrhoea and acute pelvic pain beginning in the back and spreading round the sides, and the backache is always better if they move about. In fact all Sepia complaints are better if they move about. If a Sepia patient dances vigorously all evening she will come in quite well. Sepia is better for three things – for movement, sleep and food.

All three of them have a great deal of palpitation and they are very good remedies for this complaint. Lilium Tig. has the most marked symptoms. They either feel as if the heart is grasped, as in a Cactus, and it gradually goes off – this is in a Lilium Tig. patient with all the other general characteristics, or some of them. Alternatively they feel they must bend double to relieve the palpitation, which is the reverse of Spigelia. Here again, if they do get palpitation they are apt to tell you of the imperative duties they have to do, and the responsibilities they have and all the things that depend upon them . . .

Sepia have just a mild palpitation. They sometimes feel as if the heart is going to push its way through the chest wall, but I do not consider that I have met many heart symptoms or much palpitation in a Sepia patient.

I would say that Natrum Mur. is one of the best palpitation and blood pressure remedies that there are. It is useful to remember the things that these remedies do pathologically, although I would want you to think of them as whole remedy pictures.

Another thing to remember with Sepia is its extreme usefulness in sterility. The number of cases we have had in our practice is quite extraordinary. Just a 10M of Sepia and they have started a pregnancy.

35

Comparison of
Lycopodium, Silica and Phosphorus

These three remedies provide a good comparison. They have symptoms which are similar, though in other respects they are poles apart.

Lycopodium
They are always spare, sallow, wrinkled people, from the time they are small babies. A Lycopodium baby who is very ill has nothing but lines on its face, a frown on its forehead, a very poor colour and probably abdominal pains at some time of the day. As they get older, you will find them growing above average height and nearly always with a slight tendency to stoop – a long narrow patient who stands up and then looks as though he has gone in the middle. They always have a worried expression and are difficult to get symptoms out of, simply because they are nervous of their interview and do not want to give anything away. Lycopodium never wants to give anything away, not even to his best friend. They will only give half their confidence, and always keep something up their sleeve. The result is that they are called haughty and stand-offish, but both these expressions hide the fact that the Lycopodium patient is very distrustful and insecure. I do not think you will ever find a true Lycopodium who is expansive. You can drag symptoms out of them and you find that they are great sweet lovers and will eat all the sweets in the house if they are left with them.

They also seem to be unfriendly. More than once I have heard a mother say, 'She never asks for anything, she never wants to have a party, or go out or play games. She likes to come in and read a book'. When the mother protests the child says, 'I see them at school all day and do not want to see them again'. Then there is the typical Lycopodium small boy who dreads going to school, who cannot eat his breakfast and who gets to the school gates clinging to the hand of this mother, and then is persuaded that it is really going to be all right and that he is going to enjoy it. Finally he goes in and in five minutes

133

has forgotten that he ever minded going to school.

They nearly all have digestive difficulties. Dr Borland used to call them lean and livery patients. I have two men in my practice, both businessmen, each with four other directors in the business, and they always see that they have their lunch at the proper time. If the meeting would suit the others at 12 noon, the meeting is at 11.30 a.m. for them so that they can have their lunch at 1 o'clock, otherwise they feel faintish and have to sit down, and that is humiliating. They are very nice people indeed, but if they are not well they are peevish and irritable and want to sit about doing nothing and not be disturbed. The only thing is, if you leave them in the house alone for a time, you will find them wandering around considering how they can get in touch with someone.

I had a small boy in my outpatients whose mother brought him because he was such a trial. In bed he would recite all the poetry he had learned at school and all the kings, dates and other things he could think of in a loud voice, but he would never even go to bed unless his sister of fifteen went at the same time. Not that he wanted to speak to her, but he liked to know there was somebody on the same landing. I gave him Lycopodium and it fitted him very well. He was a lean boy, thin and stooping. About three years later he came into outpatients again, and I asked him, 'Haven't I seen you before?' He said, 'Yes, you have seen me once before'. And I said, 'I remember what I gave you, too'. His mother had asked if I would please give him exactly the same medicine as last time, which I did. I saw no reason to change. He was in for higher exams and here he was shouting his facts all over the house. They are very apprehensive if they have anything particular to do.

The Lycopodium patient has not got great stamina. They get tired easily; they come home from work absolutely whacked and it is then that they want to sit down and not have anyone talk to them or interrupt them. It is one of the greatest mental fatigue remedies. It is also one of the greatest sleeplessness remedies.

I had a patient of about thirty-five who came to see me saying, 'My brother wants me to play squash with him. I have always hated games, but I feel it would be good for me, so I go out and play squash. I feel I want to die after it'. He was an exact and perfect appearance of Lycopodium, looking worried, very tall, gone in the middle, with indigestion, peevish at times, all the other things you would expect, and much better after his evening meal. It was between 5 p.m. and 7 p.m. that he felt so ghastly if he was made to play. He said, 'I feel ravenous for my evening meal, but I only take a small amount. If I take more I get indigestion and find myself pushing my plate away in the middle of a big meal'. The 4 p.m. to 8 p.m. aggravation is constant – it is a very useful point. Occasionally, remember, you get a 4 a.m. to 8 a.m. aggravation, which also is a useful point and comes into your Lycopodium. They feel slow off the mark in the morning and depressed, as if the day's work will be too much for them, especially businessmen. After breakfast things are not so bad.

I had another interesting man who came into a bed in the Homoeopathic Hospital after having had an accident. He did perfectly well: and one day he said, 'You know, I have got lots of symptoms I have not told you'. I said, 'You had better tell me them'. So we got down to an endless list of symptoms and I wrote him up for 10M Lycopodium. When I next went round the ward he said, 'I never thought I would be a Lycopodium'. He had borrowed a book and read in it that all Lycopodium patients are inclined to be close. 'I think perhaps I am a miser, because in a drawer in my desk I always keep two or three bars of chocolate, and when they are getting low I make sure before I have finished the last that I have four or five put in their place!' They are generally careful with money. They think they are not going to be able to carry on, or that it is not worth while carrying on. Some of them give up their jobs. Others, with the help of Lycopodium, manage to pull themselves together, and it is most useful for that. Then they begin to save hard. One of my greatest Lycopodium cases, as a small boy five years old, was typical. His mother said to him, 'Ian, what do you want to save money for? And he said, 'Just suppose if anything happened to Daddy and we did not have anything to live on'. Once a year Lycopodium put him on his feet, whatever was wrong.

Silica
Silica is different. No remedy looks exactly as it is written up in the books. You have to recognize the symptoms and try and see the whole picture. Silica is typically undersized, and they have very small hands and feet. As a rule they have a clean skin and quite a good colour, or their faces can be dead white and they can have sore patches around their eyes or somewhere in that region. Or again they have very cracked corners to the mouth, which will quickly give you Silica – one of those things you notice before the patient has started to speak. Sometimes there is a crack in the nose and they have a lot of nasal catarrh. They have small bones and very fine hair, but they never give the haughty Lycopodium impression.

135

They are pleasant, yielding, gentle people on the whole, giving the impression that they would give up easily, but it is an entirely false impression. The textbooks state that Silica patients have no guts. Borland, Wheeler and Clarke all said that they are people with enormous courage and an enormous capacity for work, but with a weakness in their physique that makes them at times seem to give up a thing. They are gentle and polite, as a rule – but push them beyond that point and they are obstinate and just as difficult as they can possibly be. If they think a thing strongly, then it is very difficult to get it out of their heads. It is sometimes difficult to see how the idea arose that Silica are weaklings who would give up any job and have no stamina. The reason is that if they are offered a job, they really do get in a panic over trying and failing. If they can be persuaded to take it on they do it extraordinarily well, and put everything they know into it.

The Silica child is one of the most amusing children you can have if you treat them properly. They are normally lively and friendly, but let them be mismanaged and they are frightful. I always remember a sweet little girl who had been playing with the children next door, and one of them had thrown a brick at her and cut her across the forehead. She was brought down to see me in a furious temper and was dragged with loud shrieks into my consulting room. I asked the mother to wait in the waiting room. If children like this are being troublesome I see them alone. In five minutes she was much better, telling me all about the brick that had hit her on the head and about the boys next door who were horrible when they played that sort of game. I gave her some Silica and she was quite all right. On the other hand, they can be the most miserable of children – delicate and cold. Their feet are always cold and they cannot get warm. They cannot get to sleep and they sweat profusely around the head. Their pillows are soaking and their feet too, usually with a cold offensive sweat.

In one week I had two very interesting Silica cases. The first was a girl working in a good job in an office as a secretary, who sweated so profusely that it went through the blotting paper. She had to wear a mackintosh apron otherwise it went through the back of her skirt. She put up a hand and the drops dripped off the end of it. I tried her with three remedies based on her family history. These did her no good. I gave her Thuja because of her tendency to sweat on uncovered parts, which also did her no good. Then I gave her some Silica and in one week it had all dried up. She went to live in Hong Kong from where she wrote to say that she had never had any return of the trouble, even in that climate.

Then I had a boy in his last year at school. He had bad acne but his main complaint was that he also had the most terrible sweating feet. His schoolfellows would not go near him after a certain hour in the day. He changed his socks twice but even that was not enough. I gave him Silica. Not only did it cure his sweating very quickly but it also cured his acne. (Silica is not a remedy I would use for acne as such, but he fitted into it. He was skinny, he had cracks and lots of Silica symptoms.)

Phosphorus
There are two types of Phosphorus. One is dark-haired and the other is fair-haired with a glint in the hair. Dark-haired ones also sometimes have a glint. They are usually well proportioned and their skin is always fine, but it varies in colour very quickly. The Phosphorus patient coming in looks quite flushed and a little nervous, then in a few minutes it is gone. They never perspire except for a reason. In other words, if they have taken violent exercise or have walked very fast, then they perspire. If they do, it is on the top lip and just a little on the forehead. The other thing that makes them perspire is mental exertion or nervousness. They are intelligent and cheerful and, as a rule, nice people.

Phosphorus patients have a lot of mentals. They have a tendency to fly into a passion. It is over in a minute or two and they are quite ashamed at having had it. They are never left with the resentment you get in Silica sometimes, or in Natrum Mur. They are sensitive to all external impressions. Like Sepia they are better for sleep. It is the Phosphorus patient who can sit down in an armchair and sleep and after ten minutes wake absolutely refreshed. They are better for rubbing. Sometimes when they are not well they can never 'collect themselves together' when in bed. This symptom is usually Baptisia, but Phosphorus has it too. They have a real fear of the dark, of being alone, of thunder and of dying. They fear that something awful is going to happen and are sensitive to any kind of atmosphere. They are also a bit afraid in twilight. The other thing about them is that normally they are such nice people, but when they are ill they are sometimes entirely indifferent to their family.

If they are overtired and have been working too hard, Phosphorus patients sometimes get a different set of mental symptoms – a state of mental apprehension. They get very worried about what kind of illness they could possibly have. They also get into a state about family matters and all kinds of things. I remember one boy imagined he had left a gas tap on somewhere. I rang up to enquire for him. He did extremely well on some Phosphorus.

The other thing about Silica is that if they are under mental strain and physical exertion they become quite sleepless. When they go to bed they fall into a temporary sleep for two hours. They then go over all the things they have to do, and try and work it all out. Finally, just towards morning, they fall asleep for one hour. They weep fairly easily if they are very run down, but they are never any better for it, whereas Lycopodium, if they are depressed, are better for sympathy and also for weeping. They are both sensitive to cold.

Lycopodium can have air hunger in a stuffy room and will occasionally develop a bad right-sided headache. In Silica you get a recurring stress headache starting in the back of the head. The Silica headache is one of the migraine headaches. It is a recurring headache, nearly always accompanied by sickness. It starts at the back of the neck and can go down the spine, but usually comes up over the head to the right temple. It then settles over the right eye with persistent pain on the outer side of the eye; it is much better for warmth. You will sometimes find a Silica patient applying a hot water bottle to the back of the neck. They cannot bear a cold draught. They do not want to move and they are worse for pressure, even from a tight hat. This headache nearly always goes on to vomiting and nearly always arises from prolonged mental effort and not just sudden overwork. They are also much worse for exertion.

There is another kind of Silica headache from definite mental concentration, a frontal headache. It has the same modalities as the others, better for warmth and worse for cold, worse for exertion and pressure, and is sometimes brought on by exposure to cold. As a rule it is not more one side than the other. It may go from one side to the other. I always remember going to my house and finding a colleague doing something with a hat. I could not think what she was doing and she said, 'I am just sewing a lining into my hat, I cannot bear the cold out of doors'. She wore that hat all the winter without headaches. Sometimes travelling in a train, with your seat over the wheel causing jarring, can give you a Silica headache. Another important symptom with Silica is that the ends of their fingers are apt to get sore cracks round the nails. They are unpleasant to touch, both from their point of view and yours. They go septic and become especially bad if they are working in water, with fissures in the thumb. They have rather small hands.

Now Silica and Phosphorus both have a tendency for their fingers to become cold and dead. If it is Phosphorus and they put their hands in water, within a few minutes they will feel sick, whereas if Silica comes in and puts their hands in hot water, they are warm in a minute and quite comfortable. That is a very useful point, because it is something that the patient volunteers.

The Phosphorus patient is thirsty for cold drinks and loves ice-cream. On the whole they rather dislike sweets, but they like salt very much. Phosphorus is one of the thirstiest of drugs – they drink more than average and sometimes when they are ill take long draughts of very cold water. Then when it is warm in the stomach they bring it up. Another thing about Phosphorus, particularly so in a child, is that they do not take their eyes off you. I always remember a girl of about seventeen with very bad pneumonia in a bed in King Edward Ward. I was going round with Dr Borland and she was thrilled that she was going to be seen and reassured that she was not going to die. All the way round the ward she never took her eyes off us. When I got near my hand was taken surreptitiously, just for extra reassurance. She was scared stiff. She got quite well.

Silica rather dislikes hot food. This is a useful tip sometimes. Equally Lycopodium dislikes cold food and says that Sunday night supper is enough to kill anyone.

Phosphorus is one of the great pneumonia remedies. The patient does not wish to lie on the affected side but prefers the position of sitting up against the pillows with the head a little back. That is how this girl was sitting with a jug of water beside her. They tend to get a severe pneumonia with tight chest and are very much worse if the room gets chilled or the windows are opened.

Silica on the other hand gets a rattly chest. There is prolonged coughing and catarrh. After much experience I would say that Silica is one of the best remedies there is for an unresolved pneumonia or for a chest that does not clear up.

Silica is worse in cold thundery weather, but otherwise not much affected by weather. Now both Phosphorus and Silica have one queer symptom in common. They dislike talking to people. If you say to them, 'Now go and talk to that group', this terrifies the Phosphorus patient. The Phosphorus patient is also terrified if the room is crowded, as they cannot think of anything to talk about. The Silica patient does not want to stand with a lot of people and has not the slightest desire to talk to them. It is generally because Silica dislike people rather than disliking talking.

Lycopodium can never stand tight clothing. You will find that they have the belt loosened around them. They do not like tepid or cold food, but prefer really hot food. They also prefer hot drinks to cold, on the whole. They are sensitive to noise and smells, and have dry, hot hands and dry, hot soles of their feet. A Lycopodium, in my experience, never says thankyou. When they walk to the door, their thanks is all in their handshake. Your hand is gripped and shaken with all their force. I have two Lycopodium men, and I take them half way to the front door, then hand them on to someone else to be shown out! But remember that the Lycopodium is a very faithful patient.

36

Tuberculinum Bovinum

(*Note:* In the following discussion, the remedy referred to as Tuberculinum is used interchangeably with Tuberculinum Bovinum.)

It is very difficult to give a real picture of Tuberculinum. There are certain characteristics which recur more or less every time, but you cannot give a real picture in the way you can of the Arsenicum patient. It is not a recurring constitutional remedy. If you want Tuberculinum at all you will want it once and then perhaps repeat it once more, but not within six months. One outstanding feature is that the patients fairly constantly have blue sclerotics.

Two other things they have are long eyelashes, which you would expect, and hairy backs. Very often you get a history, not of being delicate, but of quite a marked family history of T.B. sometime in the past. Like the Arsenicum patient they have a peculiar mental restlessness. It is not so much that they get up and move about, because they are apt to sit like a log and look as if they could not be bothered to talk to anyone. It is more a state of dissatisfaction – with their surroundings, with what they are doing, with whatever their condition is. They have a desire to move about, but this is really a more general desire for a change, like the child or early adolescent who gets up and wanders round the room, not because they are particularly restless but because they want a change. They want to do something else from what they are doing.

They will always be ready to travel, whatever the circumstances. They want to go for a holiday and then, in the middle of the holiday, they want to go off somewhere else. I always remember going to a young woman patient, married and with one child. She was sitting on the sofa as if she could not possibly, under any circumstances, ever get up again. I asked her, 'Do you really feel as tired as you look?' and she said, 'I feel moribund', which I thought was a very good description of how she looked. At that moment her husband arrived and said, 'Would you like to go to Paris?' 'Like to go to Paris?' she said. In an instant she was up, more or less packing, looking entirely and absolutely different.

That is very like a Tub. Bov. and in particular the slightly older post-adolescent patient. Whatever their complaint, they are better for movement. If you can make them move about they are better. Quite often these Tuberculinum cases have a history of being a good-tempered child who had definitely changed into a disagreeable, easily upset adolescent. Their mothers will tell you that they were so easy when they were small and such fun. And now, that they are thoroughly disagreeable and not at all the same, and very easily upset. The upset is nearly always that they burst into tears continually, or they get very angry.

These patients have a great dislike of mental work. From being bright children and doing very well, they suddenly feel that they cannot work or that they do not want to work. They will not settle down to it and say it tires them. They are inclined to get headaches, and make anything an excuse for not working. On the other hand their physical work is good. They can go to the garden and do an hour's useful gardening, and they do not complain of tiredness or anything. But set them down to their homework and it just does not get done.

Another constant sign is that they get the most awful aversion to people, perhaps someone they have been fond of and who is living in the same house. Sometimes Tuberculinum can make all the difference to their whole temperament.

In early adolescence it is often a good remedy for headaches. This will nearly always be in a bright, advanced child who is getting irritable, is nervous of thunder and storms of any kind, susceptible to damp, and who develops headache from work and therefore loses interest in her study. She does not mean to lose interest but says that the headache is caused by her working. This is an excuse so that she will not have to do it. On that kind of history, if they also had a hatred or fear of dogs, I would give them Tuberculinum.

These patients are nearly always musical and can burst into tears and be very upset by it. They also have a queer kind of rheumatism, worth remembering because it is rather characteristic. It is worse in damp cold. It is also worse, and I think even slightly more so, in damp heat. It is worse in a change from hot to cold, and also in a change from cold to hot. There is no other remedy where you find that symptom so marked. They will tell you, 'If I go into a cold room it really bothers me. And if I sit in the sun or go into a very hot room it can do just the same'.

There is one other thing which Tuberculinum are very bad at and that is standing. Of all the remedies, perhaps with Sulphur next, the Tuberculinum patient is worse standing. I remember a very nice girl of about eighteen, who loved nothing so much as going to a party, each time with the latest young man. But in the middle of these parties she always fainted. So she came to see me and said, 'This is no fun. I think it is standing. I think that if I could move about it would not happen'. Her mother got so worried about her that she asked if she might see a heart specialist. I did not think there was the slightest need, but I took her to one, who reported that her heart and blood pressure and everything else was absolutely perfect. You also occasionally get this symptom in young men, which is very embarrassing for them. You get it much more often in girls. I gave this girl some Tub. Bov. 10M and she did not have the problem again.

Symptomatic Prescribing

37
Emergency Remedies

LACERATED WOUNDS

In lacerated wounds the first thing I would do, really before I had thought at all, is to give Calendula, both internally and locally. I would give a 200c every two hours for the rest of the day or for twenty-four hours, and locally ten drops to a teacup of water as a compress. You have no idea, if you have not tried it, how very good it is. (Dr Tyler would have nothing else for burns, and found it very good throughout the years.)

SENSITIVE TISSUE DAMAGE

When acutely sensitive tissue is damaged, such as a nail being torn off, or a dog bite, or catching your finger in a car door, I do not think you can beat giving Hypericum, both internally and locally. I would add one word of advice: do not put on a Calendula compress with it – it does not do nearly so well as if you put on a Hypericum compress alone. It is also very useful in comminuted fractures where there are lots of bits of bone, perhaps pressing on sensitive structures, or where the fracture penetrates the joints. It will relieve in something like an injury round the coccyx, such as can arise after a bad confinement with instruments.

It used to be given as a prophylactic for tetanus, in Hahnemann's time, for people who were working in the soil. They gave a few doses of Hypericum, and very good it was. It is worth thinking of this for somebody who is constantly in contact with soil and who perhaps has cracks in the skin. On the whole I use it in 30c or 200c potency.

PENETRATING WOUNDS

A patient steps on a nail or a drawing pin. The initial injury appears minimal, but the following day there is wound sepsis. It is then that you give Ledum – do not give it too soon. I would much rather give a

144

patient Arnica the first day and wait a little to see what it does, and then give Ledum.

One recurring symptom is that the foot and leg, on the injured side, are quite cold, although the patient cannot bear to have anything hot put on. Locally they are far too hot, but they feel cold to touch. They also get a lot of twitching of the muscles round the injury and cannot bear to have it touched.

BRUISES

These are the injuries without superficial laceration, and here Arnica is supreme. A person who would like to put homoeopathy to the test could do no better than start with just this remedy alone. It is for any kind of bruise. If you fall and hit your head, in a few minutes you will have a huge lump on your head. Take Arnica and after two hours the lump will have markedly subsided.

GLANDULAR TISSUE

If the injury is to glandular tissue I find it extraordinary how it clears on some Conium. The other remedy I find very good for a severe injury to the breast – when somebody runs into something or gets hurt with a sharp instrument – is Bellis Perennis. The breast usually feels thick all round. I always give Bellis as a prophylactic in such cases.

HEAD INJURIES

Head injuries may call for any one of several different remedies. If the patient has had a bad head injury and looks dull and befuddled, I would give Arnica every time to start with. If they are not better in twelve hours and look even more befogged, I would follow this with Opium. If Opium does not do it, and you begin to be anxious about the patient, give Hellebore. Hellebore is a rare remedy, but it is good in head injuries that are not doing well and are a bit delayed in getting right again.

If, as sometimes happens, the patient has no obvious injury at all for three or four days – is perhaps not quite as bright, but really does not complain of anything – and on the third or fourth day gets a little bleeding from the ears, then you must give Hypericum. Some sensitive tissue is likely to be affected and can easily become infected.

Dr Tyler was very fond of giving Calendula 200c, both internally and externally, for scalp wounds that were not doing well. If that fails and the wound is getting still worse, and you are worried about it, do not forget Pyrogen.

There are two other remedies for head injuries, which are perhaps not quite so frequent, but which can be invaluable. These are Cicuta and Natrum Sulph. They are for what I call the more remote effects of a head injury. In Cicuta the patient is irritable and bad-tempered and cannot keep still. In Natrum Sulph. they are depressed, and have awful headaches which they tell you about, and cannot bear to sit in the sun or be too hot. There are many differences in temperament between the two remedies but otherwise the head condition probably looks exactly the same in both.

EYE INJURIES

If you get an acute inflammation, possibly with something in the eye, watering and painful, do not forget Aconite. If there is a definite foreign body which either has removed itself by the time you see the patient or needs removing, in either case the remedy to give is Coccus Cacti. (This always seems a strange remedy to me, because I connect it with coughs.) For an acute blow on the eye, causing haemorrhage of the conjunctiva, give Arnica. If the injury is more to the surrounding tissue than to the eye itself, and the whole eye looks inflamed and bluish, as if it had been injured, give Ruta. If in spite of Ruta there is more pain in the eyeball, give Symphytum.

SPRAINS AND FRACTURES

Most sprains or fractures need Arnica. They have swelling and dislike being moved. Remember that Arnica is also a wonderful remedy after an amputation. Arnica is also good for the removal of a bad wisdom tooth. Hypericum can also be useful if there is a lot of scar tissue which gets painful. If the patient is better for movement, I would give Rhus Tox.

If sprained or fractured limbs have persistent weakness, give Calc. Carb. Calc. Carb. is the chronic Rhus Tox. – it has all these bone things and will pull up the weakness of legs in a most extraordinary manner. If by chance you decide to give the patient Rhus Tox., and it does them no good at all, give the constitutional remedy, particularly if they are Pulsatilla. (You will sometimes pick a patient up wonderfully, after their first symptoms are over, by giving them their constitutional remedy.)

Arnica is invaluable for more acute things like severe fracture. I was alone one Friday night during a bad flu epidemic and was called out at 10 p.m. to a patient whom I found much iller than I expected. I did not have the remedy I wanted, so I went home and rushed up the eight steps to my front door. I left my case on the top of the steps and got the remedy, but when I came out I did a somersault over my case and broke my right arm.

Within two minutes I had taken a 10M of Arnica, and was bound up very tightly by a friend. I did not even have time to be X-rayed until the following afternoon. I can only say that some half an hour after the break, which was excruciatingly painful, I had no pain at all.

Another thing about Arnica is that it covers many other kinds of complaint. There are people who are overtired and who have had too little sleep, so that they are always tired and it affects them in various ways. There is the patient who cannot travel well, who feels sick in the train, who cannot bear to be jolted, or who feels awful flying. Such people find Arnica very useful. It is a very good remedy for ordinary fatigue, even if one is not travelling.

JOINT INJURIES

Strontium Carb. is a little-used remedy. It is like a Calc. Carb. which does not get so much pain and does not get quite so much weakness. Strontium Carb. is for a joint that has been badly injured and which you cannot use without a lot of pain. You cannot turn or move it and it is weak and stiff.

If you get a patient with a bad backache, due to fatigue or injury, and you have given them all kinds of things and think they really must be better for the next remedy, do not forget Bryonia, because Bryonia can clear it up completely.

SEPSIS

There is the question of what to do in sepsis. Boils usually clear on the patient's constitutional remedy, and if not, there are seven remedies you need to think of – Hepar Sulph., Calc. Sulph., Sulphur, Silica, Kali Bich., Pyrogen, Tuberculinum – and you may need any one of them. Then you get the sort of boil which will not heal. It just sits there and does nothing. It seems to have no life in it and goes on looking much the same all the time. There may be a slight purulent discharge but it never seems to finish it up. Give some high Silica and it will either do nothing at all or it will finish it up.

Kali Bich. is a very good remedy for boils. They are nearly always over the tibia. But use the patient's constitutional remedy if possible, for this just improves them beyond words.

A carbuncle is sometimes a difficult thing to treat, although I have found Anthracinum very useful. It produces just that kind of thing in its provings. One of the best things for a carbuncle is just plain castor oil – put it on a bit of lint. Nobody ever teaches you that.

There are other remedies to think of and they are Tarantula, Arsenicum and Rhus Tox., all of which can be of very great help.

In a cellulitis you are almost bound to need either the snake venoms or Pyrogen. A very acute peri-anal or perineal inflammation or swelling does well on Rhus Tox.

ULCERATION

Give Calendula in the sort of horrid ulcer which appears on the shin or ankle. Kali Bich. is also useful for ulcers which are sluggish with clear-cut edges and a dirty white discharge which nearly always dries on it.

If the ulcer is higher up, just below the knee, I would think of Lycopodium. It does not matter which leg. Or, if it is rather nasty, possibly a bit offensive, creeping out from the centre, and looking horrid, do not forget Merc. Sol. And always remember, in gastric ulcer and in varicose dermatitis or ulcer, to think of Carbo Veg. The best vein remedy, just taking it as a vein remedy, is Carbo Veg.

PRE- AND POST-OPERATIVE REMEDIES

Before operation you can get all kinds of reaction in the patient. One is that they are terrified of the operation and terrified of the result. Aconite will calm them in a minute or two. I do not use Ignatia much – I have never been able to diagnose an Ignatia patient correctly, but if I have a miserable, complaining patient I give Ignatia 10M frequently on the day before operation.

The third remedy is for the patient who comes in scared – not acutely like the Aconite – but just a bit scared. This person will respond well to Argentum Nit. in 10M potency.

Give Arnica beforehand if the patient is to have a tonsil operation. You do not need anything else as a rule, but you may go in the next day, having seen them eating a large supper the night before, to find that they do not feel so well and are complaining of a very stiff neck. Some Rhus Tox. will take it off within an hour or two. If you go in on the second day and find them fairly chirpy but complaining of a filthy mouth and coated tongue, Merc. Sol. will clear them up. In practice, the patient who has had Aconite first seldom needs Mercurius.

Give Arnica in the first place for a sub-mucous resection. If they have the plug out and then feel it is entirely blocked and that they are never going to breathe again, some Kali Bich. will provide relief.

We seldom see a mastoid infection nowadays. I remember being called to see a little girl of six with a temperature of 40°C and the most enormous bright red swelling, agonizingly painful, behind her right ear. She had a red face, which was most unusual because I knew that child. I rang the surgeon and provisionally booked a bed, because I did not think we could avoid an operation. He was a good homoeopath, and had worked for two years under Dr Kent.

Although it was a red face and looked hot, it was quite cold to touch, and I gave her Capsicum 10M every hour. When the surgeon arrived he said 'I shan't do an operation on this. It is going down beautifully – what have you given her?' I mentioned the 10M of Capsicum – 'Oh yes', he said, 'this will cure it', which it did.

In an empyema, as soon as you have drained it at all, give some Pyrogen because it does get rid of all the stuff that otherwise would be absorbed.

In a gastrostomy or gastroenterostomy, if you have a paralytic ileus with a tendency to distension and discomfort, Carbo Veg. 200c every two hours usually gives relief and nothing else is likely to be needed. For a gall bladder at any stage give Phosphorus.

In a case of an appendix, when you have alerted the surgeon, if the patient is able to keep still, and is not restless, give Arnica 10M. If they are restless and find it difficult to keep still, give Rhus Tox. 10M. If it is a perforated appendix and the patient is very ill, you will rather likely need one of the snake venoms, Crotalus 10M being the most common.

SHOCK

There are three remedies which come immediately to my mind. The first is Aconite, for acute shock or fright. I remember a small boy being very nearly run over by a delivery van. He was running across the road at the corner and then changed his mind and tried to go the other way, and the van missed him by inches. He was carried into hospital, so shaken that he could not walk, and he had a red face which quickly became paler and paler. The thing I have always remembered was his look of extreme terror. I gave him Aconite 30c every few minutes and in an hour he said he wanted to go home.

I have found Natrum Mur. the best remedy through the years for emotional shock. So often it is the only one needed to pull the patient up.

The third is Opium. It is needed urgently in cerebrovascular accidents and can be extremely good.

38

Depression

Arsenicum Album

Like all Arsenicums they are never placid about anything. When they are depressed they are more restless than you can possibly imagine, and when they are depressed the condition is an acute one and can become violent. Yet they blame themselves and loathe their feeling of depression, and are annoyed with the depression and with everyone and everything else. They are apt to be driven from one place to another. If it is night-time they turn and toss in bed all night. Often the depression is worse between twelve midnight and 1 a.m.

Occasionally they get suicidal from a sudden impulse. I do not normally call them suicidal, but there is always just a chance that the depression may become too much and that they may throw themselves out of a window. They have a great fear of death, so they are not really likely to want to commit suicide.

I remember a doctor who came to one of the training courses in homoeopathy. He was very keen on homoeopathy when the course had finished and went back determined to try it out. About three weeks later he rang me up and said, 'I have a man in my room at the moment and his wife is sitting with him, otherwise I would not dare to leave him. He has dashed to the window three times to throw himself out. He won't sit still for a single second. I have never seen anyone so violently depressed in my life. What shall I give him?'

I said, 'The only thing I can think of is Arsenicum. If you give him a 10M of Arsenicum I think you will find it will help, but give the first three doses ten minutes apart to reduce the risk of an aggravation. He went back the next day to find the patient perfectly all right. He never had another fit of depression. It was the acute Arsenicum, and it did just absolutely fit, which was very satisfactory.

Aurum Metallicum

Aurum is the most common and most definite of all the depression remedies. In a case of acute depression the patient is brooding and melancholy and just sits and peers in front of him and will not speak. They look extremely depressed and have all sorts of strange ideas. They think they have lost the affection of their friends and family, or that they have done something frightful, and that they are therefore feeling like this because they are to blame for it. They blame themselves for everything and get a real disgust of life. They are the patients who become suicidal.

I had an interesting patient with depression. She was twenty-four and had been in two mental homes. The main thing about her was that she blamed herself tremendously for a tragedy that had happened in the family. Her brother had died of leukaemia and for some reason she felt responsible for it, and you could not get it out of her head.

She needed constant reassurance. She never cried, although tears would trickle down occasionally, but she was not a crying type at all. Aurum is not – it is very difficult for them to cry.

I gave her a 10M of Aurum and she was quite lifted up by it. She got gradually better, from being very bad, and in between times I used to give her a 6c of Natrum Mur., because if her need had been a constitutional remedy, that would have been the one. Her depression was deeper than a Natrum Mur. depression and was covered by the Aurum.

She is now married happily with two children and comes in to see us if one of the children is ill, but otherwise is perfectly well. The only thing is that her husband finds it is very difficult to go on a holiday with her because she never likes sitting down to read. Whereas he would like to sit down on the beach and perhaps read in the sun and enjoy himself, she would never do so. In general the Aurum patient will never sit down to read. They either have to be entertained or else have something to do, and it is quite one of their characteristics.

They have a rather dusky colour. There is also one other particular characteristic about them. It is extremely hard to rouse Aurum patients to make an effort for themselves. If you do rouse them and get them to walk about in the open air, they are much better. It lifts their depression quite considerably. They say in the books that if you make the Aurum patient bathe his neck in very cold water, it has the same effect, but I have never yet managed to make an Aurum patient even want to consider doing this.

They are also apt to get bouts of vertigo, often at the same time as their depression, and walk about looking as if they are quite drunk. They stagger from side to side and look very topply. They can fall over, and if they do it is always to the left side. It is sometimes so bad that they have to lie down and even then it takes quite a time to go off.

152

They also get pains in the head on lying down and feel as if the bones of the head are sore and that they do not want to lie on them. They sometimes have eye symptoms – sticky eyes in the morning, the feeling of sand in the eyes, and their eyes usually water a lot.

Aurum patients do very well on treatment, but remember that untreated their depression can lead to suicide. When I first saw this girl she was quite likely to commit suicide, which is why I saw her so often. She would often telephone to ask if she could just run in as she was passing by, and I would encourage her to do so, rather with the idea of keeping her from committing suicide. I gave her a 10M in several doses. If you are going to use a deep-acting remedy, give it high. In case of an aggravation, relatives should be asked to keep the patient under observation.

There is another quite common type of Aurum, which is the person who comes in moderately depressed. I remember one woman of about forty-five who came in accompanied by her sister. The sister had made her come and it was she who more or less told us the story. She said that the patient was very depressed. Her younger son had always lived with her but was now going to get married. Not only that, he was going to be moved in his work thirty or forty miles away so that she would not see him, and this had depressed her frightfully.

The patient sat there absolutely silent and did not say one word. I had seen her before at other stages of depression when her husband died, so I did know her in this mood, and at that time had given her Aurum 6c. I gave her some Aurum 6c again and away she went. About a month later she came in, talking and absolutely different. She was telling me about her son's wedding, saying that it was not going to be so bad after all because either she was going to them once every three weekends or they were going to visit her once every three weekends and so she would go on seeing them. She is quite typical of a certain type who comes in with a depressed mood, probably in quite a bad phase at the time and who is picked up wonderfully by a low Aurum. I find these patients very interesting and give a lot of low Aurum.

Calcarea Carbonica

This is the remedy which is most like Aurum. It has a very acute depression and is difficult to distinguish from Aurum. When depressed, the Calc. Carb. patient will sit staring in front of him with the most melancholy expression you can possibly imagine. They have a heavy, dull appearance. They feel incapable of making any mental effort and have a great disinclination to work – more so than the Aurum who can probably be made to do a certain amount of work. The Calc. Carb. cannot, and is despondent and melancholy. You know the description in the books of a Calc. Carb. 'sitting solidly and bending pins'. This is really what they look like when they are very depressed. They will do one stupid, finnicky little thing – the last acute Calc. Carb. I saw opened and shut her bag the entire time she was with me, which nearly drove me mad.

The great contrast with Aurum is that you can actually rouse the Calc. Carb. You can even make them want to help themselves and live a more or less normal life for a day or two, although they will sink back into the same stage afterwards unless you have given them Calc. Carb. You must give them a high potency of the remedy if you are going to get them out of this depression.

The Calc. Carb. patient can rather be dominated by somebody's personality. They will also brood over all sorts of stupid little things. The Aurum patient is much more likely to brood over some sin they have committed, some awful thing that they were responsible for, and suffer under a sense of unworthiness.

Another difference is that Aurum has plenty of courage, whereas you do not feel that the Calc. Carb. patient, especially when they are depressed, has any guts at all. They have no stuffing and it is very difficult to press them into doing anything sensible. Nor do I think that Calc. Carb. patients ever commit suicide – they do not have it in them. They are terrified – the great terror that runs through all the Calcareas – of going insane. They hate going out in their depression because people will see that they are not themselves and will talk about it, and this they cannot bear.

Calc. Carb. on the whole is a much less violent personality than Aurum. You do not get them going off the deep end when they are miserable and depressed, whereas the Aurum can definitely go off the deep end if you contradict them. Calc. Carb. always have the fear, even in the child, that something is going to happen to them or to one of their friends, or to someone living in the road.

They do drip silent tears, like all the Calcareas. The tears come streaming down, although they are not obviously sobbing, and they get this awful restlessness. They can also be peevish when they are depressed, and usually there is no obvious cause.

They have often the typical sweating. One recent patient with a Calc. Carb. depression was sweating profusely in a very cold room. She said, 'It is an extraordinary thing I am not going to sweat in your warm room, but here in your chilly hall I began to sweat at once'.

They can have quite severe vertigo and it is always worse if they turn their heads suddenly. They say that everything turns with them when they turn their head. They also have a difficulty in that they cannot express themselves. They are unable to tell you what they have just done or what they have just read and can appear excessively stupid, and indeed sometimes are.

They have, of course, the generals of Calc. Carb., but remember that the adult patients can be rather thin. They can be so thin and worn-looking that you do not think of them as the pale fat-faced Calc. Carb. The patient who was so terrified of anyone noticing that she was a bit queer was very thin and scraggy. It was some time in taking her history before I realised that she was a perfect Calc. Carb., and that she would do well on it.

Chelidonium
This remedy exemplifies the depression of liver disturbance, and it is well known how depressed a really livery patient can get. They are despondent and very helpless, they tend to weep, they are more hopeless than melancholy. They get an awful feeling that they cannot cope with life, and are full of dreads that anything may happen. If they have had any worry they make it the centre of their depression and brood over it. Even sometimes when it is long past and there is nothing more to worry about they will go back and brood over it.

They cannot bear being disturbed. They are not the kind that wants someone to come in and cheer them up – they want to be left alone. You cannot get a word out of them, even from a patient who has come for help. It is very difficult to get a fair history or find out what they are grumbling about. The only bit of luck is if they tell you they have a certain amount of pain over their liver or gall bladder region, or that this area is extremely painful to touch. This is the Chelidonium pain and you find that the whole thing fits.

Cinchona Officinalis (China)
The China patient is a broken-down person who has suffered either from a prolonged illness or a prolonged worry, or who has been exposed to bad conditions for some time. The patient may have had a severe loss of body fluids, such as a severe haemorrhage, or they may have had a prolonged spell of nursing a sick person, and they can become acutely depressed. In their depression they become markedly hyperaesthetic. They cannot stand noise, or bear to have any more

worry put on to them, or even hear about another person who may also have difficulties.

I remember the case of a nurse who had worked far too long and who was worn out. She could not even bear to be told how a patient was. The depression here is really due to physical exhaustion. They get a dread of having to do mental work or having to exert themselves, and they really want to do nothing. It is very much better for them if they do not have to do anything for a while. They get more and more depressed because they feel they cannot tackle anything, and they have a horrible habit of thinking that they are either tormented or frustrated by somebody else. So they fly into an exhausted shallow temper, nothing to it. They are almost too tired to show it and this is typical of the China patient.

China is a wonderful remedy for these patients. If you can additionally encourage them to sleep for a few days, by about the third day they are different people.

Ferrum Metallicum

Ferrum is rather like Pulsatilla. It has the futile despondency of the Pulsatilla, and similarly no real substance behind the depression. Ferrum patients are tired and depressed and can be upset by any opposition, or even by advice. They weep and are so tired that they have to sit down – they are very bad at standing.

As a rule, the Ferrum at rest is always pale. They may have a slight flush, especially with a temperature, but at rest and especially when they are depressed, they are very pale, whereas the Pulsatilla at rest always has a colour. That is one of the features which distinguish between them. If they get excited they can flush up, always into a very bright flush. If there is any opposition at all, they are apt to be extremely irritable, and this will also bring on a bright flush.

I always remember a family where there were several children and where the mother was so sensitive to noise that not one of the children would have thought of eating an apple in the same room, because if they had they would have been turned out. The woman could not bear small sounds. Nobody could sit crackling a newspaper, even the sound of the pages of a book being turned irritated her. I think that is very typical of the Ferrum patient. They do not mind bumps going on outside and a terrific noise from the street.

They are extremely sensitive to cold, which is another distinguishing feature from Pulsatilla. Ferrum is a tired, irritable and very cold patient.

156

Graphites

One does not tend to think of Graphites as a depression remedy, but it can be. They are perhaps more sad than depressed, if you can see the difference. They sit down and are just sad. They sit and think of how soon their illness is going to kill them rather than being melancholy and gloomy. They then worry about whether they will go to heaven if they do die. And if they are depressed, Graphites have the marked characteristic that they cannot make up their minds. Graphites is always bad at making up its mind, but if you get a depressed Graphites you will really know what it is like.

I always remember having a depressed Graphites patient and her two sons come to tell me how very depressed she was. Her father had been a famous author and she had been left all his books. The sons said, 'We are having a terrible time at the moment because we are supposed to be arranging our grandfather's books, which are most interesting, but our mother will not make up her mind where she wants them. We spend all day having certain ones taken out and put back again'. That is very much like a Graphites. They postpone decisions and get slow and depressed and think they ought to do something positive. Their relations try to press them to do something and they do not know what to do.

Graphites patients are better in the evening. As a rule they cheer up then, if they are depressed, and sometimes you can get work out of them in the evening, and they usually sleep very well. They wake up in the morning as bad as ever, but you can gradually push them along. They are better for warmth and much better for food. Strangely enough, especially when they are depressed, they can be chilly and have at the same time a certain amount of air hunger. The only thing they complain of at night is that they are uncomfortably hot in bed. They are easily overheated by exertion. Their depression is made very much worse by music.

Lilium Tigrinum

This remedy is characteristic in that the depression is always aggravated in the evening and at night, whatever the patient's mental state. Their depression can be a sort of religious melancholia. It is not at all like Aurum – the patient never sits and stares with a melancholy expression, or anything like that. Lilium Tig. blame anyone who is around, they feel a great sense of responsibility and they must be the ones who give advice. They have always given advice to the people close to them and like to feel they are relied upon, and if they do not feel well enough to do this they get very depressed. They often have some concurrent physical disturbance which is also worse at night. Any attempt to console them makes them extremely annoyed, almost violent.

Another characteristic is that if they sit in a room at what is generally found to be a comfortable temperature they would be pushing back their coats. They are always pushing back their clothes because they are too hot. During their depression they show this aggravation from heat, and they like a lot of fresh air. Occasionally you think they may be going to be a Pulsatilla, although they are not because they are more definite characters and much more bad-tempered. I think Lilium Tig. is one of the most difficult patients you can find.

With their depression or with any other complaint they nearly always have a dragging-down feeling in their pelvic organs. They sometimes feel that everything is going to fall out of the pelvis.

The Natrum Salts
In all the Natrums there is a certain mental instability. They are either up or down, rarely on an even keel. They laugh easily and the next minute are right down in the depths again.

They have *no* sense of humour. Or, if they have, it is a twisted one, and they can make caustic and unpleasant remarks at times. They get an intense reaction to anything sad and will be in the very depths of despair after hearing about it. They all have the characteristic that if anything has upset them they dig it up and brood over it and never forget it. When they are depressed they bring up all the insults that have ever been hurled at them. When there is no definite origin to their depression, I have known Natrum Mur. absolutely hunt round for causes.

Another marked symptom is that not one of the Natrums likes to have their depression ignored. They may tell you that they do not want company or attention, but do not believe it. They make themselves the centre of interest.

They do not necessarily want people to come and talk to them but they hate being ignored. I was responsible for one such patient in hospital. Every day he would complain bitterly about his morning coffee. Either they had dropped a little into the saucer, or they had not given him enough sugar, or they had forgotten the sugar altogether. Something was always wrong and one of the nurses said, 'I can hardly bear to take him his morning coffee'. I said, 'Leave it off until I next come. I will be responsible. Don't take him coffee the next two mornings'. When I arrived I cannot say what a to-do there was about his not having had his coffee. 'But I thought you did not like it', I said. 'I thought it was always wrong and that you would really prefer not to have it'. 'Prefer not to have it! Of course I'ld like to have it. I don't like at all to be left out. I have never approved of that, and want it'.

The result was that the poor nurse, whom I had meant to help, had then to give him a bit of extra attention every morning when she took round the coffee. That is exactly like the Natrum Mur. – they demand extra attention because they feel they have been neglected.

You must not neglect the Natrum Mur. patient, however bad-tempered they are. Consider a typical case: their relations take the trouble to visit them and sit and talk to them all the afternoon. Then they go off thinking, 'Well, thank goodness, Ivy is getting better'. But when you next see Ivy she complains bitterly because the relations did not really ferret out what was wrong! They can be very angry about this and want to have it dug out.

The Natrum Mur. who loses somebody whom they are very fond of will retire into a shell. They do not want to be offered sympathy. But if you leave it out altogether and do not enquire how they are or write to them, then they resent it very much and feel hard used. For instance, having refused to go out with friends who might have offered to take them out to cheer them up, having refused a dozen times, they are then resentful that the friends do not go on ringing up and asking them out. In contrast, the Pulsatilla will weep all over you and be grateful for sympathy and pick up with it. You can get tired of their tears but they are so much easier to get on with!

Natrum Mur. and Natrum Carb. are both more sensitive to music than the other Natrums, although none of them are really musical. They may like pretty lightweight music and one is sometimes quite surprised at what the Natrum patient will be listening to.

The Natrum Ars. is the most apprehensive of all of them. All Natrum patients have their nerves rather on edge. It is an interesting experience that I think you meet Natrum patients rather particularly after shock, which is why I always say it is the greatest of the shock remedies, whereas you meet Sepia patients after years of overwork. This is just another of the useful little differences between the two.

Platina

Platinum is not a commonly-needed remedy, but sometimes there is nothing else that will touch the patient. The best way of illustrating the Platinum depression is by giving a case-history. I knew the family of this patient – his wife and all their children. One day they all asked me if I would see him, because he was so very depressed.

I have never known a man coming in with such an arrogant air. I could not believe he was the father of this rather nice family, because he was so unpleasantly arrogant. Excessive self-esteem is the main characteristic of a Platinum. They get very warped and pay undue attention to the most stupid and footling little things when they are depressed and rather down, and have minor disagreements which they magnify and brood over. This man, strangely enough, said, 'You know, I am having great trouble with my family', which I could hardly believe, because he had an extremely nice family. 'They don't treat me with enough respect'. That, and the way he came in, immediately made me think of Platinum. He could not get it out of his mind, and told me that the family tried to argue with him. I do not think they did try to argue with him; I rather imagine they tried to reason with him, but that he took it as an argument and thoroughly despised whatever they said. I gave him Platinum 10M and he became a much happier and better balanced person. He told me later that what he resented had been such stupid things and really not worth troubling about.

They are restless patients, never sitting still and moving about all the time. This man had given me a history of getting easily wrought up to a feeling of excitement and that afterwards he was quite numb and could not think properly. He said his legs or hands or other bits of him went numb for a time after getting very excited. With this marked self-esteem they also have a terrible fear of failure. Mr Dombie of *Dombie and Son* was a perfect Platinum.

They nearly always think they are going to die fairly soon and they are rather afraid of it.

Psorinum

Psorinum is another of the depressed remedies. They can be the most unshaven, miserable tramps you ever have to meet, full of fears, very melancholic and quite hopeless. They have no self-respect, or at least will tell you so, and no energy. They grumble because nobody will give them a fair deal. They are very irritable and could quite fairly be described as absolutely joyless. Moreover, even in this despairing mood, they are always hungry.

Pulsatilla

The usual picture of Pulsatilla is laughing one minute, weeping the next minute, easily cheered up, very changeable – the windflower.

But in their real depression they are a bit different. They feel they are always under somebody's thumb, which they do not much like, and that it is quite impossible for them to stand on their own legs. They will cry very easily. They think they are not going to have a chance because this, that and the other in their lives is against them, and they bring up all sorts of things which really have no bearing on what they are doing. They get a great anxiety at night, particularly when it is hot. Sometimes their anxiety at night is so great that it wakes them up. They go to sleep with that sort of anxious feeling at the back of their mind, and then in an hour or two they are awake.

With their anxiety the Pulsatilla patient is often rather tremulous, out of sorts with everything and everyone. When they are in a depression they have a way – more marked than just an ordinary Pulsatilla whom you may see at any time – of breaking out into weeping, sudden, storming weeping, especially if they are interrupted.

They can be extremely ill-humoured – much more ill-humoured than you think of in a Pulsatilla, and often without any cause. If anyone makes a remark they can take offence or think the remarks are directed at them. In this depression they will also complain that they cannot concentrate on anything and that their thoughts wander.

Sepia

The Sepia depression is important. There are two types of Sepia patient. There is the one that comes in and slumps into a chair and looks absolutely depressed, uninterested in life and very despondent. As a rule they are tallish with long backs. The other one comes in with a fatter face than you would ordinarily expect, and seems awfully stupid. As a matter of fact, they are not necessarily always stupid – they may simply be so overtired that their brain is slow and they cannot remember or decide anything.

The one that looks depressed is a resentful Sepia. They do not come willingly to the doctor. They have to be driven, and they do not like it at all, feeling that there is nothing to see the doctor about. They come in with a solemn expression and as a rule have no cheerful response to you when you greet them.

One of the great fears of the Sepia depression is that something much worse is going to happen. One of the children perhaps is ill, or not getting on well at school. They think then that the husband is going to be ill, too, and that there will be no money to keep going and that they all will be in the workhouse. They have a great fear of poverty. (The other remedy that has a great fear of poverty is

Psorinum.) When they are down and depressed they tell you, 'I can't bear people who offer help and get in the way and fuss round and that kind of thing'. They get envious of others who do not have their difficulties and who have a pleasant life, and then they can be very spiteful.

One or two other symptoms will often be present with their depression. They can get extreme attacks of anger. They may be just snappy with their depression, but they can also get real bouts of anger. If so, you will find that they are usually about times in the past when they had a lot of hardship and had to struggle, and when they had to do this, that and the other. This anger is usually accompanied by palpitation, with sweating over the whole body. They can also be very nervous and upset by the least noise. I think the Sepia patient dislikes noise more than anything else.

They have another sort of depression, one which is just so sad and discontented that they do not think life is worth living and rather wished they were out of it, and what does it matter . . . That is a slightly different picture from the usual weepy depression. Here they will weep over almost anything, and with it they are nearly always inclined to get headaches. All these symptoms are very definite ones and do not occur to the same degree in every patient. It is also not uncommon for a Sepia patient to tell you that they feel they will scream, and that they have to hold on to something.

39

Headaches

ACUTE HEADACHES

Apis
Apis has a bad headache which is nearly always from an irregular or suppressed menstrual period. It begins as a stabbing pain on first getting up in the morning and then goes on to throbbing. The patient complains that the head feels tight and is tender to touch. They do look like Apis – puffy, a bit swollen and rather congested. The eyes are bright and the conjunctivae are slightly congested. Whenever I have given Apis for headache, the patient has been damp round the head and forehead.

The pain is better for pressure. Although Apis patients are better for pressure they do not want the head bandaged, because like all Apis patients they get an aggravation from heat, as well as a certain amount of excitement and hyperaesthesia. They are worse from any movement and the pain is apt to shoot from side to side. If Apis does not seem to fit, you might consider four other remedies that are also better for pressure: these are Argentum Nit., Glonoine, Lac Defloratum and Pulsatilla.

Belladonna
Belladonna is a wonderful acute remedy for headache following exposure either to sun or cold. It also comes on from an emotional cause or shock, or else it is quite often a period headache. It is throbbing and pulsating, worse for any movement and worse for stooping. If a Belladonna patient comes in to your consulting room with a Belladonna headache on them at the moment, you find that they will sit back in their chair and if possible lean their head back, because they are so much better leaning back. They are worse for moving the eyes and worse with the head lying low. They are also worse if they have many blankets, which is significant, because a Belladonna patient can otherwise be quite chilly. It starts in the

afternoon and lasts all night. I have at least thirty patients who carry Belladonna 30c when they go to the hairdresser. One of the chief causes of a Belladonna headache is to sit under a hairdryer and then come out into a cold wind. In half an hour they will have a terrific headache.

Bryonia

Bryonia is a useful headache remedy which is sometimes overlooked. The headache accompanies an acute coryza, comes on in the morning and lasts all day. It comes sometimes from overeating the night before, although this is not its usual cause.

It is a dull, aching, frontal headache that begins in the front and extends over to the occiput. Sometimes it is neuralgic, and if so it is usually left-sided. As a rule it is all over the head. It sometimes has heat and congestion over the head but a feeling of coldness in the extremities, which is rather unusual for Bryonia. Although Bryonia has an aggravation from heat, when they are ill you can often find them asking for a blanket and rather covering themselves up. (The thought of putting on a warm cover or anything like that normally makes them feel quite ill.) There is a great increase in the usual Bryonia heaviness of the eyes and they get stabs of pain on opening the eyes. With this they have a superficial tenderness all over their head, particularly in their forehead, better for pressure, better for cold applications and worse for motion.

Chininum Sulphuricum

China Sulph. is an acute digestive headache. (Cinchona Officinalis, the ordinary China, is a more chronic headache – but they are both digestive in origin.) It starts at the back of the neck and extends to the forehead, and it can be pretty violent. There is a certain amount of dampness of the head.

The patients will always tell you that they have a tremendous lot of flatulence, because it is one of the things that troubles them. They are always trying to get up a small quantity of wind. If they sit and tell you about their headaches, they try to get up some wind all the time they are talking to you – you can see it, and they look as if they are going to be sick. All my acute China patients have always looked as if they might be sick any minute.

I always remember a patient getting up from the seat and pressing her head against the cold wall of my room. I asked, 'Does the pressure help?' 'No', she said, 'not the pressure, it is the cold that helps. It really helps to press it against a cold wall.' I had another patient who picked up a glass tumbler, holding it to her head to have something cool against it whilst she was sitting talking to me. These patients are worse if they have to turn their head much and use their eyes, and also if they have to move about in the open air.

The pain is often neuralgic and can be very acute. One of the best cases I ever saw was accompanied by a trigeminal neuralgia, and China Sulph. was the thing that cleared it up.

Cocculus

Cocculus patients always have one absolutely certain thing. They will have been through a lot of nervous strain and are often overworked. One typical patient has a very ill husband. She does not get to bed until after midnight and is disturbed at least four times every night. She has a few snatches of sleep early in the night and that is all she gets, and she has frightful headaches from sheer over-fatigue and overwork. She presents a clear description of Cocculus – she complains as if her head is empty first and then as if it is going to burst. She also complains of a thing that patients often report, and you never know where to fit it, and that is opening and shutting of the back of her head.

They are more or less worse for everything. They are worse after sleep and worse for any rough motion, like a car that is a little jolty. They are worse using the eyes and worse for stimulants. They are worse for drinking coffee, they cannot bear the smell of tobacco or anyone smoking in front of them. The smell of fat, or food, or cooking or anything like that makes them feel very poor. They are worse in a warm room and they are worse if they lie on their back because they say that the back of their head gets very tender. These symptoms are quite constant in a Cocculus patient.

Gelsemium

Gelsemium patients can have one of the worst headaches. It nearly always comes with flu, or during some acute illness, and it is often recurring and also often periodic – every few days, perhaps every fourteen days. They have the slightly flushed, heavy appearance that Gelsemium always have. They have all sorts of ocular disturbances and sometimes complain of being almost blind. They may have diplopia before the onset. (Other remedies that have diplopia or eye symptoms before their headache are Kali Bich., Iris, Lac Defloratum and Silica.) They have a boring pain over the right eye and nearly always complain of coldness at the back of the head, with shiveriness down the spine and the usual Gelsemium symptoms. They can feel rather faint and be intensely sleepy.

They are worse for motion and for light, and much better for sleep and for vomiting. If they are sick their headache probably goes at once. It usually comes on early in the day, or during the day, and does not disappear until going to bed. Another thing about the Gelsemium patient, and this is very common, is that when they first lie down their headache is almost unbearable. They do not know how to stay lying down. They wonder what they shall do and suddenly they find that it is lifting a little. And as the headache subsides, the patient passes a greatly increased quantity of urine and this is a great relief to them.

Glonoinum

The Glonoine headache is always caused by exposure to sun. It is very like Belladonna, but more intense. The face has an intense dusky redness with a feeling of heat in the head and a lot of sweating over the face. There is some slight disturbance of sight, but nothing so definite as in the remedies above. The chief disturbance of sight in the Glonoine patient is not a loss of sight or half vision cut-out, but of seeing colours when they look at things. They feel as if their head is expanding and going to burst. They are much worse in the light. They are better for cold air and cold applications. You often find a Glonoine patient sitting in a chair, holding his head so that it will not move at all, and it is a typical position for them to be in. If it is one side you see the vessels pulsating in that side and not in the other.

Iris Versicolor

Iris is not needed often. You get disturbance of vision beforehand and it is always a right-sided headache. Like other migraines it does go on to vomiting, and the vomiting of Iris is typical in that it relieves it at once. It is much worse eating sweet things, which the patients rather like and think they will have. It is worse for keeping quite still, and they want to walk about quite gently in the open air – unless it is too cold or windy, because that will only bring it on worse. I only use it in a high potency.

Magnesia Phosphorica

Mag. Phos., has either an acute neuralgic headache or else a deep headache, starting at the back and spreading all over the head. It nearly always comes from exposure to cold or from general nervous strain. It can also be started by over-excitement. It is very sensitive to light touch, whereas firm pressure ameliorates it. It is worse for cold and quite a lot better for warmth.

There is one queer and characteristic symptom. Each of my Mag. Phos. patients has had the same: the headache was very bad from 9–11 a.m. They then felt it was going to improve and were very cheered and thought it was going off. Not at all, by 4 p.m. it had come back even stronger and lasted till 8 p.m., and then it went off for good.

Nux Vomica

The Nux Vomica headache is nearly always an alcoholic headache from having done rather too well the night before. It is the headache for 'the morning after'. The patient wakes up feeling very ill, and is worse for any mental excitement. They are even worse if people come in and ask them if they would like a cup of tea or some breakfast – they are annoyed by anything that disturbs them or obliges them to answer. They are worse if they have to work. They feel very chilly and heavy in the head, and they are also nearly always constipated which makes their constipation worse for some days.

One of my colleagues stayed in a hotel in Liverpool where a man had taken far too much alcohol and had woken up with an awful headache. He gave him a 10M of Nux Vomica and later on had a letter from him saying, 'Please send me some more of that medicine. It was the most wonderful thing I have ever had. I was well in an hour'.

Sanguinaria

Sanguinaria has as bad a headache as you can get. It is very like Gelsemium and looks rather like it, and there are very few modalities to go on except that they feel rather poor and perhaps slightly giddy. I use it in a 200c.

CHRONIC HEADACHES

Aluminium Oxide

The typical headache of Alumina often occurs in what I think is a patient who is sensitive to Aluminium. It is a recurring headache, heavy and throbbing, and is accompanied by constipation. If you ask them where it is, they always put their hand on the top of their head. The patients who do best on Alumina are apt to have some epistaxis, which is useful when you get it. The headache has peculiar modalities, quite unlike any others. It is much better for icy cold applications. It is better for pressure, for walking in the open air, especially without a hat, and better for lying down. They have that strange symptom of being better for drinking cold water although they have no thirst.

Argentum Nitricum

This headache comes on from excitement and overwork. It can also come on after a journey, or after eating too many sweets. Remember that the Argentum Nit. patient is fond of sweets. Characteristically it comes on gradually and is suddenly gone. It starts with a feeling of tension and stiffness and soreness at the back of the neck. Sometimes they complain of their head being almost drawn back with the pain. It spreads over and then becomes localised in the left temple. Patients will sometimes tell you they think their headache comes from the brain, as if there is something wrong with their brain, deep inside their head. Occasionally they have a sense of nausea, although they are very seldom sick. They have a superficial tenderness of the head although they like it pressed hard, and they are worse for exertion or moving of any kind, especially stooping. They think they would like somebody to talk to, but when somebody sits and talks to them they find even the effort of talking makes their headache much worse. Like all Argentum Nit. they are better in the fresh air. On the whole they are hot.

Arsenicum Album

The Arsenicum Album headache is always accompanied by vomiting and often has a marked periodicity. The patient may say, 'Every third Saturday I get a frightful headache and can't do anything'. They give it to you like that. The pain is very intense, with throbbing and with the usual Arsenicum burning. It nearly always starts in the root of the nose and spreads across the forehead and then over the whole head. The head is rather tender and worse for touch or pressure.

The Arsenicum patient with a headache is very sensitive to the smell of food, or tobacco or cooking. They are rather inclined to think, 'A meal will do me good, so I shall have some lunch'. They have hardly finished their lunch before the headache is back again – they ought to wait until their headache stopped before eating. They often have Arsenicum mental symptoms – they are anxious, nervous and restless.

There is a contradiction about their headaches. If you catch them early they are strangely enough better for cold applications. I went to see an Arsenicum patient who had the most terrible headache that had come on about an hour before. She was leaning with her head out of the window and had a very cold flannel on the back of her head. I could hardly believe it, because her Arsenicum burning pain was always better for heat. 'Oh', she said, 'I caught it in time. If I had waited another hour then I should have been worse for the cold application.'

Aurum Metallicum

An Aurum headache sometimes comes on from sun, but much more often from rage – that is one of its main symptoms. There are a lot of eye symptoms with distortion of sight, and the upper field of vision is usually lost. They are flushed and dull and do not want to be disturbed. They look gloomy and sit in a lump, and are very touchy. They cannot bear noise, or touch or smells, or funny sounds about them which they cannot explain. As a rule the Aurum headache does not come on unless the patient is constipated.

Calcarea Carbonica

Calc. Carb. comes on from eating or drinking too much, but it is mostly from heat and cold, and there is some gastric disturbance associated with the headache, with empty eructations that are a great nuisance to them. They get congested eyes, especially the right eye, and the head is rather cold and damp to touch. The headache is nearly always in the right temple. Even describing their headache, Calc. Carb. patients sit with their eyes shut. They are worse for light, better for lying down and much better for sleep. They are worse for any kind of motion, especially stooping, or if they walk far in the open air, and are worse for alcohol. One does not always think of Calc. Carb. as a headache remedy but it can be very useful.

Cedron

These cases are quite rare, but I have needed it urgently on the few times I have used it and always to good effect. These are the regularly recurring headaches of Cedron, every two to three weeks, with a great deal of ocular disturbance beforehand. The patient has a dimness of sight. Everything they look at appears yellow, and it is usually associated with giddiness, buzzing in the ears, and – particularly helpful – giddiness on standing. It starts as a rule at about 11 a.m., lasts all that day and night and into the following night, intensifying towards the end of each day. The patient has a bad pain in the forehead, which feels distended, and this pain shoots from one temple to the other.

169

Kali Bichromicum

Kali Bich. is one of the most useful of all the headache remedies. Here again you get disturbance of sight before a headache, dimness of vision, even loss of sight. But, between the loss of sight and the coming on of the headache, there is a space when there is nothing – it may only be fifteen to twenty minutes. As a rule the pain comes on in the morning and gets worse during the day, finishing towards evening. It is usually left-sided, but not necessarily so, and is worse for light and noise.

The Kali Bich. patient cannot bear to stoop. As a rule the patient is better lying down, but a Kali Bich. pain is always worse lying on the painful side. Otherwise there is an amelioration from pressure. This sounds almost a contradiction, but it is not, because if you press, you press much harder than lying on a pillow. It is better in the open air. It also has one peculiar symptom. These patients will say they are much better for hot drinks, particularly hot soup.

Lachesis

Lachesis is one of the menopausal remedies for headaches and for all the time of the period. Exposure to heat of any kind, whether sitting in a hot room, or near a hot stove, sometimes having on a very glaring light, can all bring on the Lachesis headache. The patients have the typical bloated Lachesis appearance, with a throbbing, pulsating headache, all over the head, worse from motion and worse from stooping. During the headache the extremities get very cold. They enjoy some food and they say they feel better for it. They are always worse after sleep. If your patient has a right-sided headache, do not be put off Lachesis, because these can also occur.

Lac Defloratum

Here you always have ocular symptoms – a complete loss of sight before the pain. The pain starts in the forehead and extends back to the occiput. It is throbbing and painful and is associated with intense nausea. Patients like their head pressed, so much so that they often bind up their head with a scarf. It is worse for light, noise and motion, and is often worse during a period. There is an increased secretion of very pale urine during the headache, but – in contrast to Gelsemium – with no relief of pain.

Natrum Muriaticum

These are nearly always pre-menstrual headaches, and the remedy is most commonly needed before a period. It can also come on after a railway journey, after a theatre, after eye strain, after any mental exertion or excitement, as well as from exposure to sun. It starts in the occiput and spreads all over the head. Often you get zigzags in front of the eyes just before, or just as the splitting headache starts. If anything it is worse on the left side. It is worse from warmth, from motion, from using the eyes, and there is intense photophobia and sensitiveness to noise with it. It is also aggravated from lying with the head low, and slightly better in the open air. The scalp is sensitive and the patients quite definitely do not like to have their hair touched or brushed. They sometimes sweat profusely over the face and head just before the relief of pain.

Psorinum

Psorinum is not really looked upon as a headache remedy, and yet it can be very useful. It is always associated with eye disturbance, with dimness of sight, flickering or specks in front of the eyes. It has one useful symptom – intense hunger before the headache starts, and the hunger persists throughout. You get general congestion with acute stabs of pain running right through the head. It is worse from cold and fresh air, and the patient will wrap up the head warmly. As with Natrum Mur., if the head begins to sweat it means that the pain is going off.

Pulsatilla

The Pulsatilla headache comes with digestive disturbances and from dietary over-indulgence. There is pain in the temples and a throbbing headache all over, with marked photophobia. It is generally more marked on one or the other side, and you get, even in an adult, a flush on one cheek – the same side as the headache. It is worse in a close stuffy atmosphere, better for walking in the open air, worse for lying down, worse for stooping, better for pressure and worse in the evening. You nearly always find that the patient is constitutionally Pulsatilla when they need Pulsatilla for their headache.

Sepia

The Sepia headache starts in the occiput and spreads over the head. The pain is intense, and is associated with the period, like Natrum Mur. But it also comes on when they are tired out, after things like shopping or a long ironing session. You must then give them Bryonia even if you are quite sure that this is a Sepia patient, because Bryonia is for a headache in a Sepia patient who has become fatigued.

40

Eye Conditions

Aconitum Napellus

Here the eyes have a generally congested look and a watery, hot discharge so that the tears which run down the face feel hot. The pupils are, as a rule, widely dilated – somehow this is unexpected, but do not let it put you off. The patients are sensitive to draught, as well as to going out in the cold air, which makes them extremely uncomfortable. Occasionally they get a gritty feeling, like sand in the eyes, although more often it is a red-hot feeling, and with this they get a lot of general Aconite symptoms. They get nervous and really can be quite scared.

I always remember going to stay with a friend in the country, and we went out to look for a very special plant. As I was getting through a hedge, a small and very thin branch came back and hit me in the eye. Within half an hour I could not open my eye and it was intensely painful and very watery. I had only just started homoeopathy, and thought that for this extreme onset of wateriness I must need some Aconite. In ten minutes I had relief.

Allium Cepa

This remedy is not often needed, except in certain patients who get an acute localised conjunctivitis with burning, smarting irritation in the eyes, particularly above the lids. They have a great deal of lacrimation, all of which is bland and which can be a little bit deceptive.

I mention this because I had one patient who was bright red all under her eyes, not because of the lacrimation but because she had to mop so constantly. The eyes are sensitive to light, which causes an increased flow of tears. The patients are better in the open air, as with all Allium complaints, and worse for heat. If they have a particular complaint it is that their eyes feel as if they are being torn, and that it is a horrible sensation.

Occasionally, they get redness round the margins of the lids, with very little swelling. As a rule, there is no involvement of the iris – it is just conjunctivitis. It sometimes comes with hay fever.

Apis Mellifica

With Apis you get a sudden onset of pain and acute inflammation. The eyelids are swollen, and may actually be oedematous. They get an oedematous patch under the eyes and sometimes the upper lids swell to such an extent that they may be slightly everted. The mucous membranes can be swollen and rather like raw beef, and the vessels of the eyes intensely congested with large, bright red vessels.

As always with Apis, the patients are sensitive to heat. What they really like to do is sit over a basin and bathe their eyes in cold water. I have found that they all start in the right eye and then go over to the left. There is also profuse lacrimation and burning tears, not just burning tears running down the cheeks – they feel as if they are running down a burning surface.

They get sudden stabbing pains and their eyeballs are very sensitive to touch. Occasionally you find septic spots along the lids or styes, but more commonly it is a general conjunctivitis. The condition can also go on to corneal ulcers, with the margins and the lids all tending to ulcerate.

Argentum Nitricum

The patient has a purulent affliction of the eye, and photophobia, both much worse for any kind of warmth. They get an intense congestion of the conjunctivae, particularly marked on the inner side of the eye. It looks as if the inner canthus is going to go into an eruption, and very much as if it would bleed if you touched that part. They sometimes have some corneal ulceration, but if so, it is not deep. All the conditions are better if the eyes can be cool, so that if the patient goes out into the open air, as long as they are shaded from light, they feel much better. If the condition persists the patient has thickening and oedema of the lids.

Belladonna

Belladonna comes in for all the acute diseases, and it comes into eyes as well, with photophobia, although not quite as acute as you might expect. It has one symptom that I have not found in any other eye remedy – the eyes are hot and the pain is acute, extending from the eyes and running back into the head. The patient also has an intense throbbing headache which is worse for lying down.

The pupils of a Belladonna patient in an eye condition are mostly contracted. This is the one condition when Belladonna has contracted pupils. They complain that their eyes are not only burning and hot, but that they are also dry and painful, and that after a dry period they have a sudden gush of hot salt tears. There is marked photophobia and an intense aggravation from moving, as is usual in the Belladonna patient. You can get the lids and the whole eyes looking rather swollen in an acute condition, and it can have iritis, neuritis, conjunctivitis – any or all of them.

Chamomilla

Chamomilla has a yellowish pussy eye discharge on exposure, always in children. They are just the Chamomilla temperament, except that they are not so peevish as usual. They do not want anything, nothing is right, and everything is thrown at you. It is difficult to think of Chamomilla as an eye remedy, and yet it can be very useful.

Croton Tiglium

You find an intense irritation with the lids swollen and oedematous, and all round the lids there is a set of little vesicles – this time they are vesicles, not pimples. If it is not treated quickly, they spread outwards on to the cheek. They do not as a rule spread down the cheek. As a rule this condition is left-sided, whereas most eye conditions, if they are in one eye only, are right-sided. There is an early tendency to corneal ulcer.

Euphrasia

Euphrasia is an eye remedy that goes with hay fever. You get an acute catarrhal conjunctivitis and a lot of inflammation, both eyes as a rule bright red, with profuse and irritating lacrimation. The lid margins are very sore, and look sore. If you try to lift the lid up to see what the eye looks like, or pull it down, it will bleed.

The patient will say, 'I must rub my eyes, they feel so irritable. I feel as if pepper had been put on them. I must rub them'. And then they make an awful mess of them, because they bleed. Then they sit screwing up their eyes, making awful faces, trying to stop this terrible itching. They get a lot of tiny little septic spots round the eyelids – pimples, not vesicles – which occasionally can spread out on to the cheeks. They feel this feeling of dryness and a sharp cutting pain behind the eyes and into the head, although not quite as much as in the Belladonna patient.

If you examine their eyes you find that the vessels are so congested that they are dark, and pressure on the eyes is very painful.

Hepar Sulphuris

The Hepar Sulph. patient comes in and slumps in the chair. Everything is wrong with them – they live in the wrong place, they have the wrong friends, and so on. They are just like that and never more so than in an eye condition. They get an intensely painful eye condition with early corneal ulcers and an early development of pus. They also get a real Hepar symptom, which is that they complain that they have a feeling of pressing into the eye (comparable to the way Hepar feels as if a blunt stick were pressed into the throat). The rest of the patient quite quickly falls into the Hepar picture. They are intensely sensitive to light and cold, and get a lot of pain if you try to examine their eyes, particularly the lid margins, and if you pull down the lid you find that inside there is a little raw line.

The whole conjunctiva is puffy and oedematous-looking with a muddy cornea and deep ulceration. Occasionally they say their eyes feel as if somebody had a string pulling them back into the head.

Kali Bichromicum

Kali Bich. is one of the most useful eye remedies that there are. It has a deep corneal ulcer, tending to perforate with a sharp, clear-cut margin. The eye looks very painful, but the patient will tell you it is not painful at all, which should give you this remedy.

Like all the other Kali discharges, the patient gets a thick, stringy discharge. Another rather interesting condition is that they get acute iritis in rheumatism with associated conjunctivitis, and intense heat in the eyes. The patient emphasises his flitting rheumatic pains and has marked photophobia. The lids are always granulated and sore-looking along the margins.

Kali Iodatum

This is one of the most acute eye remedies. The patient has an acute, purulent inflammation of the eye, and the tissues, both inside and outside the eye, are red and swollen and worse in the upper lids. If the eye is touched the patient could call out with pain. Another thing is that if you examine them, however gently you pull down the lid, you get a gush of tears, followed by a most unpleasant-looking purulent discharge.

The Kali patient is very tender in the bones all round the eye – above the eye, on the cheeks, everywhere round the eye and especially on the outer side.

If one eye only is affected, it is always the right, although I have mostly seen both eyes affected to some extent, one worse than the other. And the patients explain they feel as if their eyes are pressed all the time, or as if they had a scarf round their eyes which was too tight. They display photophobia, and you can get anything from iritis to corneal ulcer or effuse purulent corneal conjunctivitis. One thing that might give a little local ease is to bathe the eyes in lukewarm water.

Mercurius Solubilis

I have found this useful after a burn on the forehead that was very near the eye. The inflammation follows when the eye is subsequently exposed to cold, and it is acute. It often arises in a rheumatic subject.

The eyes are worse for any warm application and they constantly blink because they have a feeling of irritation in the eye. The tears are irritating and make the face quite sore.

There is a green, purulent discharge from the eye, with quite a lot of acute burning pain everywhere. The patients sweat often and show other Merc. Sol. symptoms, and are much worse in the evening.

Pulsatilla

The patient gets an acute, catarrhal conjunctivitis, and there is nearly always a history of repeated styes. They are definitely sensitive, their eyes water terribly and they get a sort of pustular irritation round the lids and a profuse yellow or yellowish discharge which is quite bland, even though it looks as if it might be excruciating.

One contradiction in the eye symptoms of Pulsatilla is that the patient has relief from bathing the eyes with hot water. They scratch their eyes a lot and as a result get a tendency to more styes.

Rhus Toxicodendron

The eyes are painfully inflamed and oedematous and the lids are dark and red in colour. The patient usually complains that the eyes feel bruised and sore and that they are worse on opening, as well as for moving and turning the head. This may distract you on your way to Rhus, but do not let it, because you think they ought to be better for movement. There is a lot of discharge, usually thick and yellow.

In Rhus Tox. there is the danger that the eye condition quickly spreads on to the cheeks. The lids are sore and raw, and you get a herpetic eruption from the corner of each eye or the corner of one eye, so that the eye can be completely closed, very painful and with a gush of scalding tears. When they open their eyes the eye looks all swollen up, almost bulging forward. They get intense photophobia and are intensely sensitive to cold.

41

Throats and Influenzas

Aconitum Napellus
I rarely use Aconite for a throat because I seldom see them early
enough. The patient has stood in a cold wind and comes in within half
an hour to an hour with a painful congested throat. It will be swollen
and red, dark red at times, with acute burning pain which is worse for
any movement, worse on swallowing and worse on turning round. The
neck is always sensitive to touch. They get a short dry cough because
they feel as if their throat is closing, and they are in great discomfort.
They go faint and pale sitting up and their skin is hot, burning and dry.
They can run any kind of fever, often high with intense thirst, and their
tongue is dry and red. There is the restless anxiety which is one of the
Aconite general symptoms. As well as their restless anxiety, they are
very scared – Aconite is as scared as any remedy.

Apis Mellifica
Apis is needed much less frequently, but is an invaluable remedy. It is
an acutely inflamed and painful throat. An Apis and an Aconite throat
are both bright red and rather shiny-looking, but the Apis is more
glistening than the Aconite, often with oedema of the uvula. The
throat and mouth are dry and burning. They get a sharp stinging pain
in the throat on any attempt to swallow, and nearly always get a lot of
swollen glands, and the glands are highly sensitive to touch. They
cannot bear anything tight round their neck. The pain is worse for hot
applications and worse for a hot drink. The tongue is red, scalded,
swollen and raw-looking. With the Apis picture, you often get rather
swollen lips.

It also has a time aggravation in the middle of the afternoon, rather
unexpectedly. They are not only worse for local heat, they are worse in
a hot room, in front of a hot fire, after sleep, and much worse for any
solid food, which they simply cannot take because of the stabbing pain
it gives them.

Two other things go with the Apis sore throat. One is a marked urticaria. If I have got an urticaria with a sore throat I should think immediately of two remedies, the first being Apis. (The second is Dulcamara.) The other thing with their sore throat is a generalised soreness in the joints and all over. During an attack they are quite thirstless, which is surprising, and they look chilly. They are shivery and rather shaky, and you are inclined to wrap a blanket round them, but in a few minutes they are feeling much worse. They feel quite ill and throw it off. As a rule their face is either puffy and red and swollen, or pale and swollen. Occasionally it is oedematous.

Quite often their tonsils ulcerate and they show a sort of bright red mark round the margin. This is characteristic of Apis – I do not know any other remedy in which it occurs. They are generally very distressed.

Baptisia Tinctoria

Baptisia is one remedy that cannot possibly be left out. The patients tend to be very ill. They have a certain amount of offensiveness of the mouth, which Baptisia can always have in any condition, and this is aggravated in a flu. They have a typical tongue, with a white coating and red papillae showing through, and then this tongue rapidly becomes dry, with a red streak down the centre. Later still it will be dry and cracked, and tending to bleed. They have a foul throat which you think must be very painful, but they tell you to your surprise that it is painless. They can also have a dark red, almost purplish throat, and this one is usually painful.

They can only swallow fluids with great difficulty, feeling as if the throat is being held and constricted outside. They have a tendency to gland enlargement, although not so marked as in Baryta Carb. They have no obvious thirst. On the other hand, if a drink is there, they will probably be quite pleased to drink it off. The patient with a Baptisia sore throat has a lot of aching, always aching in the part lain on. They cannot get comfortable in bed and move about the whole time. As with every Baptisia complaint they often feel as if part of them is lost, perhaps with the legs disconnected somewhere else in the bed, and get very agitated about this.

Baryta Carbonica

Baryta Carb. is much more common, and I consider it to be one of the greatest throat and flu remedies. It has a recurrent very sore throat. In each case they probably tell you that they have walked in the open and that they have got their feet wet. Baryta Carb. is very susceptible to getting wet feet and having perhaps to sit in wet shoes. They often tell you that 'this brings back my throat every time'. They have a raw, scraped feeling on attempting to swallow. They feel as if there was a plug in the throat and that they cannot swallow past it without acute pain. Also, that it is worse on empty swallowing, although they do not like solids either. The only thing Baryta Carb. can live on is a little fluid taken fairly frequently. The voice usually goes hoarse, and the patient gets quite a lot of blisters on the tongue and a lot of salivation.

I have never yet seen a patient needing Baryta Carb. without glands in the neck. They always have swollen glands and often have chronically enlarged tonsils. You look at their tonsils when they are apparently feeling quite well and they are still chronically enlarged. They are chilly patients who want to be covered up, and are described in the books as being soft, flabby, bloated, pale people without much stamina, although they are not necessarily always like that. Another symptom I have seen many times is a swollen upper lip.

Baryta Carb. patients get an offensive foot sweat and this can be a gift, just to confirm the remedy. They get a lot of cracking in the ears, a sort of flapping noise and unpleasant sensations, which are always worse on chewing or eating and better lying down. They also get eruptions round their ears – not a generalised urticaria. Occasionally they get an inflammation of their parotids. That rather comes and goes, and is not there all the time.

Sometimes, when you have given Baryta Carb. 10M to these patients and they have done well on it, they still come back in six weeks with another throat. They get depressed and you do not know what to do, so you repeat the Baryta Carb., thinking that this is about as long as it lasts, but this time it has no effect. In that case, put in a few doses of Psorinum 10M. It can be of the greatest value in a recurring Baryta Carb. throat that suddenly stops responding.

Baryta Muriatica

Baryta Mur. is seldom used for a throat, even though it is an effective remedy. It has a right-sided throat, very painful, which feels like a lump in the throat. It usually has a large tonsil, particularly on that side. The patient is thirsty, with dry lips and an offensive mouth and some glands, and a marked aversion to all foods. They feel rotten and do not want anything at all to eat. The pain is much worse on swallowing, especially as the throat is peculiarly dry, and except for water, everything they try to swallow just sticks. As a rule you will not need Baryta Mur., but you may have a patient with a lot of throat

179

symptoms as well as glands, and you think they are Baryta Carb. but they do not quite fit – fifty per cent of them will be Baryta Mur.

Belladonna
Belladonna is one of the remedies you can tell mothers to give when they ring up and say their child has a sore throat, does not feel well, has a bright red face, a high temperature and all the rest of it.

It has one curious symptom, which is a very sore throat where the pains jerk about a bit. They jerk out to the neck or up to the head. The patient cannot bear to be jarred, and gets a real spasm of the throat on attempting to swallow. It is almost as if somebody had clutched the throat. It is a horrible sensation which comes on even when they lie quite still. It lasts just a few seconds and then goes again. At the same time, strangely enough, they have a constant desire to swallow – it does not matter what happens, they want to swallow in spite of this choking spasm, and they get much more flushed as they try to do so. They often have dilated pupils and are also thirsty, although you will find that they do not like water very much – what they really like is lemon juice. Occasionally you get the front of the tongue with a coated centre and red all round the coating. Sometimes you get a strawberry tongue, which you would expect, because Belladonna was the prophylactic for scarlet fever that Hahnemann found. The neck is tender to touch and talking makes the pain worse. You can see the patient wince when they talk to you.

Calcarea Sulphurica
One thinks of Calc. Sulph. as an acne remedy or a skin remedy or behaviour remedy or anything else, but it is also a great throat remedy. It has the characteristic that it is apt to push out infection. The whole mouth is dry. As a rule the front of the mouth looks quite clear and clean. But if you make them open their mouth a bit wider, the whole of the back of it is coated yellow, with a lot of yellow secretion which they cannot get rid of. They get pain on swallowing and a tendency to ulceration of the tonsils, and a rapid involvement of the glands of the neck.

Again, there is this feeling of fullness and choking, quite often a sort of air hunger, and a thirst for cold drinks or fruit. They are all worse for hot things to the throat. They are not easy patients to deal with, because they do not want to be asked questions – they do not want any kind of disturbance. They are fat and pale and soft, like Calc. Carb., but at the same time nearly always have a rather rough, red skin like Sulphur. They really are a mixture of Calc. Carb. and Sulphur.

I used to think that one never saw quinsies nowadays, but one Christmas I was haunted by them. Everyone I met was either developing a quinsy, or had a quinsy which was going to be opened that morning, or had a quinsy which would not discharge properly and which was giving them awful trouble, and Calc. Sulph. was the remedy I used. It made the stuff pour out, instead of taking ages. The one patient who took an antibiotic felt far worse than the others. If you think of it as an acne remedy you will not miss it as a throat remedy – here is something to push out and this is a remedy that will do it.

Causticum

I do not normally think of Causticum as a flu throat remedy, although I have seen cases that needed it badly. They all started off with a dryness at the back of the throat, a scraping feeling going on to rawness, with a tickle and a dry, irritating cough. They had a paroxysm of coughing and at the end brought up a little expectoration, but could not get the mucus moved. It was somewhere at the back and after a great effort they finally had to swallow it. That symptom comes very much into Causticum. All cases were accompanied by hoarseness, made worse by talking, one of them with a complete loss of voice.

Some of the cases had frequency accompanying this throat, and one of them had slight incontinence on coughing or sneezing, particularly in one of the paroxysms of cough – another very good Causticum symptom. It was a cold spell at the time and they were all worse for it. But, when it rained the next day, I was surprised to find that they were all of them better. (Causticum is a remedy that is better in the rain and so, to a lesser extent, is Hepar Sulph.)

Chininum Arsenicosum

China Arsenite is one of the worst throats you can see, verging on a diphtheria. You think – this will be gangrenous before I turn round. The back of the throat is inflamed, with a horrible putrid smell, and feels on fire. As a rule there will be a dark, brownish exudate.

The tongue is characteristic. If you see it early enough, you get a thick, yellow slimy, shiny coating. Then it goes dry and tends to crack. There is nearly always a swelling of the gums, sometimes even ulceration, and they bleed and look horrible. You would think the patient would have a bad taste with the state of the mouth and the smell from it, but they do not. They have a bitter taste – it is not putrid to them. They are always trying to clear the throat – there is so much mucus sticking round the back that they try to clear it, which is agony to them, although they probably will not get it clear. The lips are bluish and cracked, and the patient has a thirst for cold drinks.

They are chilly patients and very sensitive to draughts. They have all the anxiety of Arsenicum Alb. Thus China Arsenite has the temperament of Arsenicum Alb. and the throat symptoms of both remedies. They are restless, irritable, and weak. They are very ill and really feel they cannot do anything, and with their weakness they have a tendency to develop quite a marked tremor. They get a general aggravation after sleep. They nearly always also get a change in their pulse – it is irregular or rapid, usually both, like an acute septic condition.

Crotalus Horridus
This is not often needed, but you must bear it in mind when you see a septic throat. The patient looks bluish and ill, with purplish and often very painful lips. Often they tell you that the lips feel numb. They get a yellowish tongue and have a tendency everywhere to cyanosis.

Crotalus Horridus patients are fuddled all the time because they are so frightfully ill. One such patient of mine felt she was shut in somewhere against her will and spent her life trying to escape, which is a feature of Crotalus Horridus behaviour. They get early epistaxis – a trickle of dark, fluid blood which does not clot, and their tongue is bright, fiery red, rather as if it had been polished. They get a lot of salivation, and that is nearly always blood-tinted too. They also get a sort of mouldy, sweetish odour. Even on opening their mouth they feel as if the throat is going to go into a spasm at any minute, and they are quite frightened.

They are worse after sleep, like all the snake venoms, and wake feeling suffocated. During these throats they are very apt to dream of dead people. With a sore throat the Crotalus Horridus patient nearly always has digestive trouble. Their stomach gets out of order and they are liable to have an offensive diarrhoea of dark, watery stools. The patient himself is weak and tremulous and looks ill, and the extremities become puffy. They also have a tendency to develop purpura.

Dulcamara
In a Dulcamara throat you nearly always have a history of chronic post-nasal catarrh, and there is a typical rheumatic sore throat in cold wet weather. They go out and catch a chill and then they get an onset

of their sore throat. They are specially sensitive going from a hot to a cold atmosphere, which will often start off the chill. They get herpes round the mouth and a dry, rough tongue and want a lot of cold drinks. They very often get a stiff neck with the throat, and an early development of urticaria. I do not think I have ever seen a Dulcamara throat without an urticaria – I would not give this remedy without an urticaria.

They are better if they move about a bit – they say their neck unstiffens and that their skin is better too. They are hoarse very early in their tonsilitis and they get a tenacious, frothy yellowish exudate at the back of the throat. It always looks like soap. They practically always get some lumbago with their sore throats.

The Dulcamara patient can become untypically confused – they are muddled or get the wrong word. If you have known them beforehand, you are quite surprised. They get a certain amount of earache with their sore throat, and complain of icy cold feet with a general burning heat. I always think of Dulcamara as a red-faced Calc. Carb.

Gelsemium

The Gelsemium throat has one or two marked characteristics. You get the dull, slightly bluish, heavy-looking patient who has waves of heat alternating with waves of chilliness. They complain that they are thoroughly tired, and also sometimes very giddy, with the generalised aching pains of the Gelsemium acute illness. If you feel the face of the Gelsemium patient it is quite damp. They are anxious with their sore throat – more anxious with a sore throat than with any other Gelsemium complaint. They sometimes develop an acute fear of death, which I have only found in a throat, not otherwise.

They get a horrible taste in the mouth and the tongue feels numb. When you ask them to put it out it is quite trembly and has a thick yellow coating. Although they have horrible-looking tonsils and quite obviously have tonsillitis, they complain of pain in their neck and their ears rather than in their tonsils. It is worse on swallowing and much worse for a hot drink. With all this they are quite thirstless.

Guaiacum

The Guaiacum throat is an unusual one, but you do sometimes need it. It comes in the early stages – you get a sudden acute throat and think of giving Belladonna or Aconite or one of the acute things, when it really needs Guaiacum. The patient has a congested red face with the sore throat and is depressed and indolent. If you let them they would

183

prefer to sit about and do nothing – they often forget what they wanted to tell you: 'Oh, there is something I wanted to tell you but I forget what it was'. And you never get it out of them.

They nearly always have dilated pupils and are thirsty for cold water. One thing which I do not think you find with any other remedy is that with their sore throat they get a pain in the back of the neck. You do also get a certain amount of joint pain sometimes, which is worse from heat. If they have this pain in the neck you find them holding their neck, or they may put a shawl round so that they have some support to the neck. They have a definite aversion to milk, and a slight desire for sour things.

Hepar Sulphuris

Hepar Sulph. also has a recurrent sore throat. A patient will tell you, 'One of the things I get is a sore throat on every provocation', and they do. It is not quite the same recurrent sore throat as Baryta Carb. because it is not just 'getting my feet wet will bring back my throat'. It is a recurrent sore throat and they get it perhaps two or three times a year. They are hypersensitive people who cannot bear disturbance or touch. They are irritable and chilly – this is one of the chilliest remedies. They also get that most horrible fishbone sensation in the throat – as if a fishbone was sticking in hard somewhere, not necessarily in one place.

I find that this remedy is always needed in a flu epidemic. After an epidemic one year I found that I had used it in half the cases, although that was unusual. It is always needed for the tracheitis that can occur in a case of flu. The patient may have been in contact with flu and escaped it. Then there is a cold spell and they go down with extremely painful tracheitis. They describe the fishbones or blunt pins or something like that sticking into the throat, setting up a dry, hacking, painful cough. You have only to see them having a paroxysm of cough to know how painful it is. After the tracheitis they go on as a rule to a bit of a sore chest up at the top, not otherwise throughout the chest.

They get a tendency to a formation of pus – it is an old quinsy remedy too. Often it is common for the Hepar patient to get a little ulceration at the corner of the lips and a painful crack at the centre of the lip. It cracks again when they talk and then it is most painful, with an offensive mouth. They do not stand pain at all well. Anything hurts them – they cannot open their mouth, they cannot move their head, they cannot even put out their tongue without it hurting. They have a stabbing pain on swallowing. They get a foul septic-looking mouth and very offensive breath. They tend to sweat, with the sour, typical Hepar smell and it does not relieve them a bit.

They are greatly comforted by something nice and warm wrapped round their neck. They are so chilly that I have had the greatest difficulty through the years examining certain Hepar patients. If you uncover them to listen to their chest, they pull half the blanket over them before you have had time to start. They will not put a hand out of bed if they can help it. They are covered with sweat and keep the blankets up to their necks. They are also the most snappy patients I have ever met. I remember going to see a very nice girl of about eighteen whom I had known since she was ten. I went in, looking forward to a nice friendly greeting. Not at all – she was furious with her mother for sending for me. I would want to examine her and why should she be examined, and this, that and the other. I gave her Hepar Sulph. without much examination and she was infinitely better the next day.

Lac Caninum

The Lac Caninum throat is affected on alternating sides. It may start on the left and go to the right, or vice versa, or go from side to side. The tongue has a white, silvery coating, and in a case of tonsillitis you will find this same silvery exudate on the tonsils. They are very painful and sensitive to touch, worse on swallowing, and the pain tends to radiate up to the ear. The patient has probably always had an aversion to milk, but this aversion is even more pronounced when they have a sore throat. Another useful point is that if you have a girl who gets a sore throat with every period, it can only be one or two remedies – either Lac Caninum or Dulcamara.

They are fair, gentle people who weep easily. At the same time they can be irritable. They are frightened of being alone and frightened of the dark, and generally rather nervous. They get very thick saliva, which is difficult to get away – often they tell you that they are worse swallowing saliva than if they were taking semi-solid or even solid food. The reason is that it sticks about the mouth and they cannot get it moved, whereas solid food they can shoot down somehow. The Lac Caninum patient is usually hungry in acute illness. It is one of the remedies that has distressing and persistent dreams of snakes, and I have met this in its throat symptoms. Another curious symptom is that the patient sometimes feels as if he is floating in air. (The other remedy which has the sensation of floating in air is Thuja.)

Lachesis

The pain of Lachesis is always left-sided and very acute. It radiates into the ear on swallowing. The throat feels swollen and almost as if it is going to close up. The patient cannot bear anything tight, even up the spine at the top of the sternum, and loosens everything round the neck. It is worse after sleep as well as from hot applications and hot drinks, and it is also worse for liquid food rather than for solids. (One of the Lachesis symptoms is worse for liquid food, especially warm food.)

You also get a purplish, swollen, inflamed appearance of the throat, and ropy saliva round the back of the throat. It gets worse during sleep and the patient finally wakes up more or less choked. Sometimes they like a cold thing wrapped round their throat, and cold drinks. They get swelling outside and inside their throat – the neck is often quite swollen – and frequently get a bad headache with the throat.

They cannot bear to sit in a hot room or to get too hot. They are restless and tremulous, with a lot of hot sweating, and are nearly always a jealous sort of person.

Lycopodium

I think you always get a Lycopodium throat in a Lycopodium patient – it has so many of the general characteristics of the remedy. It tends to be right-sided. It is worse for cold drinks or cold food, and has either a 4–8 p.m. or 4–8 a.m. aggravation. The throat is often worse after sleep. The tongue is dry and often swollen and the throat gets sore very early. The patient looks like a Lycopodium – anxious, and a bit lined and sallow. They nearly always have flatulence and eructation and all the typical symptoms with their throats, and a dry, putty-coloured tongue without much coating. There is also one other useful point – I have never yet given Lycopodium to a throat patient who did not have toothache as well.

Mercurius Solubilis

Merc. Sol. is a good throat remedy, although perhaps not so commonly needed as it once was. You get a dark red, swollen throat, if anything somewhat worse on the right side, and very offensive, with quite a lot of superficial ulceration. The patient complains of a lump in the throat and says it is difficult to swallow, and that the pain tends to radiate into the neck – all round the neck, not so much to the ear. There is a nightly aggravation. They break out into a hot drenching sweat, which makes them feel much worse and aggravates the pain.

I always remember standing at the bottom of the bed of a man with a real Merc. Sol. throat. He had an acute Vincent's infection and every sort of Merc. Sol. symptom you could possibly want. He would sweat profusely, which made him feel worse and complain bitterly, and he would push down all the bedclothes with a sort of tremor. Later you would see him dragging up the bedclothes with the same tremor because he got chilly, and this went on all night. They have a great thirst for cold drinks, an early tendency to pus, a greasy, slimy saliva and their mouths are offensive. This man had a very bad haemorrhagic throat. They become muddled and talk slowly, and do not know what they are saying, and are suspicious of what you are doing. If you ask the patient to put out his tongue, the tongue too is tremulous.

Mercurius Cyanatus

A boy of eighteen once came in with the most awful throat and mouth I had seen for a long time. I took a throat swab as well as one from between all his teeth to see if he was really growing Vincent's everywhere. He had a thick yellow exudate round the back of his throat and his mouth was terrible. He had been to the dental hospital and brought a note to say, 'We think we should take all this boy's teeth out'. I thought this would be ridiculous and gave him some Merc. Cyanide. In two or three days he was a different boy. I gave him some more to keep for whenever the throat got bad again and he needed it occasionally over the next three years. Then I changed it to Crotalus Horridus with good effect and made the mouth look better too – it helped the gums more than the Merc. had done.

Nitricum Acidum

Nitric Acid has a throat very like Hepar Sulph., although it has some things that are different. The patient is extremely sensitive to touch and has the same sort of excruciating pain. They do not like being examined, and dislike having to open their mouth or put their head back or move the neck in any way. If they are just sitting in a chair or lying in bed, the pains come and go, but if they are trying to do something, or move about or eat, then they get very bad pain for a while. It radiates to the ear more than in Hepar Sulph., and the throat, when you look at it, is more oedematous in appearance – this is one of the things that put you on to Nitric Acid. It has a bad smell – worse than Hepar Sulph., which just smells of sour sweat and the perspiration smells unpleasant too. This patient gets a lot of stringy, rather unpleasant saliva which is difficult to move. Their tongue is coated and yellow but they are quite thirstless. They often have ulcers or sores at the corners of the mouth, and the whole of the lips tends to crack, more than in Hepar. They are extremely irritable, although not more so than the Hepar, which would be difficult.

Phytolacca

Phytolacca is a common acute throat – darkish red, if anything worse on the right side. The uvula gives it to you directly, because it is practically oedematous. The patient feels knocked out and yet is entirely indifferent to what happens to him. They get pain and dryness and a burning heat in the throat, and are worse for any hot drink. There is pain at the root of the tongue, which is much worse if they have to put their tongue out, extending into the neck and nearly always up to the ear. They always have a lot of swollen glands, and will tell you that they are quite unable to swallow. The tongue is raw and scalded-looking. It has a yellow streak down the centre and a definitely yellow coating, with a lot of stringy saliva about.

The patient is exhausted and restless with a generalised aching in the bones and joints and often an acute backache. With these specific symptoms it is valuable in influenza. It makes them feel that they cannot rest or sleep well – they have to move about, not that this helps them. Phytolacca is perhaps one of the illest of all the throats. It is a hot weather thing with an aggravation from heat. They complain of waves of heat, wishing they could get away from it. They sweat on the face, and then have a cobweb sensation over the face when it has dried on them. (The other remedy that has a cobweb sensation is Graphites.) The pain may start in the chest and spread up to the throat. It is a useful remedy sometimes when you are stuck and think that the patient must be a Pulsatilla, but does not respond at all to Pulsatilla.

Psorinum

A Psorinum throat is just like a Baryta throat which recurs. It arises in the typical Psorinum patient with the dry, rough, nutmeg-grater skin, with the tendency to acne, often with an untidy, dirty-looking appearance and a cold sweat which is slightly greasy to touch. They are anxious and melancholy, and very much afraid they are going to die. If they are children, they get peevish and irritable towards evening and cannot sleep in the early part of the night. They may have weak eyes with the tonsillitis – chronic blepharitis – and they look miserable little things.

There is a scalded, raw feeling in the throat and a tendency for the upper lip to swell and for the mouth to get very sore and dry. There is some salivation, although not a lot, and it is tough and offensive. Like all Psorinum patients they are sensitive to cold and worse from cold, and nearly always with a throat they have some generalised aching pain. If they run a temperature they get marked skin irritation and probably some skin rash. It is one of the remedies for recurring quinsy.

42

Pneumonia

Lycopodium

A lot of us are apt to think of Lycopodium as a chronic remedy which, on the whole, it is. However, you can get a virus infection that needs Lycopodium very badly, although not until after the third day. If you have not cured the infection by the third day with an acute remedy, you might very well need Lycopodium.

These patients are not usually flushed in appearance. The face is pale, almost yellow, distressed-looking and wrinkled, and they look very ill. Another thing you notice is a pinched nose and often also the flapping of the alae nasi, not synchronous with the heartbeat or breathing. This may not always be the case, but there is invariably twitching in some muscles of the face, more often round the eye than elsewhere.

A very ill Lycopodium patient is difficult to nurse. Nothing pleases them – they want their own way and are resentful if they do not get it. The iller they are, the weaker they are, and the more peevish and irritable too. They have a fairly characteristic sore tongue. They often tell you that when they put it out it is stiff and very sore, and that it often has painful vesicles which spread out on to the lips. These are not patches of herpes – they are really vesicles. The patient dislikes being left alone, although they like somebody quite near. They do not want to be talked to, they cannot bear to be contradicted, and they are very sensitive to noise.

Their cough is characteristic. It is a short, dry cough with little expectoration but, when it does come up, it is either saltish or bitter, and the patient complains of it very much. The sputum usually looks purulent or blood-streaked, and occasionally just rusty. It mostly originates from the right side, but it may come from either side.

There is often some kind of gastric disturbance with the cough – distension and discomfort and a horrible taste in the mouth. The aggravation time is, as usual, 4–8 p.m. However, in a virus infection, it is commonly also 4–8 a.m. They have rather a marked lack of

190

thirst. If they want anything it is hot drinks, not cold, because cold makes them feel awful. They sweat very little, although in a virus infection, when they are very ill, they do so more than usual.

You usually find coarse râles over the whole area. They tell you that their sore tongue extends back and gives them a tickle in the throat which brings on their coughing. Their coughing is not exactly a paroxysm, it is more this short, dry cough. If anything, they are more irritable in the morning and become a little more placid and easier as the day goes on. Lycopodium patients in general like to be propped up when lying down.

They are restless in their sleep and wake in a state of fright, which you would not expect from them. They nearly always dream. They will tell you they have had an awful night, that they dreamed they were in a frightful accident, and although they were not hurt themselves they were involved in it. While you are percussing them you get little local twitches over the chest, which you would not see if you were not actually touching them.

Mercurius Solubilis

There are two remedies for pneumonia in an alcoholic patient. Merc. Sol. is one (the other is Rhus Tox.). The patient is deadly ill and you do not expect them to get through. They are soaking with sweat. They have a general tremor, more marked in the hands, and they are uncomfortable – they are either too hot or too cold. The Merc.Sol. alcoholic will push the clothes off the bed because he is too hot. A few minutes later he will drag them up to his neck because he is too cold.

The mouth also is typical. As a rule the tongue is pale and swollen and teeth-marked, and it feels greasy. It may be unpleasant to feel, but it is very useful. Although it is nearly always whitish you can get it going brown and sore, and looking inflamed. There is also a lot of salivation.

You will never find a Merc. Sol. patient lying on the right side, regardless of where their lesion is. They lie on the left side and the pillow is soaked with their saliva. Perhaps in consequence they are violently thirsty and want quantities of cold water. They also have paroxysms of cough which go on and on until a small quantity of offensive sputum is brought up. The whole mouth of the Merc. Sol. patient is offensive.

They usually have a swinging temperature and are very shaky and restless. They are often too ill to complain, but if they do, they tell you they have a feeling as if the chest is going to burst. They also have a marked metallic taste, which you rather expect from Mercurius. They are worse at night in every way, and have a delirium in which they talk incessantly and very rapidly.

It is important to compare this picture with both Baptisia and Lachesis. The Lachesis patient usually talks on and on, but it will be about something. The Baptisia mutters and mutters, and not about anything. But the Mercurius patient just chats as hard as he can, at a terrific rate, and it is very characteristic of them.

Phosphorus

Phosphorus is one of the greatest of the chest remedies. You need it early, in the first twelve hours. The inspiration, when the patient has got the attack, is short and catching and very painful. They have clear skin with a reddish flush, dry and hot, and occasionally sweaty. Ill as they are, they still look like Phosphorus, alert and intelligent, and they usually answer your questions however bad they feel. They are scared stiff – they think they are going to die and will be thankful if you stay beside them for a few minutes and perhaps hold their hand, just to reassure them that they are not going to die. They are not quite so acutely anxious as Arsenic, but nearly so. They fear solitude and death and all kinds of other things, including thunder. They must have a light on at twilight.

Their tongue is usually dry, with just a slight coating, and the lips are also dry and they complain of it. They get a dry, short, hacking cough which sounds painful, but it is not so much pain as a feeling of weight in the chest which is very unpleasant for them, and it is always worse whenever they cough. They say it is more commonly right-sided although it can be either side. The pain is always over the affected area and can be quite distressing. They can get bright red sputum in the early stages, with a lot of distress on breathing in.

They do get a general aggravation lying on their left side, although they are more comfortable lying on the unaffected side. The Phosphorus patient, as a rule, is another one who likes to be propped up. The typical position is with the head up and a little bit back on the pillow, and the chest cases nearly always take up that position. Occasionally they get pleurisy at the same time.

Pulsatilla

There is no reason why a virus infection should not need Pulsatilla. It is more in the late autumn or early spring, when you get Pulsatilla pneumonias, and they are the typical Pulsatilla patient, mild and gentle and yielding, and doing what you ask them to do.

Although Pulsatilla can look congested ordinarily, here there is an increase of their usual appearance. They get a marked general aggravation from heat, as in all Pulsatilla cases. They get a feeling of tightness and a hot rawness in the chest and are not at all well. They are worse at sunset and at night, and worse lying down – they want to be propped up a little, like Lycopodium, because they get respiratory embarrassment when lying down. They have marked air hunger. The few Pulsatilla pneumonias I have seen have all been apical, and severe.

They get a dry, teasing, irritating cough with sputum that is difficult to get up, and they usually get it up by gagging. They vomit much more often to get up the sputum than the normal case of a chest infection, and when the sputum comes up it is tough and yellow and blood-streaked, as a rule. It is rather like the typical Pulsatilla catarrh – one of the things that makes you think of Pulsatilla is the yellow colour of the sputum.

They get intense dryness of the mouth and like a bit of lemon to suck or something rather sour just to have by them. They drink very little, and a cold drink will bring on a spasm of coughing, so they avoid it. They get a lot of pain in the chest – a typical Pulsatilla pain that wanders from place to place. It can be quite sharp, and the patient may complain bitterly about it. They are better lying on the unaffected side. They have a white coating to the tongue, and often a rather unpleasant mouth, dry and hot. Even with their thirstlessness you think they must be thirsty with a mouth as dry as that, but they insist that they are not.

You have to remember to compare Pulsatilla with both Ipecacuanha and Antimonium Tart. Ipecacuanha has more nausea but they can all have rather similar gagging. All these patients are much worse if they are too hot, but I think it is really only the Pulsatilla patients who get this kind of effect with a viral pneumonia.

Rhus Toxicodendron
One does not often think of Rhus Tox. as an acute virus infection, but it can be very useful. There is nothing very typical in the Rhus Tox. acute appearance. The patient is very ill. They are distressed and restless and full of all kinds of fears. The extraordinary thing is that they get a marked relief from all their symptoms from moving about, even moving about in bed. They also have an unpleasant metallic taste, rather like the Mercurius patient. The taste is one of the things that puts you on to Rhus Tox., because you cannot fit them into

Mercurius. There is no sweating, they have no tremor and no twitching, but they have this relief from moving.

They have also a typical acute Rhus Tox. tongue. It is usually coated, with two red streaks down the sides, and has a fiery red tip. Sometimes you do not see much of the red streaks, but you do see the fiery red tip. Otherwise, the whole tongue is red and hot and sore, and rather unpleasant for the patient. They have an intense thirst for cold drinks. They get rapid, shallow, difficult breathing and stitching pain in the chest, anywhere. There is a septic element about their virus infection. They get a septic kind of sputum – not much, rather like the Mercurius but not offensive. This is one of the differences. They ache as much as any remedy, and they move because they get a certain amount of relief from it.

They have a nightly aggravation with a low type of delirium and extreme restlessness. With the delirium they have a queer delusion that they are either going to do important and strenuous mental work, or some very strenuous physical work. It may be that they feel tired because they move about so much.

Senega

The patient gets into a serious state of intense illness very quickly. In twelve hours they are in a desperate state. They cannot bear to be examined or percussed because they say percussing hurts them. Sometimes the chest wall can be swollen in the less muscular areas. They also have the most tough and gluey sputum of any remedy. It hangs about the back of the throat. They get it half way up and then they swallow it. They get it up and then it sticks to the teeth and the mouth and they cannot get it out. Senega is often needed in emphysema when the patient gets a cold or a bronchitis or a virus infection.

They are better for gentle moving in bed. On the other hand, movement brings about a spasm of coughing so it may not actually be worth it. They are very sensitive to cold air, and a paroxysm of coughing comes on immediately if they sit in any draught. It is surprising how much there is in the chest when you listen (the râles are all over the place). When it is unilateral it is more commonly right-sided than left, but in fact both lungs are generally affected together. When both are involved the patient is worse lying on the right side. They are drowsy and congested and certainly look a bit muddy. One has to remember the comparison with Mercurius and Baptisia, because they all share certain similar symptoms.

Sulphur

Sulphur can be badly needed, but in contrast to Senega, late in an attack. It is much more like Lycopodium, coming in after the third or fourth day. The patients are misleading in that they look collapsed and pale and chilly, and absolutely lack reaction. They feel stifled, as if they have a load on their chest, and are quite sure they are going to die. They want to keep perfectly still. It is easy to remember this when you think that they are the chronic of Bryonia. They do not want movement or disturbance or to be spoken to, and they just lie there with this muffled, collapsed, dusky appearance.

Sometimes they look dirty, as the Sulphur patient always can. They sweat a good deal – their sweat is general and there is nothing particular about it. They have a feeling of burning pain in the chest, and get waves of heat on the slightest exertion. If they have to exert themselves, even to be washed or sit up, they feel absolutely done in afterwards. They feel as if they are going to faint, and sometimes do so. They are worse after sleep, as with all Sulphur conditions, and they are very thirsty for large quantities of cold water.

Although these patients are generally cold and collapsed, when they need Sulphur for a virus infection they can get very hot hands and feet, even though the body is cold. They have patches of beginning resolution in the lungs, as a rule, because it comes so late in the attack, and possibly they are beginning to clear up. But they themselves are so collapsed and ill that they must have some other remedy, and Sulphur comes in very useful then. It is needed for a septic type which starts as an ordinary case which you think is going to clear up well, and you are quite satisfied for a day or two. You then find that it is not clearing up and the patient is very collapsed, and here it works to great effect.

43

Asthma

I divide the following series of cases into three groups: children's cases, adults with a family history and adults without a family history.

CHILDREN'S CASES

The first was seen by me at the age of seven and a half. She had a history of bronchitis since infancy and had developed asthma at the age of five. There was no family history but her grandmother had bronchitis and there was tuberculosis on the mother's side. There was a history of nettlerash in the patient at the age of two. Since she started asthma the attacks had been so severe that she had had to have injections of adrenalin. It was the child's dread of injections that made the parents try homoeopathy. The attacks of asthma started about midnight and got increasingly worse during the night. The child had an exhausted appearance with a dull bluish flush during the attack, and occasionally sweated over the chest and head, mostly on the chest. She had to be propped up with the head thrown back, as she felt she could not get enough breath, and was made definitely worse by even leaning over to the left. Her respirations were over 60 per minute and her temperature about 38.5°C. There was very little sputum at first and the chest was full of wheezing sounds, going on to bubbling râles and often crepitations at the left base as the attack subsided. She had an asthmatic-shaped chest.

Her nose and throat were investigated and she was tested for sensitiveness to eggs, dust and feathers, with negative results, and nothing in the way of food seemed to upset her. She was fond of meat and salt and was seldom thirsty. She always sneezed a great deal in the early morning. Generally she felt the heat and could not stand a hot room, but she was also sensitive to east winds. In herself she was a thin, pale, rather reserved child – silent and placid as a rule but apt to be irritable and restless when not well. She was started on Tuberculinum Bovinum 200c in October and seemed to improve on it up to the following February. In April the mother was given Spongia 6c to keep by her, for use if the child started wheezing at night. She then gave about six doses at two-hourly intervals and said that it frequently checked an attack.

The next year the child started badly and I saw her in three acute attacks. I had an autogenous vaccine made from her sputum and a nosode of the 30th potency prepared from it. The only use I found from that was that it checked a cold effectively. I then saw her in another bad attack in which she was struggling to get her breath and kept holding on to her chest at intervals, as though she felt it had no air in it. She complained of being too hot, and I gave Natrum Sulph. 6c every two hours. Why I had not given this before I cannot imagine, as she had always been a warm child with a desire for salt and more marked signs in the left lung, and her mentality fitted the remedy.

After two winters with almost complete relief, her nettlerash began to return and she was given Psorinum 30c. After that she had a threatening attack of asthma in October for which Natrum Sulph. was immediately given, and it did not develop. She was now able to be at school without a break for the first time in her life. Subsequently she had an episode of influenza with a temperature of 39.5°C for which she was given Gelsemium 10M. She was wheezy for two hours only and then had Natrum Sulph. with immediate relief.

The next case is a girl now fourteen and a half. I first saw her at the age of seven. She had a history of having had asthma for three years for which she had been attending hospital. She had large tonsils but owing to her chest condition, a persistent wheeze and a TB family history, operation was not advised until she was much older. The child was thin with dark hair, blue eyes, long lashes and a tendency to fine hair on the back. She stood with her shoulders hunched up, but there was no actual spinal deformity on examination. She was a chilly child but could not stand great heat either, rather scared and inclined to weep if she was looked at, and particularly frightened of what one was going to do to her. She was fairly easily cheered up if depressed.

She disliked fat but was not easily upset by food, and as far as I could ascertain it did not make the slightest difference to her asthma. She had a poor appetite as a rule.

The actual attack came on at any time, usually with a rise of temperature. It lasted at least twelve hours and left her with a wheezy chest and a good deal of phlegm. She had a yellowish nasal discharge also, and at the time was never fit to attend school.

She was given Tuberculinum Bovinum 200c to begin with, and at the end of a month seemed better in herself and was eating better. She had not had a bad attack of asthma, and if anything was less wheezy. She had one repeat of the remedy after six months and seemed definitely better. She then had a series of acute asthmatic attacks and was given Pulsatilla and Tuberculinum Bov. with some definite improvement, particularly from the latter, but she was never quite free from the wheeze. Two years later she seemed so much stronger in every way that she started school, but at least twice each term had to be away for a week or two at a time for attacks that were much milder but still a great handicap. In that autumn she seemed in every way so like a chilly Pulsatilla that she was given Thuja 10M and never had an attack of asthma since. The wheeze cleared up and the Thuja was not repeated.

Her subsequent history is interesting. She had one complaint left, which was persistent catarrh in the nose and throat and a tendency to tonsillitis. During the next two years she was given Mercury 10M for acute tonsillitis with rapid recovery from the acute symptoms, but the throat was so unhealthy that I sent her to see an ear, nose and throat surgeon. Tonsillectomy was advised and performed. Her catarrh steadily cleared, there was no sign of asthma and she seemed very well. A year later she complained of headache one Sunday afternoon and by evening her temperature was 40.5°C. She was given Gelsemium 10M. On the Monday her temperature was still the same, her headache was almost intolerable and she was developing marked photophobia. There were no other signs. The next day she developed slight neck retraction. She was admitted to hospital and given Glonoine 10M. This alleviated the headache slightly and gave a temporary slight fall of temperature but it went up to 40°C again at night and the next day Glonoine CM was given. Later she showed signs of a typical meningitis, but no lumbar puncture was done as we considered it would militate against the chance of recovery and the diagnosis was obvious. She wanted cold applications to her head and had a dull heavy purplish appearance, twitching of the limbs and an accentuation of her previous symptoms. She was given Sulphur 10M and very quickly showed a change. Her speech became temporarily clearer, and during the evening she demanded boiling hot applications to her head and became very chilly. Her temperature went up to 40.5°C and she was wandering. One day later she was given Psorinum 10M with an immediate drop in temperature and a rapid recovery. She had a slight relapse and 39°C temperature the following week. A 1M of Psorinum settled it finally. The three remedies which did her the most good were

Tuberculinum Bov., Thuja and Psorinum, and I often wonder whether she should not have had Psorinum from the beginning.

A third case is that of a boy aged nine. I saw him first at the age of six with an asthmatic family history and typical wheezing sounds all over his chest. He got definite attacks of asthma, always starting with a sudden onset actually during sleep. He would wake up in a sudden fright, distressed and choky, and he always dashed out of bed trying to get his breath. There was very little sputum.

He was a fat, pale, flabby child, with an almost emphysematous chest, easily frightened of everything and waking in terror even when free from attacks. I could not trace anything that started the asthma. I gave him Calc. Carb. 10M on his general symptoms and make-up and he improved very much in every way. His chest became clearer, he slept better and improved in colour but his asthmatic attacks remained just the same as before, although somewhat less frequent. In the autumn of the next year I gave him Sambucus 10M during one of his bad nightly attacks on its very typical history. He was quickly better and did not have another for nearly a year, then only a slight one, and the Sambucus was repeated. I examined his chest subsequently and there was not a trace of wheezing and he needed no further remedy.

Another boy, aged eight, had quite different symptoms. I first saw him at the age of four with a history of asthma following every cold and a great tendency to catch cold. He was a fair, pink-skinned little boy with blue eyes and long lashes. He had spots periodically but otherwise had a clear skin. His chest had the asthmatic shape that I associate with most of these children, apt to be thick through the upper part but with no deformity of the spine. He had a certain amount of wheeziness almost at any time, with definite sudden attacks of asthma, from no cause that could be traced, coming on about sunset, with marked dyspnoea, and going on into the night. After one of these bouts he would fall asleep towards morning and wake with his chest full of râles and a troublesome cough. The attacks were apt to be worse in the spring and summer. I gave him Pulsatilla 10M six times in close succession every four hours. He never needed any other remedy. The Pulsatilla was repeated at more and more infrequent intervals during the next two years.

In some children's cases I have found a disconcerting lack of symptoms to prescribe on, and in others such a contradiction of symptoms that it was not possible to perceive an indication for any particular remedy. Many of these were cleared up entirely and others helped in varying degrees by Natrum Sulph. 10M. One marked exception who did not respond to this was a child to whom I gave Phosphoric Acid 10M on her entire lack of interest in things. To my surprise, it cleared up her asthma entirely although I had only expected it to bring out symptoms to indicate more clearly her correct remedy.

ADULTS WITH A FAMILY HISTORY OF ASTHMA

These are the most difficult type to deal with because of the element of suggestibility which is so commonly present. I feel that members of this group, which really should also include cases of children in whom a family history is a prominent factor, need something in addition to the homoeopathic remedy, and that only with the correct remedy, a little extra patience, and the exercise of a good deal of common sense can they be put right. I am certain they can be cured whether the origin of their asthma is physical or psychological.

The first of these was a woman aged forty-three. She had a history of asthmatic attacks of many years duration and said that all her family on both sides were either wheezy or asthmatic. She had been de-sensitised in the previous year with no benefit at all. When I saw her she was always tight or full and distended in the chest, as she expressed it, and could never reckon on more than one good day in every four. A definite asthmatic attack was brought on from smoke, dust or being near a gas stove. She was not affected by fog or in any way by weather but was rather better for air generally. The attacks were worse in the early morning and lasted for a short time after rising, and left her feeling tight for the rest of the day. At other times she got an attack immediately on rising, which got increasingly worse until about 10 a.m., then gradually subsided, still leaving her tight. Often it was very difficult to get up the phlegm, and it was thick and stringy when it did come up. She was hoarse after the attacks and the cough became almost croupy in sound as it subsided.

She was nervous, particularly of thunder – nervous alone if not well, inclined to get fits of depression about her health, and then was always better left alone to get over it. Otherwise she was cheerful and good-tempered, She was small and thin and often inclined to look a little mottled and bluish in the cold. She nearly always felt rather bad on Sundays, but whether from the effect of extra cooking or having her husband at home was not divulged. Her appetite was variable and she was afraid of eating chocolates or fatty foods.

She had fine rhonchi all over her chest. She could not stand too much heat and had very poor circulation in her hands in the cold.

I tried to work out this case but it did not come through to anything definite. I muddled along until I gave Kali Sulph. 10M in spite of the patient's morning aggravation time. She was so very much like it in other ways and it covered the symptoms of her attack – the type of sputum and hoarseness after – better than anything else I could find. She was steadily better and only had one bout of asthma since that, following influenza and bronchitis. She was then greatly helped by Natrum Sulph. and Sulphur in finally clearing the influenzal bronchitis, but needed Kali Sulph. again to control the asthma. The worst she had thereafter was a return of the old tightness once every two or three months.

The next case was a brother of the last patient. I first saw him at the age of forty-one. There was the long asthmatic family history. His own history dated back six years, when he developed acute bronchial asthma after a chest cold. He became, from that time, very breathless. He was given an anticatarrhal vaccine two winters running, with no effect – in fact, he was rather worse the second year.

Since then he had been getting asthma with increasing severity. The attacks were always worse each weekend and were probably brought on by gardening. Food seemed to have no effect. He was very fond of salt, rather fond of sugar, and liked his food reasonably well flavoured. He was irritable, and better alone if depressed. He was rather nervous about his health and somewhat restless generally.

He felt the cold winds keenly but did not think that weather actually affected his chest. His attacks were worse in the early morning, often about 7 a.m., but quite frequently came on at night, starting between 10 p.m. and midnight, or after, and his wife said he had a sort of head tremor in his sleep until the attack woke him up properly. I gave him Arsenicum Alb. 10M. He had two attacks the following two weekends but thought they were more quickly over than usual.

The Arsenicum Alb. did not alter the frequency and the next attack was as bad as ever. I then found out that he wanted air in an attack but was never cyanosed. Also, that he got a good deal of flatulence which aggravated the attack and that it was preceded by offensive breath and a very unpleasant taste. He became quickly exhausted and inclined to sweat with his asthma. He was always hoarse and particularly chilly for days after the paroxysm. Sometimes he complained of irritation of the ears and wanted to bore them out. His cough gradually became moist with a fair amount of watery sputum as the attack went off.

I gave Carbo Veg. 10M. He was very much better afterwards and had no further attack until three months later, in spite of continuing his weekend gardening as usual. He then had another dose of Carbo Veg. 10M. I did not see him until a year later when he came just to have his chest checked, as he had been doing strenuous digging and was nervous that it might start up his asthma. I found his chest quite clear and gave only Sac. Lac. He said he considered his asthma cured and had had no sign of it for well over a year.

The nephew of this last patient and son of the previous one was starting the family asthma and was very scared. He had had two definite attacks when I saw him. On the symptoms I was able to extract, which were very few indeed, I gave Natrum Sulph. 10M. That was two and a half years ago and he has not had any further hint of the trouble.

ADULTS WITHOUT A FAMILY HISTORY OF ASTHMA

The first case was a woman of twenty-four. She was a typical asthmatic, nearly always short of breath, and her constant complaint was that she had a load on her chest with a paroxysmal cough. She was extremely sensitive to cold, and any draught was apt to bring on an attack. She had a dry wheeze all over the chest. She was never irritable but got frightened about her health and rather down during a bad bout of asthma. The attacks were unaffected by food but were aggravated by talking, and unless she was well she had a curious flat, toneless voice. She was thin and clear-skinned but always had a peculiar bluish-grey colour when at all breathless. She was fond of salt and was thirsty, but had no other definite food tastes. I gave her Phosphorus 30c and she was soon better. Her improvement continued and she was free from asthma for three years.

The following year she got wet and chilled and caught a cold, leading to bronchial asthma and an evening temperature. She was given Phosphorus 30c, with quick improvement, and came back the following week. I think then that she should have had a 200c of Phosphorus, but instead she was given Sulphur 200c and for weeks after I could do nothing at all for her. I mention this because I have had other cases of asthma where a dose of Sulphur seemed to check all improvement and prevent anything else from working for a time. I followed with Phosphorus, without the slightest benefit in this case, and she got so ill that I went to visit her at her home. She was sitting up in bed with obvious air hunger, unable to stand a hot room, and markedly cyanosed. She was at her worst from 8 p.m. to 10 p.m. She had no thirst in the very acute stage and her chest was full of bubbling râles, worse on the left side. She had quantities of stringy green sputum and was inclined to sweat from coughing.

I gave Kali Sulph. 10M repeatedly, with marked relief, but it did not hold. Two days later she complained of pain in the chest and was worse lying on the left side. She had the same stringy green sputum and began to feel sick. I gave Natrum Sulph. 10M and she seemed relieved for a few hours, but was then as bad as ever and started vomiting greenish fluid. I gave Ipecacuanha 10M, with very little effect. She was then admitted to hospital and given Drosera 10M. This instantly relieved the asthma. Her sickness cleared up and she began to eat again, but she was left with a severe paroxysmal cough. This remained much the same until she was given Phosphorus 10M. She then began to mend at once and has needed nothing else since.

The last case was a man, aged forty. He had a long history of asthma from boyhood but no family history. He was a thin, withered-looking person – irritable, full of fears and very chilly. In his attacks of asthma he had a raw feeling in the chest and a sensation of acute constriction. He described it as feeling as if the chest got tighter and tighter until he felt he would never get a breath. He was not cyanosed during the attack, nor very restless. His worst time was between 1 a.m. and 3 a.m. I felt pleased with this history. The man looked and sounded so like the typical Arsenicum patient, if only he had been more restless. In spite of this point I gave Arsenicum, with no effect.

Dr Borland described Cactus as very similar to Arsenic – almost as full of fears and having the exact sensation of tightness on the chest that the patient described, but without cyanosis, and said that this might be taken as a distinguishing feature from Arsenic. The Cactus patient is also more silent and much less restless than Arsenic, as he is made worse if he moves much. I gave this man Cactus with relief, and it was over a year before he came up for a repeat. He had been perfectly well between.

As a homoeopath I feel strongly that every case of asthma – whether there is a marked nervous element or not – is a potential cure.

44

Five Lesser-known Respiratory Remedies

Aesculus Hippocastanum

Aesculus has been described as a remedy for old men who live too well. They are fat, short-necked, red-faced, cyanotic types. They have a venous congestion all over and a great distress of all their symptoms immediately after a meal. They get muddle-headed and short of breath. They often get upset with a headache, with a sort of fullness and tension. This is worse when they have a bout of coughing, and worse from motion, and they are depressed and miserable to live with. They do not feel at all well and are rather peevish – you have a sort of sympathy with them and wish that they would do something about it and not think of themselves all day. They are worse in a stuffy room, and much better if they go into a draught of cold air. The cough is short and they say they have persistent stringy mucus in the upper chest.

Hydrastis

Hydrastis is for the old, broken-down, chronic bronchitic who tells you, 'I have started my bronchitis again. I know it is going to last for the next four months'. They often tell you that it is going to last longer than you think it will. They get a tremendous lot of thick ropey mucus, often rather yellow in colour and very profuse if they go out into the air. It almost stops when they are in the house, which is a very useful symptom. At the same time, their nose gets blocked. They are easily discouraged and always think, with their ropey phlegm and cough, that they are going to choke. The cough starts with a feeling of irritation. Very often when they are walking about, you can more or less hear them rattling. They also get a certain amount of pain in their arms and legs.

204

Kreosotum

Every year I have half a dozen cases wanting Kreosote. They have a cough which is nearly always due to bronchitis during teething, or due to bronchitis which accompanies a summer diarrhoea. They have typical blotchy, discoloured, red faces. I always remember a girl of twelve whom I always thought of as a most pretty little girl. She came in with a blotchy red face and I hardly recognised her. She had running from the eyes, her cheeks were quite sore where the tears ran down, she had cracked lips, her mouth was cracked at the edges and she looked a mess. She told me she got very easily worked up, with anything making her excited. When she felt worked up she was apt to weep, which made her excoriation much worse, and she pulsated all over for at least an hour after getting excited. The cough is always worse for hot drinks and better for cold drinks.

Another distinctive symptom is the subjective smell of tar, which I find in every patient to whom I have ever given Kreosote. They have a coated tongue, sometimes brown, and they are extremely sensitive to music. They feel unsafe with music because they cry copiously. Kent said that there are three things to be remembered about Kreosote. One is the excoriating discharges, and the second is the complaint of pulsations all over the body, when they get worked up and excited. The third – which I have never met – is profuse bleeding from small wounds.

Mucor, Aspergillus, Penicillinum

I treated a woman of seventy who complained of wheezing and coughing. She lived in the country and was very definite about the time of year, saying it always began in September and then was gone after Christmas. I thought it might be the moulds on the trees, and gave her a remedy called M.A.P., which is made from the three moulds that occur on trees in the autumn: Mucor, Aspergillus and Penicillinum. Within a few days it had done her a great deal of good.

Rumex Crispus

I find Rumex a useful remedy, especially in the autumn. You know the kind of patient who says, 'I have just had another virus. I had one in October and got on quite well, and now I have had another virus and feel worse than I felt all winter'. There is nothing particular about their facial appearance, except that they look miserable because of their barking, irritating, miserable cough. They tell you it comes from an irritation just below the larynx and that the rawness is much worse if they breathe cold air. In fact the cough is worse in any change of atmosphere. They also get copious catarrh. This comes away with a watery fluid which, as the cough goes on, becomes thick and ropey and difficult to remove.

They often complain bitterly about a cold east wind. Two patients had a violent attack of coughing in front of me and both of them put their blanket over their head while they coughed. This is a Rumex symptom. They are worse when they move about, are worse for coughing and they get often an intercurrent diarrhoea. They get some rheumatic complaints with it. Everything is worse from cold and worse from movement.

45

The Circulatory System

ACUTE CARDIAC FAILURE

There are three remedies that you ought to think of for acute congestive heart failure. These are Arsenicum Alb., Antimonium Tart. and Carbo Veg. They will see you through most of the acute heart failures with irregular palpitation, often violent and mostly at night.

Arsenicum Album and Antimonium Tartaricum

The patient wants to spring out of bed, and with this gets the terrible anxiety which is always found in the picture of Arsenicum. The Arsenicum patient nearly always complains of a great feeling of chest oppression and constriction round the chest, as well as all the Arsenicum general symptoms – the acute anxiety, sweating, restlessness, extreme pallor and great distress. As a rule they want incessant sips of water. It is an interesting point that Arsenicum will only pull up the patient – as a rule it will not see them through.

For many years, I looked after an old lady with an extremely bad heart. She used to get sudden collapses when she would become absolutely pallid and be scared stiff. Arsenicum was marvellous. Before I was out of the house she had got relief, and would then be able to go on for long phases. But the great thing about the Arsenicum was, unless it was followed up, usually with a 6c of Antimonium Tart., she would fall back within a week or two and send for me again, quite probably in the middle of the night, in a condition of extreme distress. The low potency to follow is not necessarily Antimonium Tart. I can remember another case distinctly where the second remedy was always Sulphur.

In Antimonium Tart., in its acute stage, there is not nearly so much sweating. Nor is there so much anxiety as in Arsenicum, and not nearly the same degree of distress. They do not look pale – they nearly always look rather dusky, with a sooty appearance round their nose, and rather sunken. Whereas Arsenicum patients want constant sips, Antimonium Tart. patients feel much worse after a drink and do not as a rule want to be offered one. They do not have the same feeling of awful constriction as in the Arsenicum, but are hopeless and miserable about their condition. Their hearts are so bad that it has a tendency to go on to oedema of the lungs with a very bubbly chest. Antimonium Tart. fingernails are often bluish, even though the patient may not have the dusky facial appearance. They are much worse in a stuffy room, although they never want to be fanned or have a stream of air blowing round them.

One marked characteristic is that they keep deadly still, in contrast to the Arsenicum patient who is always moving something. The old lady I referred to, in her Arsenicum acute stage, would sometimes spring out of bed even though she could hardly stand up. In her Antimonium Tart. stage she wanted to keep absolutely still – never moved. I give a high potency for an acute stage which could not be anything but Antimonium Tart.

A newly-qualified doctor once asked if I would come immediately to see a man who had just been admitted to one of the wards. When I got there he was the most horrible colour, dusky and sooty and absolutely still. They had offered him something to drink, which made him feel awful and thoroughly upset him. The young doctor thought he was dying. I agreed and said, 'Listen, the one thing that might save him is some Antimonium Tart. Give it very high and give it every quarter of an hour for the next two hours'. He was so miraculously better the next morning. This doctor gave Antimonium Tart. to everybody who was admitted for weeks – I had great trouble in making him think there was any other remedy you could possibly use.

Carbo Vegetabilis

The third acute remedy is Carbo Veg. The patient is completely worn out, mentally and physically. If you feel them, the whole surface of their body is cold and clammy – they are usually quite covered with sweat. However, if you feel their nose, you will be surprised how icy cold it is. They are characterised, when you first see them, by their acute air hunger. They are always better for having the windows wide open and plenty of air blowing on them.

I remember admitting a patient into hospital who had had six broken ribs and at the age of eighty-five insisting on being flown back from Italy because she wanted homoeopathic treatment and could not get it there. She was seen by our orthopaedic man who strapped her up and she got on very well, taking various homoeopathic remedies, mostly Arnica, and went home. Just at the end of the time she had a nurse, and when the nurse was out she thought, 'I am nearly well. It's absurd for me to wait for the nurse to come in to put on my dressing gown'. So she pulled herself into her dressing gown and collapsed, and when the nurse came in she sent for me hurriedly. I arrived to find the woman more or less dying, with practically no pulse, absolutely covered with cold sweat. I sent her to hospital in an ambulance, and when I arrived the orthopaedic consultant said, 'Brave old lady, it's a pity she is going to die'.

It was a bitterly cold day and she had all the windows open. She was an icicle to feel, and was lying with the door open and in a complete draught. I thought there was just a chance to pull her round, although I rather doubted it. I sat by her for an hour, giving her a teaspoonful of Carbo Veg. out of a jug, every five minutes. By that time her pulse was beginning to improve, her sweating was going off, and she was getting generally a little warmer.

She did live, to the age of ninety-three or four. She flew back to Italy again, and did everything she liked. She always carried Carbo Veg. because if she thought she was going to collapse and be absolutely worn out, or if she was beginning to sweat and her hands were icy cold, she would take a few doses of it.

CARDIAC FAILURE OF SLOW ONSET
Lachesis
Lachesis always has one quite constant symptom. In their heart condition they cannot stand any pressure at all and everything has to be loosened up. They cannot stand the bedclothes being too heavy, or having things around their neck, or their pyjamas tied tight round their waist or anything like that. They have a sense of great constriction in their chest and feel awful.

They also have various other symptoms. You can tell the Lachesis patient directly you see them because they are so purplish-coloured. They have purple lips, a rather mauvish face and bluish-red hands. They cannot stand the heat and they get a suffocating feeling after falling asleep, waking up with a cough that racks them. In heart things Lachesis always has a tremor. If you ask a Lachesis patient to put out his tongue, it trembles and so do his hands. They complain quite a lot of numbness in the left arm and hands, and are always worse lying on the left side. They also have the general symptom of Lachesis – the patient nearly always thinks his food is being poisoned or that somebody is trying to do him down or that there is something happening. They are very suspicious.

Laurocerasus

Here the patients are very blue, quite different from Lycopus which is pale. They have pains in the heart region and very often put their hands to the heart, as if it helped, and their heart is slow and very irregular. They are intensely breathless after the slightest exertion.

We had a patient for years with very marked emphysema, a very dilated hypertrophied heart, and not at all in a good condition. He used to go to the city by train and then had to walk five minutes to his office. When he arrived at his office, everyone thought he was going to die. When we first saw him, we took him to a heart specialist who X-rayed him. He said he was one of the worst emphysemas he had ever seen and thought he had a very short life ahead. We gave him Laurocerasus. He always took one tablet before he left home in the morning and another before he got out of the train, and he arrived really quite respectably at his office. The other remedy he took, which did him a lot of good, was Antimonium Tart., because he used to get a cough with a lot of bubbling phlegm. We took him back four years later to see the same heart man, who could not believe in the improvement that there was in his chest since he last saw him. He said that even his emphysema was better. He did very well and went on for years.

Lycopus Virginicus

This is rather an unusual remedy, but when you do want it you want it badly. It is always an irregular pulse. The patient is probably pale rather than cyanosed and will tend to have a cough with a sensation of throbbing in the head and in the neck. A positive symptom of Lycopus is an intense feeling of activity in the chest. The patient tells you their heart is beating to such an extent that they feel the whole chest is active. They are also worse when they lie on their right side, as a rule. The other marked symptom is a great desire for food and particularly for the smell of food.

Naja

Naja is much the same but has even more numbness, as well as marked stabbing pains through to the scapula. It also has a pronounced swelling of the hands. I never think of Naja unless the patient comes in with her hands very swollen. They have very few mental or general symptoms. You do not get any of the suspicion of the Lachesis. They have a certain amount of tremor.

ANGINA

Aconitum Napellus

Aconite will give enormous relief in a first attack of angina, especially if the patient is terrified, where they get such very bad pains and beg you to help. However, I have never found a case where Aconite is effective in a second attack. It just gives relief in the one first attack and then you must go on to something else.

Arsenicum Album

This remedy is for angina in a broken-down patient, with pain rather like in Cactus, with a tightening of the chest and a feeling of constriction – never quite the tight band round the chest, but pretty bad. They look waxy, distressed, wrinkled and restless. They are frightened and chilly and they always describe one thing in their angina, which is that their pains are burning, like all Arsenicum pains. The pain is sometimes referred to their neck and even into the occiput.

Cactus Grandiflorus

After the first attack, the greatest standby in an angina pain is Cactus. The patient is always afraid of death, not that they are going to die immediately, but that the condition is going to kill them. That is one of the things they tell you. They get a very tight sensation in the chest – always a sort of squeezing of the heart which travels laterally on both sides. It gets worse and worse and feels as if there is a tight band being screwed on to their chest, making it tighter and tighter. And they always feel, at that stage, especially if it goes on, that it will stop the heart beating at all. There are no radiating pains in Cactus. They suffer violently and are in great distress.

I always remember a patient aged seventy who came with a note from her doctor, saying that she had had one attack of angina and that there was the question of whether she had had a coronary. The doctor thought she had had an inferior infarct and that she would only live at most a year – but would I mind looking after her? As a matter of fact, she lived for twenty-two years. She had two more coronaries in that time and had nothing but homoeopathy. She used to ride her bike, and died at the age of ninety-two. She always carried with her a 200c of Cactus in liquid form. If she thought the pain was coming on and it began to get tight and squeezing throughout, she would produce her bottle of Cactus and put ten drops in her hand and lick them up. She always did this and thought it was wonderful.

She also used to take Latrodectus occasionally when she got a sort of chronic pain down her left arm, and she used to do well on Spigelia when she got attacks of palpitation. Constitutionally she was a Pulsatilla. I used to give her Pulsatilla 10M, sometimes, and she would go on for months.

Latrodectus is not often needed, but it has pain through to the left axilla.

Lilium Tigrinum
This remedy has a heart constriction rather like Cactus. The patients are terribly hot and badly want air. They are depressed, but not terrified. They are also far less afraid than any of the other anginas, but they are awful to nurse or look after! Instead of being terrified they are weak, unreasonable, intensely irritable and give their families or whoever is looking after them a bad time. Like Lilium Tig. generally, they think that everything depends on them and that they must be better soon, that the family cannot get on without them, and that they are certainly going to the workhouse very soon if they are not there to see to their financial affairs. Men very seldom need Lilium Tig. It really is a woman's remedy.

Spigelia
Spigelia has a typical stabbing pain in angina. It starts at the apex and goes through to the left shoulder and it will move down through the left arm. It is the only other one that has the same degree of numbness as Naja. If possible they always like to lie very much propped up and a little bit on the side. Any movement aggravates them, brings on the pain and makes it worse, and the pain itself is very much like the Naja pain.

Spongia Tosta
Spongia is another anginal drug which is very useful at times, with marked symptoms. The heart feels as if it is getting bigger and bigger, that it is swollen in the chest, spreading up to the neck. Both the patient and the neck get very congested – they get a severe pain in the chest with this feeling that it is getting larger and larger. They get a marked aggravation from lying down, and then quite choky with the pain. They are extremely chilly and any draught increases their pain.

They get a rather strange numbness, in that the numbness is only in

212

the fingers. It is never in the arm as in Naja and Spigelia. I find that nearly always the lower extremities too are numb, which does not happen in either Naja or Spigelia. If only one side is numb, whether hands or feet, it is always the left side.

APOPLEXY

The chief remedy is Opium.

Opium

The patient is characterised by a violent delirium or else by a sort of stupor. When they are delirious they have staring eyes, a bright red face, talk about all kinds of things, and constantly see masked figures standing at the end of the bed, or somebody crowding around the room – even when they are awake. In the other type, where they look intoxicated, they are absolutely stuporous. They lie, sometimes with their eyes open and usually with a very red face, just taking no notice of anyone.

One of the best cases I ever saw was in a man who had every kind of drastic illness in the twenty-two years I looked after him. There were six occasions on which he got something which was considered to be fatal. This was one of the occasions and it occurred at a time when he had to do a very great deal of extra work. He came to his wife one morning and said, 'I have got the most appalling headache'. She looked at him with alarm because his face was bright red, which it never normally was and he looked awfully ill, and while he was still talking to her he had to sit down. Before she could turn round he had become unconscious. She got a man in from outside and between them they carried him up to bed, where he remained unconscious, still with this very red face.

His wife telephoned to ask me to come, saying that she had also asked a consultant physician and the family doctor to be present as well. We all arrived at more or less the same moment. The specialist examined him very carefully and found his blood pressure to be 240/140. He said, 'I think he has had it. I don't find any actual sign of a stroke but he has obviously had a cerebral catastrophe and I think he won't live more than forty-eight hours'. He asked me what I would like to give him and I replied that he should first tell the nurse what kind of regime to follow for the night and I would then tell him what I would like to give him. So, he suggested a little jelly and fluid but did not prescribe any medicine.

I said I wanted to put a homoeopathic dose of Opium straight on to his tongue. To which he replied, 'How pleased my mother would be. She was such a great homoeopath'. Whereupon I put a dose of Opium 10M on his tongue. All three of us left at twenty past four, with the nurse having been given all the instructions. I left a bottle of Opium granules and asked her to put a dose on to his tongue every two hours. A little later the nurse was arranging everything for the night, and very busy, when suddenly a voice said from the bed 'What about dinner?' So he had his dinner, and got completely well. The local doctor, with whom I became very friendly, went in to see him every day. When he said, 'You are doing wonderfully, aren't you?, he got the reply, 'No thanks to you. Please don't take any credit for it'. That is the sort of thing you can do. He lived for another ten years.

Afterwards he described the pain. He said the pain in the head came on like a sort of pressure on the temples, so acute that he did not know what to do and could not have done any work or talk to people. All he could think of was to get into the house where he could lie down. With the onset of the attack he also had very contracted pupils. Prior to the attack he had had extreme constipation, although, as far as his wife remembered, he had never been constipated before. Only with great trouble could he get anything away from his bowels at all. And when he did it was only a series of black balls. It occurred to me that this fitted so perfectly with Opium, which is one of the most constipated remedies in homoeopathy. It is also characteristic that the patient does as a rule pass rather hard, small balls. He was all right again within a few days.

There is one other point which you find in the Opium patient, especially if they had their Opium and have got much better. If they are coming to a time when they perhaps need one repeat of the remedy, a few weeks later, they will complain that they feel as if dust had been shot into their eyes and was still there, and that they could not get rid of it. This man had just that problem. At first, when he was getting better, he also had very drooping eyelids, which Opium has too, but that went off quite soon. He complained of the dust for some weeks and it never quite cleared. I then gave him a second dose of Opium 10M, after which it cleared up entirely.

46

Some Diarrhoea Remedies

There are many remedies for diarrhoea. The ones below are an ABC of some of them.

Aconitum Napellus

Aconite is not used very often but you do need it for diarrhoea resulting from exposure to cold and chill, from fright, and occasionally from overheating in the summer. The patients get a great deal of sweat, especially when they are covered up, very often with nausea and vomiting, mucus vomiting to begin with going on to bile, and a horrible taste in the mouth. As well as that they get abdominal distension and tenderness with a dry tongue, frequent small and intensely green stools, with some tenesmus before and during stool, and mucus and blood if it goes on. They are very much relieved after an action, although their stomach symptoms persist.

Aethusa Cynapium

This is an invaluable remedy for summertime diarrhoea from excessive heat, predominantly in babies under eight months. Sometimes it comes during teething in a hot summer, sometimes from overfeeding, and the onset is sudden. There may be diarrhoea alone but there is often some meningismus with it. They look really ill – pale and collapsed – and they get dusky and twitching and rather frightening in appearance. There is no thirst. It goes on to intense sickness and complete intolerance of milk unless you stop it in the first stage. You then get a white glairy, frothy mucus being vomited, often so violent that it is followed by prostration. Now the stool is often green mucus, nothing else, and goes on losing its green colour until it is just mucus alone. If it goes on longer it becomes blood-stained.

Aloes

Aloes is a remedy which is often left out at times when thinking round the acute diarrhoea remedies. It comes on in hot weather as a rule, or sometimes from sitting out in the chill of the evening during a hot summer. In adults it can be due to food poisoning. Occasionally it can be due to too much beer on a hot evening. (It is useful to remember that you can get a real Kali Bich. diarrhoea from beer.) Aloes symptoms can also be caused by anger. In appearance they are rather like the Sulphur patient, and they are worse for heat and much better if they are cool or cold. They have a hot, dry, dusky skin with intense heat and irritation of the feet, often worse in the very early morning. They are irritable and hate to be disturbed.

They have an intense red tip to the tongue (the other remedy which has that is Veratrum Alb.). The Aloes tongue is red, dry with thirst, and they complain of a bitter taste in the mouth. There is a lot of abdominal distension, with gurgling and flatulence, and quite often very marked tenderness in the liver region. They get a central colic which is worse for further bowel action. Their diarrhoea comes on after moving or eating, and the pain is worse if they move. The Aloes patient gets a lot of pain on passing water, which is useful to remember. (The other remedy that has diarrhoea and pain on passing water is Muriatic Acid.)

Aloes has a rather mixed yellow stool which is streaked with green or mucus, sometimes involuntary, with an enormous amount of flatus. Frequently the patient thinks the bowels are going to act, but there is a tremendous amount of hot flatus without any bowel action at all. They get tenesmus before and during an action. The diarrhoea is so explosive and bad that it can give rise to an acute attack of piles, leaving much soreness from excoriation around the rectum. Aloes (and Phosphorus too) lie with their legs wide apart to avoid pressing them together because it is so sore round the rectum. They are better for cold applications, and worse for any kind of ointment that may be applied.

Antimonium Crudum
This is a rare remedy which may be overlooked in diarrhoea. It comes either in hot weather or from chill, often from bathing in cold sea water or else from excessively cold drinks in hot weather. Although both these are Arsenicum Alb. symptoms they do not apply, because in all other respects the patient looks like Calc. Carb. They are pale and flabby, and mentally not at all unlike Calc. Carb. – depressed, useless. Even small children do not play when you expect them to – they just sit about. They are entirely thirstless and they have a thickly-coated tongue, generally white. They also have a terrible

tendency to snuffles; in fact it is the snuffles and the cracks around the nose which provide the clues to Antimonium Crudum.

The vomiting is just as marked as the diarrhoea, violent and bitter and worse for any food or drink. The patient's intense nausea is not made any better by the vomiting. The bouts of diarrhoea are often accompanied with a degree of prolapse. (The other remedies which have prolapse after diarrhoea are Pulsatilla, Phosphoric Acid and Podophyllum.)

Antimonium Crudum can get any type of stool but it is always profuse and offensive, with an intense cutting pain in the abdomen before stool. They are extremely exhausted after stool and have a lot of tenesmus which hangs on for some time and makes them feel very miserable.

Apis Mellifica

Apis is always a hot weather remedy in all its complaints. The skin is dry and hot, the patient is mentally fagged, their attention wanders when they are giving you their history, their speech is rather thick and it is altogether difficult to get hold of their history. They have a dry mouth, the tongue is red and shiny and they are thirstless, even though the tongue does not look as if they should be thirstless. They are irritable, often very restless, and they have some vomiting of bile. If it persists at all they get a puffiness – blue and slightly puffy hands. They get intense abdominal pain with their diarrhoea, and the abdomen is distended and so tender that they cannot strain at stool. As a rule they lie with their knees drawn up. They are worse from motion, worse for any kind of warmth, like all Apis complaints, and worse in the morning. They describe the stool as large, formed and hot, starting yellow and becoming green, and then streaked with mucus or slime. It is also painless. Occasionally it is large and watery, and sometimes offensive.

Argentum Nitricum

Argentum Nit. diarrhoea usually arises in children who have been recently weaned, or it may just be due to pure funk. If it comes on in hot weather the patient is chilly during the actual diarrhoea, although still craving fresh air. The patients are thin and wrinkled, looking rather like Arsenicum Alb., and they have a great tendency to chronic conjunctivitis. They have a dry mouth and dry lips, sometimes with stringy mucus in the mouth which they cannot get rid of, and which hangs down rather as in Kali Bich. They are weak and tremulous and may stagger about or sway. If they are children they may be unable to sit on your knee, but sway as if they are going to fall off. They have a lot of flatulence with marked eructations, but no relief. Their diarrhoea is always made worse if they drink. They often get intense nausea with the diarrhoea, but not vomiting, and they have a general abdominal tenderness which is better for pressure. The stool is green mucus with very little faecal material in it at all. It is accompanied by a quantity of offensive flatus, occasionally by a cast of the rectum, or else the stool is blood-stained mucous diarrhoea, and painless. You get a little colic beforehand but no urge to stool.

Arsenicum Album

This diarrhoea arises from chill or very cold drinks. It comes on in children during teething or sometimes from excessive eating of fruit. In adults it comes on either from food poisoning, alcohol or malted liquors. It will not work unless the patient has the Arsenicum make-up – the wrinkled, frightened appearance, the restlessness and all the fears. The remedy is characterised by great prostration which is worse from any exertion. This is particularly marked from the diarrhoea. It is worse in the early morning and early afternoon and the lips are dry and cracked, or they can be pale or bluish-black with a tendency to bleed – the lips can look horrible in an Arsenicum patient. They are intensely thirsty for sips of water – they never take a long drink but want constant sips. They are inclined to vomit after food or drink – the vomit is burning like all Arsenicum complaints and can be anything from mucus to blood, and they get this diarrhoea after food and drink.

They get prostrated after having their bowels open and perspire profusely. The stool is generally offensive, although not if it is just mucus. It can be any colour and is fluid and watery as a rule. It is usually scanty and frequent. There is redness and excoriation around the anus, which you would expect with the Arsenic make-up and all the symptoms. There is also a certain amount of colic before the bowels act and a burning pain in the rectum during and after. They are chilly while they are having diarrhoea.

Capsicum

Capsicum children are homesick. They never want to be sent away, and if they are, they develop diarrhoea, even some weeks after. They resemble a Calc. Carb. in appearance, but the Capsicum child nearly always has a bright red face, puffy lips which tend to crack, and with the diarrhoea nearly always has difficulty in passing water. The stool is fairly frequent, small, dark, slimy and with some mucus, and a certain amount of colic and flatulence beforehand. If the patient gets thirsty they have severe tenesmus – if they are not thirsty they do not have it so much. And because of the tenesmus after stool one is apt to give them either Mercurius or Nux Vomica, which does not do them half as much good as one dose of Capsicum would have done.

47

Urinary Tract Infections

The remedies described in this chapter are all of great value in treating kidney and bladder complaints. They also have important constitutional symptoms which need to be considered at the same time.

Berberis

Berberis is a most important remedy. It is difficult to give a mental picture of the patient. They change and alter and can be anything. But they do have a certain amount of mental dejection over their complaints, and will often tell you that this makes it difficult for them to think. They have an aggravation period from about 4 p.m. until they go to sleep at night, whenever that may be. Another strange symptom is that, in twilight, dogs and people in the street look much larger than they really are. They will also often tell you, 'I have a most unpleasant feeling towards evening, as if my head is becoming larger'. They get quite severe pain in the head, in no particular place – now here, now there – and carrying with it a peculiar cold sensation in the right side of the head. One other constant head symptom is the feeling that they are wearing a cap.

Berberis patients are contradictory. They are chilly in the morning and complain about it, and describe a sort of creeping chilliness which goes all over them. Then, in the afternoon, they get too hot and complain equally about the heat. They sweat extremely easily on exertion. After midnight, they nearly all sweat.

Many remedies for the kidney and bladder also have a marked gouty diathesis – all sorts of queer pains, and very useful it is in some of these. They usually also get a troublesome dry nose with little discharge. In the middle of giving you a kidney history they can suddenly tell you that their nose is uncomfortable and they would like you to do something about it.

They present with a sickly expression and dry lips, but there is otherwise nothing very constant about their appearance. Their mouth is dry and sticky and has a kind of frothy saliva which looks like cotton wool or, more often, a sticky saliva that looks like soapsuds. This is a great indication for Berberis.

They have typical pains. It is quite common for a patient to tell you that they have an awful pain just under their right costal margin. They point to it and say it is acute here. 'Does it move at all?', 'Oh yes – it radiates either through to the back or down the front'. Whether they have kidney or bladder trouble, or gouty trouble, the pains start in one spot and radiate. They can wander about but always come back to that one spot.

A few years ago I saw three patients all in the same month. They gave a history of pain in the kidney region which was intolerable to pressure and which radiated down to the upper aspect of the sacrum, and thereafter to the front of the upper leg. They felt very ill. I referred two of them to a kidney specialist for an opinion. He diagnosed them as having renal stones and suggested that I give them an antispasmodic for the pain spasm. I said I would do this only if my homoeopathic treatment did not relieve the pain, to which he agreed. The first patient responded well after being given Berberis. The second patient, who was the worse of the two, was also given Berberis and responded well after passing a minute renal stone. She got quite well and never had another stone. I then saw a man with the same trouble who had been seen by the same specialist, who suggested that I may wish to use my 'homoeopathic stuff' rather than his antispasmodic. This I did with equally satisfactory results. Two little stones were produced. He made a complete recovery.

Renal stones of small diameter, and hence capable of passing down the ureter, are often extruded into the bladder after Berberis is used. Given in 30c potency every four hours for relief of pain it is a very effective remedy.

Especially with kidney problems, Berberis patients often get a constant desire to have their bowels open. The stools are characteristically burning and light in colour, and rather sticky. They get sticking, digging pains in one kidney, worse on pressure. These pulsate or 'tear' after rising in the morning, and radiate somewhere. The whole back gets affected. If they stoop they very often cannot get up again. As a rule they have a better spell in the afternoon. They often get burning pain in the bladder, too, which also radiates, and pain into the ureter, especially from the left kidney. There is a burning in the urethra, especially in female patients, worse during and after urinating, and lasting quite a long time. The urine is pale yellow, with a transparent gelatinous sediment which floats about. On the other hand, you can

221

get a clay-like, mucous substance which settles at the bottom. I have also seen a sort of mealy white sediment in Berberis patients.

There are various symptoms that go with their kidney trouble. There is often a puffy swelling of the left spermatic cord, worse on walking, and also a drawing and burning on sitting, with pain radiating into the testicles – now one side, now the other. In the female there is a sensation of burning and soreness in the vagina, which can be very sensitive and cause great discomfort.

One thinks of Berberis as just a kidney remedy, or a bladder remedy, and it is too easy to forget its odd pains – these are very important and are sometimes the symptoms you prescribe on. You get a lot of stitching and shooting pain in the neck and back. They complain of coldness round their shoulders, just at the top of their back, in the neck. They point to all these regions and tell you what the pains are like. Sometimes they get stiffness in the back which radiates round to the abdomen. Even without any kidney troubles they get a certain amount of pain in the loins and kidney regions which runs across the back, and occasionally down into the pelvis and thighs, and even down to the calves. They can be stiff and almost lame with this.

Then you get odd pains in different special spots – for example, a kind of paralytic pain in the shoulder where you cannot lift the shoulder, with a weakness and paralytic feeling in the arms and legs. There can also be a heaviness after the pain, sometimes lasting for days, and this is where you get the gouty complaints. You get things like pain in the right knee, moving down to the ankle and into the foot. Often the legs feel heavy. They have to drag them round, and when they walk have a sensation as if their legs were not moving freely. Most Berberis pains are worse for rest. They are better if the patient is standing or walking about. The pains have this tendency to choose one toe or, say, one joint or one small part.

On the whole, Berberis has less skin complaints than kidney and bladder complaints, but it does have them and they are very useful to confirm that this is the right remedy. These are single, sticky, red pimples anywhere on the skin which come up and look quite angry. As a rule they are single, although they can also be in groups.

Cantharis

Cantharis is the follow-up to the bladder symptoms of Causticum. This is a wonderful remedy for kidney and bladder complaints, with rather more serious infection than even a bad cystitis. A typical Cantharis patient is characterised by burning inflammation, which gets rapidly worse. It is no good ignoring the patient – they want something done, and done quickly. When they are ill like this they are very peculiar. They have extreme anxiety with any acute condition. They may scream or lose consciousness. They may be extremely peevish. They have a definite afternoon aggravation, very often with a delirious, semi-violent state at this point.

Cantharis patients do not look happy – as a rule they look as if they are suffering intensely. They have a disgust for food and often an urgent unquenchable thirst. They may bring up masses of frothy mucus.

They get a lot of distension and burning and tend to get diarrhoea. Their chief bladder symptoms are cutting, contracting pains in the kidney region, with an urge to urinate, and a history of it getting worse and worse. As a rule the kidney area itself is quite tender to touch. You get an irritation of all the urinary organs and constant, violent pains in the bladder, with tenesmus. Only a few drops pass at a time. Patients have to go constantly but feel they cannot empty their bladder properly. They often pass bright blood and get this burning, cutting pain through the whole of the urethra into the bladder before, during, and after micturition.

A woman came to see me with a temperature of 39.5°C. She had a rash on her hand, with blisters coming up, and looked so ill that I took her into hospital. Never in my life have I heard anyone who could sing so many vulgar songs or use such frightful language. It is characteristic of the Cantharis patient. You will meet it quite often in a person who really needs this remedy. She had an awful rash which spread all over her hands, which became quite swollen. It did not exactly crack, but it oozed matter from everywhere under the skin. Tests were carried out on it and all sorts of different germs were found. It then began to spread and she got it round her eye and on her face. I gave her some Cantharis, with instant effect, but the point is that she then said, 'I believe that this medicine is going to be what I need for my bladder'. Not having thought of her bladder I asked her what was wrong with it. 'I always have some kind of infection going on and when I go on long journeys it hurts intensely to try and pass water and I suffer misery. Sometimes I can't pass it at all, but sometimes I could scream with the pain I get right down to the opening of the bladder.' She now travels as often as she wants to, but always carries a 10M of Cantharis with her. At the same time as she needed Cantharis, with this rash on her hand, her hair began to fall out excessively. I thought she would lose it all but this problem also cleared after the Cantharis.

223

The other thing about Cantharis is that it is one of the great skin remedies. It is a remedy for erysipelas. When you get these horrible patches of erysipelas with blisters and little vesicles and a high temperature, and the patient feels very ill, Cantharis can completely clear it up. It is also the best remedy in the world for burns.

Causticum
Kent described Causticum as full of contractures of muscles and tendons, but not quite so full of contractures as Cuprum. It can have a very definite picture. The patient is melancholy with a lot of anxiety, especially before sleep, even in children, who may not be able to get to sleep. Their moodiness is tiring and they are often quite unfit for the next day's work. On the whole they are peevish and disinclined to work. They can be persistently silent and just sit and not speak to anyone, and not even answer questions. They can also be inattentive. If you are telling them something which they are not interested in, their attention wanders away in the middle.

Causticum is also one of the great vertigo drugs. When the patients feel giddy they are inclined either to fall forwards or sideways, but never backwards. The Causticum giddiness is much worse in bed. Directly they lie down they feel giddy, and they think they will be better if they sit up. However, they are no better if they do sit up and so they go on being giddy. If often comes with a period and is worse from stooping. It may go off in the afternoon and the patient can be quite free from it.

The Causticum patient nearly always has some kind of eye symptoms. Either it is dryness in the morning, which is very common – with weakness of the eyes and stiffness, burning and stinging and some photophobia – or they feel a pressure of the eyes as if there were sand in them. It is most uncomfortable and they cannot bear to touch them. There is also itching in the eyes, particularly sometimes in the lids, and twitching of the eyelids, and they suffer from the typical Causticum inclination to close the eyes. If you look at the patient they have a disinclination to open the eyes, almost as if they will not open and something is keeping them shut.

They get intense lacrimation – always worse in the open air and, sometimes, in a fairly cold room. They blink and get flickers before the eyes and are constantly brushing away tears.

They also get a certain amount of deafness – Causticum can be very good for a case of deafness, nearly always because of damage to the auditory nerve, and it will help enormously.

Causticum is the most useful of all the urinary remedies so long as the patient has some of its acute sensitiveness to cold. It is certainly the most useful of all the plain cystitis remedies. When it gets a bit more complicated, or is a pyelitis, you will want some other things. The patient tells you they get a great urgency to pass water without being able to pass anything at all, and then they may be sitting about or talking to somebody and have an involuntary passage of water about a quarter of an hour later. That is a common symptom. They also get involuntary micturition on coughing or sneezing, or doing anything strenuous, and involuntary dribbling. It is also quite the best remedy for paralysis after an operation when the patient cannot pass water. There are other remedies, such as Staphisagria, but on the whole I find Causticum the most useful here. They also have a funny symptom which occurs quite often, which is a shooting pain in the rectum when they try to pass water and find they cannot. The urine can be quite dark brown and the cystitis can be accompanied by leucorrhoea.

Causticums have a lot of hoarseness, cough and sore throats, and if they talk much or try to sing or anything like that, the cough is apt to come on badly. They feel as if there is a raw lining to their larynx, so they cough and cough and try to bring up stuff – they bring it so far and then have to swallow it. It can be very useful when this arises in flu. They nearly always lose their voices and get very breathless when they are walking fast or taking too much exertion. There is more rattling in the chest than you would expect, with phlegm that will not come up.

Causticum patients have a lot of problems with their jaws and mouths. I remember having a girl with a rather bad tooth, but the thing that really gave her trouble was that she could not open her jaw in the mornings. She got quite a lot of pain in it and the pain went up to the ear, and she felt as if her teeth were too long and that they interfered with her eating. You can get a lot of shooting pain in the teeth from exposure to a cold wind. After many years experience, I think it is the best remedy of all for a facial paralysis. It is also a great remedy for a stiff neck. The patient who rides in a car on a cold day with the window open, and comes in with a stiff neck, will nine times out of ten respond to Causticum. Remember one other thing about Causticum – they are better in the rain. They cannot bear dry, cold weather.

They are very restless. At night they cannot get into a quiet position and they get up and move about. Causticum was one of the chorea remedies, and the restlessness in bed was one of the symptoms on which one gave it. They have a tendency to pimples, especially to warts on the nose. They are not big warts and they are usually quite white, but they are there and often make the patient think he must do something about it.

Clematis Erecta

Clematis has only been partially proved. It is characterised by two signs – eruptions and urinary symptoms. How often these two things go together. There is one strong mental symptom which makes me give Clematis if I see it – they cannot bear being alone. (They almost equally dread having company, so where are you? It is very difficult, but this is what they tell you.) They are irritable, angry, rather fretful, and hate to admit that they dread to be alone. If they have to be alone for very long this mood is followed by great apprehension – sometimes a lot of weeping, homesickness and trembling of the whole body, and they weep until they are exhausted.

You seldom see a Clematis patient without some sort of eruption. The most common one is severe small, itching crusts in the scalp. They are quite upset by this because they cannot get rid of it. You sometimes get vesicles and ulcers in the skin, but the most common place for a Clematis rash is the scalp. As a rule the rash is fairly dry although they can be moist. There is another curious symptom – a pustular rash round the loins. It is tender to touch. They are ashamed of this rash because it looks horrible and will not show it to you, if possible, but they may do so because they are rather worried about it. They have small spots in the face and elsewhere, which may possibly suppurate.

They also have toothache. It is very satisfactory when toothache is relieved by homoeopathy, and Clematis is one of the remedies that help. It is the type of toothache that is quite unbearable on lying down at night. It is all right in the day but at night it is awful. One strange thing is that these patients either draw in cold air, as cold as they can find it, or they drink very cold water, both of which you would think would increase their toothache. There is one other odd thing – they get swelling of the inguinal glands very often and these become sensitive while they are walking. These are also worse in bed.

Clematis patients have definite urinary symptoms. At the beginning of urination they get a burning sensation, and they tell you that the pain sticks in the urethra for quite a long time after they have passed water. The other complaint they make is that they feel there is constriction in the urethra and the flow is very slow, and for that reason they cannot get their bladder quite emptied.

I do not know a bladder or kidney remedy that has not got some kind of skin eruption among its symptoms. Not always very bad, but it is rare to get none.

Sabal Serrulata

As a general rule one uses this remedy chiefly for any stage of enlarged prostate – and it can be extremely useful. They get funny, unusual feelings – they tell you they are confused and that they cannot remember anything, and say they get quite annoyed unless people leave them alone so that they can think out what they want to do. You often find the reason is that the patient's mind is simply concentrated on his complaint. They tell their families that they had better go away and die alone – very depressed and down. They get pain and aching in the head, going into both temples – usually worse on the right side – and a lot of vertigo with the headache. Often they give you the wonderful symptom that the pain starts at the root of the nose and goes up into the head – or that the pain is in the base of the brain and runs down to the mid-cervical region. It takes rather a definite route.

They have various, quite individual, urinary symptoms. They get a painful urination, which in girls and women is connected with ovarian pain. They complain that the bladder feels too full, that when they start to urinate it is extremely painful and that they have a feeling there is a block in the meatus. Sometimes the water is absolutely scalding to the patient and they get a lot of smarting, lasting quite a time after it. They very often have to get up at night – it is a satisfactory thing when they come back and tell you that they used to get up three times or so and now never get up more than once, if that. One symptom that is complained of quite constantly is that the testicles are tightly drawn up and painful. They get despondent and irritable – they do not just dislike sympathy, they get furiously angry if anyone sympathises with them. Very often, with their enlarged prostate, they get constipation.

They nearly always sleep badly. They think there is some unknown danger ahead and would rather be awake to face it. You never can make out what it is but this symptom comes up again and again. If they sleep well their pains are definitely better. They do have skin eruptions – not so markedly perhaps as other remedies – either on the hands or on the face, sort of eczematous patches. There is nothing very definite about them except that you wonder why they have any skin eruption at all.

Sarsaparilla

Sarsaparilla is a bladder rather than a kidney remedy, again characterised by urinary complaints and skin troubles. The patients have no special appearance but they complain of a headache or throbbing in the sides of the head, often with a sinking sensation that is better at rest and worse for motion. Most of their symptoms are worse for walking, for motion, and much worse for going up and down stairs.

I think of Sarsaparilla if there is a rash on the eyelids, because I have found this so frequently. Often the base of the nose and the eyes are swollen as well. They usually complain about one nostril being stopped up and very uncomfortable. They look poorly and old-looking and wrinkled, and they nearly always have some sort of eruption on their face and forehead, which makes them look even worse. They get scabs on their face – the description in some of the old books is that it looks like crusted milk – which is exactly what it does look like.

They have poor appetites. Their food tastes bitter, or sometimes sweetish; at other times it tastes metallic, all of which they find equally unpleasant. They also have a sinking, empty feeling almost immediately after food, and a definite distension after a very little food. The Sarsaparilla patient is always better on a cold diet and worse for warm food.

If they are thirsty it is for water, which they drink a great deal. They pass very little water or they pass frequent pale urine. They get a lot of pressure and tenesmus in the bladder and sometimes pass a white, thick, turbid stream with a lot of mucus. Sometimes they want to urinate urgently and then find they cannot pass any. Often there is such burning during micturition that it almost stops it, and all they get is a discharge of a sort of elongated flakes and no proper urine at all. It can be turbid, like clay water, and quite often it may be red, or else you can get a lot of gravel. There is always a burning on passing water. Occasionally, when they cannot pass water because of the burning pain, they get a slight incontinence of urine which is worse in the day and worse when the urine is very highly coloured. In really bad cases you get scalding in the urethra. The white, turbid appearance of the urine should make you think of Sarsaparilla because, if you do hit it and it is indicated, it is a very quick-acting remedy.

Terebinthina

I was always told to remember three things about this remedy. First, the tongue – a typical, smooth, red, shiny tongue with no papillae showing at all. The second is an excessive tinkling in the ears. The third is drowsiness. Even in the middle of their pain, in the middle of giving their history, they can actually fall asleep. I like to feel that when I am going to give Terebinth, these three are all there.

They also look half-intoxicated. They are queer people, full of pressure in the head, and they have a fear of getting epilepsy, even when there is no possible reason in their family history for such a fear. They get a dull headache and sometimes have a feeling as if there is a tight band round the head, and their voice sounds unnatural to them. They get this tinkling in the ears, and will say quite often they cannot tell the direction from which a sound is coming. This is unusual, because if you do ear tests on them they are quite normal – it is the direction they cannot tell.

When they feel ill they are often hungry and thirsty, which surprises you. They get rather a tight feeling in the upper abdomen and chronic liver complaints. This is accompanied by distension and gurgling and a certain amount of tenderness in the upper abdomen, all of which are better if they move about. The pains, on the whole, go from left to right across the abdomen. They are nearly always constipated.

They have a queer symptom in that they get a sort of pressure on the kidneys when they are sitting down, which is relieved immediately if they move about. They often have a burning pain on passing water, and have a frequent desire to do so. They really do not get any peace – they go into a spasm on any attempt to urinate, and there is a diminished secretion of urine. Occasionally they can get a profuse flow of urine and then, often, a deposit of mucus. The urine is thick and muddy-looking with some haematuria – alternatively, at that stage they can get a lot of blood, very little urine, and constant dysuria.

They get a clammy sweat in bed at night. It is also said to be a good remedy for children who fly into passions without warning.

48

Rheumatism

I am more and more convinced that a constitutional remedy can work for the worst rheumatism. On the other hand, you may not always be able to find it. There are many patients who present with various symptoms of rheumatism in one or another part, to whom a local remedy may be given, with great help.

Aurum Metallicum
Aurum is a more useful remedy for rheumatism than many people realise, a rheumatism which jumps from joint to joint. It often occurs in the ankles and the feet, which are particularly painful. Patients inevitably say they cannot lie down with it, especially when they have it in any of the upper joints – they have to sit up in bed and usually have to bend forward. (If anyone told me this in a pneumonia I would think of Kali Carb., not Aurum.) They are bluish as a rule – the reason they cannot lie down is partly because they get so breathless. They are very despairing and nearly always tell you that they feel their heart beating and that it feels too rapid.

Cadmium Sulphuricum
I use this remedy for patients who are getting pains at the top of the spine. I am always surprised at how well it works, especially if they point to one particular part and they say that that is what hurts them.

Calcarea Carbonica
A man of about fifty refused conventional treatment for his very bad rheumatoid arthritis. Everywhere was affected, with the wrists, ankles and shoulders the worst. He was chilly, with cold, clammy hands and was apt to sweat a lot round the face and head. He said he felt awful in the cold. He had a great craving for eggs – if you asked him what he would like to eat, it was always some eggs or an egg dish. He lived in terror of what was going to happen to him, above all whether he was going to be able to carry on his work and keep his family. I gave him

Calc. Carb. 10M – he improved very quickly and in two months was able to go back to his job. About twelve years later he came back, because he was just starting to be threatened by his old trouble, which I find is a constant thing in rheumatism. They want a repeat of their constitutional remedy, in a high potency.

Calcarea Hypophosphorosa
Calc. Hypophos. is for hands, fingers and ankles which become very painful and which cannot be moved. It is effective if you can give it early in a patient whose pain is beginning in the base of the thumb or in the fingers.

Causticum
Causticum is a useful local remedy when somebody complains of having rheumatism in one part, particularly in the articulation of the jaw – the patient suddenly cannot move it. They may or may not have a stiff neck with it. They may even have a slight facial paralysis or tendency to facial paralysis if they have stood in a very cold wind. It is always a cold dry day that will have caused it, and they are better on a rainy day.

Drosera
Drosera is a remedy to remember when patients say, 'I've got pain all down my legs', 'I've got a pain right down my shinbone', 'I've got pain in all the bones in my arms' – a drawing, shooting pain which is a sort of stitching pain when it gets into the joints. I have found it more in ankles than in any other part. It starts in the shin, goes down into the ankle and stays there. The ankle feels as if it was dislocated when the patient tries to walk. These patients always complain that the bed is too hard – they cannot get comfortable and they cannot get their ankle into a good position because the bed is too hard. (Arnica is the other remedy where the patient complains that the bed is too hard.) They nearly always get severe night sweat all over, and yet they are shivering when they are at rest.

Dysenteriae Composita
One of the best cases I ever saw was a man who was wheeled into outpatients in a bath chair. He was completely invalided with the arthritic changes in most of the joints, and had not been able to move for a long time. During his interview he said, 'I don't know whether it has anything to do with it, but I have never been well since I had

dysentry at the age of sixteen'. I gave him one powder of Dys. Co. 30c and was very pleased because in a month he walked in on two sticks. He eventually walked in without any sticks at all and went back to his full work. He never had anything but the one dose of the remedy.

Ferrum Phosphoricum

As a rule Ferrum Phos. pains attack between the shoulder blades. The patient has to get up in the night and walk about to ease the pain because it hurts so much and they cannot get off to sleep again. (The other two remedies that get up in the night and walk about are Pulsatilla, which gets up every night because they are too hot or better for moving, and Rhus Tox.) Moving eases all three of these and they get back into bed and probably go straight to sleep.

Ferrum Phos. patients are cold and a bit irritable – nice people but certainly irritable. They do not like being touched, because it aches. In all their complaints, whether it is a pneumonia or a bad cough or the end of a flu, or rheumatism, they have a singularly uncoated tongue.

Medorrhinum

Medorrhinum has definite and unambiguous modalities. Somebody wakes up in the morning, or comes in from being out of doors and getting chilled, and finds by that evening that they have pains in several joints. Although the pain starts in several joints, it settles in only one, and this is the key that your remedy is Medorrhinum. It settles in one point with severe pain which is worse on movement, most often in the knee, ankle or wrist. At this stage the patient will also have a certain degree of sciatic pain, and the pain goes down their legs to the ball of the foot. If the patient says they have pain in the ball of the foot I always think of Medorrhinum. It is another of the remedies where patients stick their feet out of bed (like Sulphur and Pulsatilla).

Natrum Phosphoricum

The pain is often lumbar, with heaviness and weakness in the arms, always worse in the right wrist or right elbow and sometimes shooting in the neck over the right shoulder. If the pain is in the wrist, it will characteristically move into the palm of the hand or into the fingers. If the patient gets this right-sided rheumatism it is often in their writing hand and they cannot write. Their right elbow is also apt to get very bad. They are depressed and worried about this and think that they are soon going to be chronic invalids.

Natrum Sulphuricum

Natrum Sulph. has stiffness, mostly on the outer side of the left leg and left forearm. It is a sort of compression, as if there was a tight band round the left elbow. The patient may complain of his left elbow being very painful, as if somebody was boring into it all the time.

Nux Vomica

Nux Vomica is a great rheumatic remedy and very similar to Causticum. The patients are chilly, and in the rheumatic line they are most apt to get lumbago, coming on from cold. They get acute spasmodic pain and are usually annoyed because they have to sit up in the night in order to turn over. They are worse for motion and dread it. They dread it quite as much as the Bryonia patient, except that Nux is a very chilly person. They are worse for draught and worse for cold. They are better for warmth and hot drinks. A Nux Vomica patient will tell you how very much better their lumbago is for a good hot drink – it is rather a good tip. They are worse in dry weather, especially dry cold weather – Nux Vomica likes rain.

Pulsatilla

This is well known for rheumatism, and if it is the patient's constitutional remedy it can clear them up completely. The Pulsatilla I mention here is the Pulsatilla for single joints, particularly the knee joint. The patient is much worse for a hot bath, although anything hot, even sitting in a warm room, is likely to be unbearable. They may say they have to get up at least twice every night to walk round in order to be able to get off to sleep again. Here I would give three doses only of Pulsatilla 10M.

Radium Bromatum

I use this remedy at least once a week in the winter for patients who have a consistent pain in their backs. Rhus. Tox. would probably relieve then in an acute stage, but they still get spine pain in the lower part of their backs, coming along to one or both hips and not relieved by pressure or heat, and the desperate chronic pain goes on and is a great worry to them. This is one of the occasions where I use Radium Brom. 10M once a week for about six weeks.

Rhododendron

Rhododendron is similar, but with certain differences. I always find that it is needed for an unexpected cold spell in early summer when the flowers are out. A cold, windy, rainy beginning of June is the kind of weather that brings on the complaints that respond to Rhododendron. The pain shifts about all the time, even more than in Rhus Tox. In Rhododendron, the pains are inclined to go from above downwards. If they are in the shoulder, the next day they are in the ribs or hands; or they are in the legs and the next day they are down in the feet.

Rhus Toxicodendron

Rhus Tox. is one of the most common of these remedies, and is for a cold, wet-weather rheumatism. The patient has a tearing sensation round the joints, or even in the joints, and is very restless. The pains move from joint to joint and are worse when the patient first moves but definitely better when they get going, especially if they can continue to keep busy. They are often better for warm, dry applications – they like a nice hot pad put on their back.

Sanguinaria

Sanguinaria is a great shoulder remedy. I have not given it often for anything but shoulders, usually the right shoulder rather than the left.

Thuja

Thuja is another knee remedy. You can get a patient with rheumatism in just one knee. The remedy has marked characteristics – you get profuse sweating on the uncovered part. If the patient happens to sleep with one arm out of bed, it is soaking wet. All round their neck it is wet. Their feet can be wet. Sometimes the sweat is oily and offensive.

I use the following six remedies for children.

Aconitum Napellus

A child may come in with a violent shrieking pain somewhere, perhaps after standing out in a cold dry wind or getting chilled. They have a very restless night and feel miserable. Many of these cases that come on suddenly and are bad with restlessness clear up with a few doses of Aconite.

Actea Racemosa

Actea Racemosa, also known as Cimicifuga, is a less common but very useful remedy. The child has an acute crick and pain in the neck, due

234

to standing in the cold. They cannot turn the head. It always comes on in wet, cold weather. A curious thing is that the patient will tell you that if they get pain in one shoulder they get pain in the opposite knee, and this is a good symptom for Actea. Pain on opposite sides of the body: one shoulder and the opposite knee, one knee and the opposite ankle, even one side of the neck and the shoulder on the other side.

Aluminium Oxide

I find Alumina useful for a child who complains of pains in the shoulder blades, or pains in one shoulder – no particular cause, but quite bad pains which everybody thinks are rheumatism. In these circumstances it is also prudent to ensure that the patient's food is not cooked in aluminium utensils.

Bryonia

There is another type of child who gets one very stiff joint. I remember one girl getting a very stiff shoulder. It became red and swollen, and she was unable to put it up very far without acute pain. All she wanted to do was prop it up on the table and sit quite still. She was irritable if people talked to her or even asked her what her shoulder was like, and she also had an extremely white-coated tongue. On that I gave her about eight doses of Bryonia, only a 30c, which cleared it all up.

Kalmia Latifolia

Kalmia is for wandering pains which start, say, on the shoulder. If it starts on the shoulder it moves down the arms and then to the hands. If it starts at the top of the leg, which it sometimes does, it moves down the leg. Then it will come again, perhaps in the elbow this time, and move down to the fingers. The pain moves constantly and always moves downwards. It does come and go quickly, and reminds you of Pulsatilla. The one thing that I have found fairly constantly in the young who need Kalmia is that they complain their heart palpitates.

Natrum Phosphoricum

Natrum Phos. in children is for stiffness and tightness of the muscles. They often feel as if the tendons in their legs are shortened and draw them up behind their knees. Their limbs can be weak and rather heavy. The pain is frequently concentrated in either the right wrist or the right elbow. I find it has a special effect for that area, above all the right elbow.

49

Sleeplessness

Aconitum Napellus
This is valuable in an acute chill which brings on restlessness, mostly in children. They cannot settle down and are excitable and afraid they are going to die, and you can get them to sleep with Aconite. I would use a 30c every night.

Chamomilla
If the Chamomilla child sits down he is very sleepy and if he lies down he cannot sleep at all. If he does fall asleep he wakes with violent pain which prevents him going back to sleep again. He has the real Chamomilla temperament, wanting to be carried round and the parent paces the floor at night with him. It is particularly early in the night that these children are so sleepless – they may get up and walk about. Older children will, as the night advances, fall into a natural sleep and sleep until morning.

Cocculus
Cocculus is invaluable in people who have been nursing someone for a long time, who have had to be up every night and who are completely exhausted as a result. They then go to bed and cannot sleep. They tell you quite rightly that they are much too tired to sleep, even when they have a chance to do so. They become irritable and find themselves a bit inclined to be giddy.

Coffea
Coffea does not always work, but every now and then one finds it very useful. The patient's mind works and they plan and arrange things and there is just no sleep in them. They are very sensitive to any kind of emotion and love nothing better than what they call a pleasant surprise, whatever it may be. Then there is a bit of a crisis and they cannot sleep. It is particularly useful for coffee drinkers who sometimes get through a big ordeal and are then very much on the verge of a breakdown afterwards.

Lycopodium

Lycopodium is my favourite sleep remedy. The patient is unable to fall asleep, although once they are asleep they are all right. Lycopodium children keep the whole house awake at night because they cannot get to sleep and they recite their poetry and sing their songs. Their minds are very active and they cannot forget the work of the day. They can get some restless dreams. It is a great remedy for teenagers who are working hard for examinations and then go to bed and find they cannot get their work out of their minds at all. They feel rather poor in the morning, and as a rule sleep badly for several nights at a time.

They dream a lot when they do go to sleep. Ask them what they dream about and I have never yet met a Lycopodium who could remember. They are often wide awake by 4 a.m., and if they dream between then and breakfast time their dreams are more easily remembered, often of wild animals and things they are really quite nervous of. They do not sweat, and the more sleepless they are the more anxious these dreams after 4 a.m. will be. They talk and laugh in their sleep occasionally. It is the ambitious boy's sleeping remedy, although I have also seen several girls who needed it.

Nux Vomica

The Nux Vomica patient is apt to be sleepless after mental strain, as well as after any abuse of coffee or alcohol, or even tobacco. They are apt to study late at night – 'I could hardly get down to my book, I was so sleepy during the evening. By about ten I woke up and did two or three hours work'. Commonly they wake between three and four in the morning with a very active brain, and they may or may not get up and work. If so, it is usual for them to get back to bed by about seven and be dead asleep at eight, and very hard to rouse. If their sleeplessness is due to worry, it will be about anything on earth, but not about themselves.

Pulsatilla

The Pulsatilla patient is not always sleepless, but they can get phases of not sleeping. They are worse in a warm room and sleep better if they are able to move about before going to bed. They are not thirsty, but they always think a cold drink makes them feel better if they are sleepless. When all is well they always have a sort of pink and white complexion and look plump and cheerful, but they become rather mottled-looking if they are really sleepless. The other thing about their sleeplessness is that they are inclined to eat too much. Any over-rich food, as with all the other Pulsatilla complaints, will wake them.

Rhus Toxicodendron

Rhus Tox. symptoms come on in the cold and in the open air, particularly when the patient is perspiring. They get fearful at night and all their mental symptoms become worse at night. They are irritable and restless, which is the typical Rhus Tox. picture, both in an acute or chronic state. It is common for the Rhus patient to get up and make quantities of tea in the night and walk about the place. They can also be sleepless from pain, and Rhus is, of course, one of the rheumatic remedies. The pains are worse from keeping still – another reason for the Rhus getting up in the night to move, which also sends them back to sleep.

Thuja

The Thuja patient is persistently sleepless. They are very restless and talk incessantly, especially by moonlight, or so they tell you at times. If they go to sleep, they dream of dead people. Thuja is quite commonly needed for sleeplessness after vaccination or re-vaccination.

50

Dreams

The remedies in this chapter relate to conspicuous and repeated dreams, ones that patients tell you about every time they come to see you, and which really are part of the trouble of their lives and a great trial to them. These are the dreams where patients say, 'I wouldn't mind if they were ordinary dreams, but I do get the most frightful nightmares'. Then you ask what they are about and by Jove they are unpleasant. Or, they get such busy unrefreshing dreams that they cannot rest, and it is very useful to know them. I am not counting the dreams that patients like to tell you because they have been to an analyst.

Arnica

Arnica is one of my favourite remedies. One does not think of it as an important remedy for dreams, but it is.

The dreams are not so horrific as some of the others but they are there nevertheless. As a rule the Arnica patient will tend to be very drowsy all day. They cannot sit in a chair and think, oh well, let me go to sleep and get it over. They go to sleep in the early evening, for an hour or two, and wake up with a red face and hot head, and they feel quite afraid of going to sleep again in case these physical symptoms recur. They get anxious dreams and unrefreshing sleep. It is one of the remedies that dreams quite constantly about animals – that they are being chased by animals. They wake up very fussed and can feel quite giddy.

I had two Arnica patients whom I very seldom saw, two young men. Both had occasional episodes of dreaming that they were being chased by a black dog that was going to bite them. In fact they loved dogs – this is the point, they were not in the least bit afraid of them. They would wake up as if it were true, and as if they were to blame. That is very characteristic of the Arnica dream.

They also dream another thing – that they cannot make up their mind. Here they have a situation which they must make decisions about, and yet they cannot do so. They wake up and take some seconds to realise that it has nothing to do with them.

They talk and groan in their sleep, and occasionally will be so anxious that they pass an involuntary stool and urine. Occasionally they do dream of death, of people being drowned or injured, but in my experience not nearly so often as where they are responsible for something and have not done it. They are the typical Arnica patients, rather red-faced and feeling the heat; the bed is too hard and they do not want it to be jarred, and they feel bruised all over.

Arsenicum Album

The patients who want this for dreams are usually like the Arsenicum patient. They are restless and anxious and chilly and they hug the fire. Acute Arsenicum dreams are often characteristic. The common ones are of some great sorrow they are going to have, some great care they have to carry, or else that they may be in great danger. Occasionally they can dream of fire and being shut in in the dark, and then they wake in a terrible fright. The last patient I saw who had acute Arsenicum dreams was very wheezy round midnight and had all sorts of Arsenic modalities, sipped cold water every few minutes, never drank it down and was chilly and all the rest of it.

She had all these kinds of dreams and woke with acute palpitation and in an awful fright, and it took her three-quarters of an hour to settle down.

Aurum Metallicum

The depressed Aurum patient is very restless and at night she worries over herself. In her dreams there are nearly always serpents and snakes. Quite commonly she will dream she is hungry. If she is not too sleepy she will get up and have some food and feel much better and usually goes to sleep. But she does not always get up and can occasionally dream of corpses. (There are really only three remedies that dream of corpses. Calc. Carb. is the chief one. Thuja is another and Aurum is the third, although more rarely.) She also dreams that she is in an awful argument that will never end. It goes on and on and nobody ever finishes it. She gets very upset and depressed by this going round and round and feels she is not fit to be alive, and what should she do. She longs to be out of life and this is when the Aurum patient can commit suicide.

240

Calcarea Carbonica

This is one of the most common of the dream remedies. The Calc. Carb. patient is terribly troubled by dreams. It is one of the children's dream remedies. They shut their eyes and go to sleep and dream that people are standing all round the bed, and this scares them stiff. They are sensitive, nervous children anyhow, always thinking that something is going to happen to them or their friends. As a rule they eat well and have the characteristic Calc. Carb. symptoms. They are fond of eggs and are nearly always constipated. It is characteristic of the remedy that patients feel much better when they are constipated.

The children have night terrors, waking up with the feeling that they are seeing faces. They dream the very constant Calc. Carb. dream of seeing corpses. It quite worries me at times to hear a child say that she saw dead bodies lying all round the room. Adults may also say they can smell the corpses. They do really have dreams quite bad enough to make them shriek out in the night.

Chelidonium

This is another, less common, remedy where I find the patient has a lot of dreams. It is the Chelidonium patient who gives you a description of a loss of appetite, how he no longer fancies his food, how he is off meat and cheese, and that he wants very hot drinks. That if he can get the right food, he likes it hot and then feels better. They get prolonged hiccoughs, sometimes lasting for two or three hours, a lot of distension and rumbling, sometimes with the feeling as if a string was tied very tightly around the waist. They have always a tendency to constipation, although a real Chelidonium patient can have a sort of mucous diarrhoea last thing at night and then very constipated, hard, difficult stools in the day, bright yellow. They yawn, they are lethargic and they get very sleepy and then they find they cannot sleep. And, if they do sleep it is unrefreshing and full of dreams – that is how they always describe it.

Every patient to whom I have given Chelidonium for dreams has dreamed about their business. They can also dream of horrible things like corpses and funerals, but business is always more prominent. Occasionally they may dream of falling down and being killed, or else get a horrific dream of being buried alive. But these are not nearly so common as their plain, rather worrying dreams about their business, that they have not finished it, that they have not added everything up, that they have not put the papers in the right place, that they will not be at the meeting on time. (The other remedy which has this kind of dream is Bryonia. Bryonia have one other dream, according to the books, which I have never met. I think that I should have dreams too if they told me about it – of lice clinging to their shoulders.)

Pulsatilla

Pulsatilla is a remedy with all sorts of odd dreams. You might even say visions, although that is not the right word except that you can have a Pulsatilla patient who can see a ghost at any moment. They get a lot of confused and rather unpleasant dreams. One patient says she starts off dreaming something and in the middle of the dream finds she is dreaming something quite different, and then goes back to finish the first one. She is full of all kinds of fears and cannot go to sleep because of them, and dreads having to see strangers, or having to be pleasant to people, especially when she is in what she calls one of her dream-phases. She only gets the dreams for a few weeks at a time and then they will go off for quite a while.

Sepia

Sepia patients do not have so many special dreams, but if they do they will be about arguments and quarrels or things that worry them. They are always worse at the menses.

Thuja

Thuja dreams can be horrible. They dream of corpses or the smell of corpses. I am always slightly careful when I ask what their dream is about, in case I make them nervous of them. Another Thuja dream is of falling from a great height. There is always danger of some kind when they are dreaming – they are going to be killed or they are going to do something very risky. Sometimes they describe a funny thing, as if they are being held down in bed and cannot move, not even a toe. This can last up to two hours, and they think, here they are in this vice. Then it goes, just as quickly as it came, and they think it could not have been anything after all. These dreams can arise in any constitutional type after vaccination.

51

Mental Handicap

CONGENITAL CASES

A boy aged four was brought to out-patients suffering from constant snuffles and bad nights because of a wheezy cough. His father's first wife had died of acute TB and a step-sister, aged fourteen, was dying of the same complaint at the time. He had one other step-sister with a marked TB diathesis. His mother was a chronic alcoholic and he was a poor weedy little boy who could talk very little. He smiled vacantly round and had very limited intelligence. He was admitted to hospital on account of his chest and was found to have a positive Wassermann.

No amount of washing would make him look anything but a dirty bedraggled little urchin. He was given Sulphur 10M to start with and his snuffles improved slightly. He was then given Lueticum 10M and his snuffles became much worse, with a greeny-yellow discharge. His tonsils swelled up and he could hardly breathe. On reflection I feel that it was too soon to have given a nosode. He was given Kali Iod. 10M, with immediate relief. The child completely changed and within a week or two looked better and brighter and his nose and throat were almost clear. He subsequently had his tonsils removed as they showed a tendency to swell with every cold. After the operation he got acute broncho-pneumonia which to my surprise cleared up with a few doses of Kali Iod. 10M, given to help the nasal discharge. I then gave him Natrum Sulph. 10M and found him already improving. His Wassermann was negative when it was next taken a few weeks later and, within a few months, his health and intelligence had improved beyond recognition, with every indication that he would be able to lead a normal life.

The second case was of a girl whom I first saw at the age of two. She could not walk because her legs seemed to be double-jointed and would bend any way, and she was not able to talk. She was a sweaty, unhealthy-looking child with a flat-bridged nose. She did not look mentally alert. I found her Wassermann strongly positive but the test done on both her parents was negative and they had never had any treatment. She was given Calc. Carb. CM and in two months came back already standing and attempting to walk. Her whole mentality began to develop normally and for six months she was left on the single dose of Calc. Carb., with definite improvement all the time. At the end of that time she could walk alone.

She was becoming abnormally quick about money and was talking fairly well. At that stage she was given Lueticum 10M. Shortly after that she developed acute tonsillitis and was given Mercurius 10M, repeated. Within a few days of that she seemed to take another leap forward. Her interest in money continued and she could count pennies and deal them out before she understood anything about figures at all. She had scarlet fever with albuminuria and adenitis at the age of five and cleared rapidly on Calc. Carb. again. She is now seven, and a recent X-ray shows signs of old epiphysitis.

CASES DUE TO BIRTH INJURIES

I am often tempted to look upon these as impossible to help. However, the following two cases are instructive.

The first was a boy aged two. His mother gave a history of having had seventy-two hours labour followed by a very bad confinement and instruments. She immediately showed me the scars from the instruments on the boy's nose and forehead. He was weak on his legs and unable to walk or stand alone. He had no idea of talking and made a kind of muttering sound only. He was acutely nervous, and I soon learned to move gently if he came into the room, as he would quite suddenly yell the place down if I made any unusual movement. He was given Natrum Mur. 10M and the first thing that changed markedly was his speech. He would mutter and then seem to listen and, quite often, would laugh at the sounds he made. By the end of six weeks his muttering was occasionally understood by his mother and he was beginning to walk. In that way he was therefore better, but he developed a habit of being constantly sick, particularly if he were left alone or was being carried downstairs. I gave Borax 10M, with great improvement, and until September he progressed steadily.

Then he got a sudden violent squint, went very thin, could not walk and screamed incessantly for two days. I again gave Natrum Mur. 10M and, in a few days, he was reported to be 'fine again'.

In November he had a return of the biliousness, with a cold and sore throat, and was rather tottery. He had Baryta Carb. 10M for the throat, and it cleared rapidly but left him as nervous as before. I went back to Borax 10M and by his third birthday he was talking pretty well. He walks perfectly and has entirely changed in appearance and everyone remarks on his astonishing memory.

The other case in this group is of a boy, first seen in June at the age of one year. He was the first-born of twins after a very bad confinement. He had convulsions when he was three days old and again later. When I first saw him he could not sit, hold anything or hold his head up. He had never been able to take any solid food, as it seemed impossible for him to swallow. He could not be taught to be clean in his habits and was apparently blind. He was sent to the eye department and the report was that he had double optic atrophy. He was given Baryta Carb. 10M. In September, four months later, he could sit alone and keep his head up, but otherwise was much the same. In November he was not well; he was actually choking over his food and would not tackle solids and had thick mucus in his nose. I gave Kali Carb. 30c and, in December, he had started to take a little solid food. In December I gave Lueticum 10M and did not see him again until February. He had then just got over flu, and was skin and bone. He could not sit or hold up, or swallow, and I gave him Baryta Carb. CM. He was much better after that, and in spite of setbacks from colds and an acute attack of diarrhoea in the spring, he was standing, eating quite well, walking a few steps with help, and learning to be clean in his habits.

In October, to my great surprise, he picked something up off the floor in out-patients, although I had always regarded his eyesight as more or less absent until then. He also walked quite well with someone holding his hand, but walked sideways.

In January the following year he was better still, and at just three years of age could feed himself, and stand and walk anywhere holding someone's hand. He could also see a certain amount.

'INDUCED BACKWARDNESS'

This heading needs explanation. I consider that every normal child has an expectation of success or failure in every subject he tackles or skill he seeks to attain. This expectation is usually exerted quite unconsciously, and only if the child is thwarted or pampered unnecessarily will his expectation develop along the lines of failure. Then, although he may be really normal mentally, he may become stupid and seemingly below the average in intelligence. He may thus turn out to be rather dull and backward all round, or his expectation of failure may be confined to particular branches so that he cannot tackle games, swimming, or some special subject in learning. I have an example of exactly what I mean.

The patient was a boy, first seen at the age of ten. He was originally seen because he had put on no weight at all for a year, took no interest in food except in sugar and salt, and was getting on very badly at school. His headmaster had written to say that he was 'peculiar' and should have a firm hand. His nerves were dreadful and had certainly given rise to the term 'peculiar' as he was, indeed, a strange contradiction. He would revel in a thunderstorm, but a shot from a pistol at school would fill him with abject terror. It did not matter who was near. He did not at all mind when the boys at school hung a placard on his back with some insulting joke about himself on it. In fact, he did not even bother to remove it, but no amount of persuasion or threats would make him face the swimming bath or water.

He could not stand still for two minutes and would 'prance', to use his mother's expression, up and down by the hour, or he would run round in circles and move his hands and arms in a twiddling movement, much to his parents' disgust. He developed a stutter in front of strangers or if he was nervous and would then make grimaces. To quote from his headmaster's letter: 'He is terrified by a sudden noise or the expectation of one and he plays up constantly to the reputation he has of being peculiar. He has an unusually good memory and is good at mechanical things but he cannot tackle any problem in any subject and will sit idle for hours rather than ask for help'. He advised various things for him, but nothing very helpful; it was rather a condemnation of everything else that had been tried than anything constructive.

His mother made valiant efforts to understand and help the boy and, at the same time, emphasised his peculiarities. His father lost his temper over his twiddling gestures and wanted him to be a manly boy, and so also emphasised his peculiarities. The parents also disagreed in his hearing about his doings and occupations and general behaviour, so that I think they induced a type of backwardness in the boy which need not have been nearly such a bugbear had it not been so mishandled.

On physical examination he was a fairly average-looking boy of ten, but clumsy in his movements. He had a marked tendency to develop moles on the face and elsewhere. He found some difficulty in looking at anyone for long a time, and had a nervous, chatty, manner, particularly in front of strangers. He had a narrow chest and poor expansion, but otherwise was not organically unsound. I found his knee jerks very much accentuated and a tendency to an ankle clonus.

This boy was given Thuja, with very great improvement. By the age of fourteen he was getting on well and had caught up in his school work. He still found difficulty in facing noise but that was becoming less and less marked. Although his reflexes were still accentuated they were less marked than they used to be. To my great interest the moles on his face were also much improved.

I give the above case in detail because it is typical of many that I have seen, and because these patients are so much in need of help. All of them have been labelled stupid, peculiar or backward, and all have derived great benefit from homoeopathic treatment.

Materia Medica

The art of equating the homoeopathic remedy to the totality of symptoms presented by the patient requires a working knowledge of the homoeopathic materia medica. A great deal of time and effort can be spent in searching the larger publications for the less common remedy characteristics.

The materia medica given here is compiled from the teaching of Dr Blackie. It displays her unique gifts of clinical observation, her wide experience in homoeotherapeutics, and her ability to describe the essential characteristics of a remedy in a practical way.

F.J., C.E.

Aconitum Napellus

An important remedy following shock or fright. Patient is restless, and may show degree of panic. Distress accompanied by tremulousness. Look of terror. Frightened. All hyperpyrexic states are accompanied by offensive foot sweat.

Eyes. Pupils as a rule are dilated. Eyes are very sensitive to draughts and cold air. Change of atmosphere in a room can aggravate eye conditions. Local feeling of grit in the eye. Generally may feel hot or cold.

Throat. Painful, red, congested and swollen. Tends to be a darker red than found in most throats. Burning pain worse for movement, worse for swallowing and turning neck. A feeling as if the throat is closing. May have very short croupy cough. Restless anxiety. Flushed when lying down, pale and faint on sitting up. Skin dry, burning and hot. High fever with intense thirst. Tongue dry and red.

Diarrhoea. Due to exposure to cold or chill, overeating in summer, or fright. Nausea and vomiting with diarrhoea. Mucus vomiting which later turns to bile. Horrible taste in mouth. Dry tongue. Abdominal distension. Frequent green small stools with tenesmus present before and after stool. Tenesmus is relieved by bowel action whereas stomach symptoms are not.

Aesculus Hippocastanum

Old men who live too well. Fat, short-necked, red-faced and cyanotic types. Venous congestion all over. All symptoms are worse after a meal. Muddle-headed after eating, often accompanied by dyspnoea. Headache worse after coughing. Feeling of tenseness and fullness which is worse for movement. Peevish, depressed, miserable and difficult to live with. Worse in stuffy rooms and better for draught of air.

Aethusa Cynapium

Summertime diarrhoea from excessive heat, teething, or overfeeding in hot summer. Sudden onset often with meningismus. Pale collapsed child, may have dusky appearance and twitching. Thirstless. Intense sickness with intolerance of milk. Vomitus is white, glairy frothy mucus. Diarrhoea starts as green mucus, later becoming bloodstained.

Allium Cepa

Coryza in which clear nasal secretions are acrid. Excoriation of external nares and upper lip. Eyes show acute localised conjunctivitis. Burning smarting irritation in eyes, particularly above upper eye lid. Bland excessive lacrimation. Feels as if eyes are being torn out. Sometimes redness round lid margins, very little swelling present. Iris never involved. Better in open air.

Aloes

Diarrhoea in hot weather or chill of evening during hot summer. Food poisoning in adults. Over-drinking of beer on hot evening. Many Aloes symptoms caused by anger. Appearance of patient rather like a Sulphur. Hot dry, dusky skin with intense heat and irritation of feet. Irritable. Hates to be disturbed. Worse for heat. Better cool or cold. Worse early morning. Tongue red and dry with intense red tip. Thirst with bitter taste in mouth. Abdominal distension with gurgling. Flatulence. Tenderness over liver. Central abdominal colic, increased by action of bowel. Diarrhoea comes on after eating or physical movement. Pain is worse for movement. Dysuria may accompany diarrhoea. Yellow stool streaked with green or mucus. Sometimes involuntary stool. Enormous amount of flatus. Tenesmus before and during stool. Explosive diarrhoea. Excoriation.

Aluminium Oxide

Contented, alert intellectually and competent. Can change in mood from being lively and full of assurance to an attitude of marked timidity, with marked morning dullness, improving as the day goes on. Very contrary. Can take things the wrong way and weep. The patient may easily become confused, taking things in slowly and answering slowly. Impression of mental dullness. Boring. In whichever mood, they are less good in the morning and improve as the day progresses. Children are peevish, whining and obstinate in general. Pale or greyish tint to skin. Often have pain in shoulders or scapulae.

Eye complaints. Digestive disturbance. Head symptoms.

Chronic Headache. Recurring whenever constipated. Heavy and throbbing, worse on vertex with sensation of weight on top of head. Often profuse epistaxis which relieves headache. Pain better for ice applications, pressure, walking in open air with head bare, lying down, drinking cold water. No actual thirst.

Antimonium Crudum

Diarrhoea in hot weather or from chill, especially sea bathing, also from excessive cold drinks in hot weather. They look like Calc. Carb., pale and flabby. Mentally like Calc. Carb. Depressed, useless sort of people. Small children do not play but sit around completely thirstless. Tendency to snuffles. Cracks around nose. Thick coated white tongue. Vomiting is as marked as diarrhoea, is violent and bitter, and is worse for food or drink. *Intense* nausea. Profuse offensive stool. Cutting pain in abdomen before stool. Marked tenesmus. Rectal prolapse may occur.

Antimonium Tartaricum

Acute cardiac failure. Cyanosis, either involving whole extremities or else being confined to fingers or toes. Patient hopeless and depressed. Drinking increases distress. Worse for heat. Air in room must be fresh and still. Early oedema of feet and ankles. Thick-coated white sticky tongue. Feeling of fullness in chest with râles very marked. Sooty appearance round nose. Patient keeps deadly still.

Apis Mellifica

Hot weather remedy. Flushed puffy face. Bright eyed. Dampness or actual sweating of head, particularly the forehead. All symptoms markedly aggravated by heat. All pains markedly worse for movement and walking. Symptoms attended by excitement and usual Apis hyperaesthesia. Aversion to hot rooms.

Eyes. Sudden onset of symptoms with rapid signs of acute inflammation. Sudden stabbing pains. Eyelids swollen and oedematous. Oedematous patch under the eyes, which look sore. Swelling of upper lids may cause eversion. Mucous membranes look like raw beef. Vessels of eye intensely congested, with large bright red vessels spreading over the eye. All symptoms start in right eye and spread to left. Profuse burning lacrimation. Feel as if burning tears are running over burning surface. Better for bathing in cold water. Occasionally there may be styes.

Acute Headaches. Often accompany suppressed menses. Start on rising in the morning. Violent stabbing pain of sudden onset. Congestion in head which feels full and throbbing. Skull feels tight. Scalp extremely tender. Whole head is sore. Pain better for pressure although cannot wear anything tight around head. Headaches associated with emotion or excitement. May be brought on by sudden check of catarrh by conventional nasal spray.

Throats. Very acute painful inflammation. Glistening and oedematous. Oedema of uvula. Throat and mouth dry and burning. Sharp stinging pain on swallowing. Cervical glands swollen and very tender to touch. Cannot bear anything tight around neck. Better sitting up. Pain worse for hot applications and hot drinks. Tongue red, swollen and raw-looking. Tonsils may ulcerate, and red margin shows bright fiery line. Red or pale puffy face, may be oedematous. May have urticaria with throat infection. General soreness over whole body. Worse mid-afternoon, after sleep, in warm room or by fire. Thirstless. Shivery.

Diarrhoea. Skin dry and hot like all Apis complaints. Mentally fogged. Attention wanders when giving history. Speech thick. Dry mouth. Tongue red and shiny. *Thirstless.* Irritable and restless. Puffiness with bluish appearance. Intense abdominal pain and may vomit bile. Distension so marked as to be unable to strain at stool. Lies with knees drawn up. Worse for movement, warmth and early morning. Stool large, hot and yellow with mucus and slime. *Painless.*

Argentum Nitricum
Chronic Headache. Caused by excitement or mental overwork. Occasionally after a journey. Often confined to left side. Pain comes on gradually, and suddenly eases off. Starts with feeling of tension,

(*continued overleaf*)

Argentum Nitricum, continued

soreness and stiffness at back of neck. Feels as if head is drawn back. Spreads over head and localises in left temple. Nausea. Feeling of soreness in brain. Superficial tenderness of scalp, but headache better for pressure. Worse at noon time. Worse using eyes, for motion or exertion (talking, stooping). Better in fresh air. May occasionally be due to eating sweets.

Eyes. Purulent, painful afflictions of eyes. Intense photophobia which is worse for warmth. Marked congestion in inner side of eye. Inner canthus red and swollen. Sometimes corneal ulceration. Better if eyes are kept cool in open air or shade.

Diarrhoea. Usually in children who have been recently weaned, or else may be due to pure funk. May come on in hot weather, and during the actual diarrhoea the patient is chilly and craves for fresh air. Thin and wrinkled child. Dry mouth and lips with stringy mucus in mouth which is difficult to get rid of. Weak and tremulous, and may stagger. Children sit on knee and sway. Flatulence with marked eructations which do not give relief. Nausea without vomiting. Diarrhoea worse for drinking. Abdominal tenderness better for pressure. Green stool with little faecal matter. Very offensive flatus. Occasionally passes a cast of the rectum. Mucus may be bloodstained. Painless diarrhoea.

Arnica Montana

Virtually specific for muscle injury. Used also pre- and post-operatively and for extraction of teeth. General fatigue and exhaustion. Tired travellers. Patient feels bruised all over, and if lying complains that bed is too hard. Worse for being touched or even approached. Useful in cardiac states with bradycardia. These cases often have chilly body and hot face and head with a cold nose.

In a general way they tend to be drowsy all day but cannot sleep in a chair. Go to sleep in the early evening for an hour or two and wake up with red face and hot head. Night sleep is unrefreshing – they dream constantly about animals or being chased by wild animals. Talk and groan in sleep and may have involuntary stool or urination. Dream also of death and drowning.

Arsenicum Album

Appearance of a rather thin build. Pale sunken face often lined, may be swollen in the evening with swollen eyelids. They look anxious, worried and fearful. Very alive people, rapid walkers. Are fidgety when sitting and have quick movements. Definitely 'on the spot' people. Too much energy to put on fat. Fine skin and fine hair with a tendency to sweat. Some may have coarse skin, rough and unhealthy-looking with cracks. Children may develop quickly. Precocious and nervous. Fine skins which flush easily. Very chilly patients who hug the fire – must have heat.

Mental. Afraid of everything. Mental anxiety with sadness. Tell their history punctuated with anxiety and worry. They do not sit down calmly and wait for you to talk; they have a tale to tell and straight off start to tell it. Think they have something definite and seriously wrong with themselves which cannot be cured, hence have a feeling of hopelessness and despair – not really worth telling history, recovery impossible. Never placid. Tend to violent depression with marked restlessness, and may show suicidal tendencies. Blame themselves for the depression and become irritable and annoyed. Occasional suicide from impulse, although they usually have a marked fear of death. Self-pity very marked. Depression also leads to weeping and agitation. Fear of failure or of losing money. Covetous of other people's possessions. Have desire for possessions rather than a fear of poverty. Not only fear for themselves but for other people, relatives etc. When under stress become impulsive and get distressing thoughts which may also lead to severe depression. This stage may be helped by just talking to someone whom they can trust. Advice may nevertheless offend. Very capricious and fretful. Easily find fault with everything. Over-sensitive to all surroundings, smell, touch, hair being combed, but particularly to all circumstances in which they live. Finicky and fastidious about personal appearance, house etc. The 'Gold-headed Cane'. Admire beautiful things which they wish they possessed. Very intelligent. May be finicky about health and worry about imaginary diseases, and seek advice from one doctor and then another.

Particularly afraid at night and panic when alone. Worse around 1 a.m. to 2 a.m. or 1 p.m. to 2 p.m. Worse in darkness – ameliorated if there is a light. Bad sleepers and awake around the times stated. They are then restless and move around and walk, make tea followed by more walking.

Headache. Marked periodicity. Chronic headaches often alternate with rheumatism. Pain intense, throbbing and burning. Often starts at root of nose and spreads over whole head. Hair of scalp tender to touch

(*continued overleaf*)

Arsenicum Album, continued

and pressure. Pain is better for cold applications and then very much worse a short time afterwards. Pain is also worse for movement. Neuralgic type of headache which is always better for heat. Hypersensitive to smell of food and tobacco, and headache is increased by it. The heachache will recur if food is taken while the headache is subsiding. Headache may be worse after lunch and worse into the night. The chronic headache is always accompanied by vomiting. Slightly ameliorated by fresh air.

Diarrhoea. Brought on by chill or very cold drinks. In children during teething, or excessive intake of fruit. In adults, food poisoning, alcohol and malted liquors. Lips pale, dry, cracked, bluish with tendency to bleed. Skin may be wrinkled. Intense thirst for sips. Marked prostration. Vomits after food and drink. Vomitus is burning. Prostration and sweating after bowel movement. Worse early morning and early afternoon. Stool offensive and liquid, any colour and scanty as a rule. Very frequent stool. If mucus only then not offensive. Redness and peri-anal excoriation. Marked abdominal colic before stool. Burning pain in rectum during and after stool. Very chilly after stool, which may be accompanied by fainting.

Food. Very sensitive to anything which is not quite fresh. Sometimes has a definite desire for sour foods, especially when acutely ill. Can like fat very much or have an aversion to it – but usually has some definite attitude to it. Upset by watery or juicy fruits, melon and pears, which tends to cause diarrhoea. Not good on a vegetarian diet. Upset by iced foods in hot weather. Desires coffee and quite often milk too. Many complaints worse for alcohol.

Stomach. Anorexia usually associated with depression. Loathes food and smell of cooking. May cause vomiting. In cases of acute illness, thirst for small drinks satisfies their needs. Easily upset by fatty or greasy food. Gastric pain aggravated by taking food.

Pain. Generalised burning pains, better for warmth and wrapping up. All secretions are acrid and excoriating, and may cause some degree of pain.

Influenza. Excoriating watery nasal discharge. Sneezes from one spot of irritation in nares. Worse for changes in weather. Chest soon involved. Putrid sputum, although may have unproductive hacking cough. Generally feels chilly and is worse from draughts. Hugs the fire. Restless and anxious. Complains of a feeling of ice cold water (or boiling water) flowing through vessels.

Acute Cardiac Failure. Mental distress with extreme fear and anxiety. Mental and physical restlessness. Constant thirst for small sips of cold water. Weight and constriction of chest. Feel they cannot get enough air into lungs. Feeling of impending doom. Complains of feeling cold and is cold to touch. May however complain of burning pains in chest. Grey, pinched and wrinkled lips. Possibly severe dyspnoea. Response to Arsenicum is quick. If no response within fifteen minutes then patient is *not* an Arsenicum.

Dreams. Great sorrow, or is in great danger. Fire. Shut in the dark. Very vivid imagination. Wakens from sleep in terrible fright.

It is quite common for Sulphur and Phosphorus patients to require Arsenicum Album in acute illness.

Aurum Metallicum
In acute depression is brooding and melancholic. Sits and peers in front of him. Will not speak and looks extremely depressed. Strange ideas. Patients think they have lost affection of friends or family. Real disgust of life. Can become suicidal and blame themselves for everything. Find it difficult to cry. Need constant reassurance. Prefer to be left alone and often find difficulty in rousing themselves or in making any physical effort. When roused they have to be busy or even entertained. Have rather a dusky colour. They are better moving in open air. Vertigo may be present and they stagger from side to side. They may fall over – always to the left side. Brood over some sin which they have committed. Sense of unworthiness. Violent if contradicted.

Chronic Headache. Caused sometimes from sunshine and rage. Eye symptoms precede headache, upper half of vision impaired. Feeling of soreness on the surface of the cranium, worse for pressure. Eyes often agglutinated in morning. Feeling of sand in eyes, with lacrimation. Flushed, heavy dull appearance. Does not want to be disturbed. Oversensitive to touch, smell and noise. Associated with some degree of constipation.

(*continued overleaf*)

Aurum Metallicum, continued

Rheumatism. Moves from joint to joint. Ankles particularly affected. When in upper joints, patient is unable to lie down, sits up in bed and bends forward.

Dreams. Of snakes, hunger, corpses. (Only three remedies dream of corpses – Calc. Carb., Thuja and Aurum.) Dreams of argument that will never finish.

Baptisia Tinctoria

An exaggerated Gelsemium. Dull red face, dusky, drugged, besotted look. More intensified than Bryonia or Gelsemium. Swollen face with heavy eyes. Looks almost comatose. Acute illness, usually of rapid onset, patient very ill. Required often in toxic cases of influenza, particularly with sudden violent diarrhoea and vomiting with collapse. The so-called 'typhoid state'. In cases of influenza, mouth and throat are very foul with boggy, purplish, swollen throat, with ulcers which are painless. May affect ears. In throat infections the soreness is not in proportion to the appearance. Glairy, offensive, horrid mucus. Great difficulty in swallowing solids. Great difficulty in breathing. May get a good spell of sleep early in the night, then is awake muttering until morning. Tongue coated, dry and red with offensive mouth. Patient cannot feel tongue. In chest involvement there is spasmodic suffocative cough with dark sticky sputum, which is difficult to expectorate. Often cannot breathe deep enough to expectorate. There is dyspnoea with a feeling of oppression in the chest.

In acute illness there is a dull headache, not as severe as in Bryonia cases. Mental confusion. Does not know where he is. Feels as if there are two separate parts of himself in bed and he cannot get them together. Wants to go home when he is at home. Picking and pulling of bedclothes. Befogged. Confused as to who people are and what they are discussing. Hot, moist, clammy skin. Resents being covered. Body tender to touch. Says that bed hurts and in spite of toxicity is restless and always moving to find comfortable position. Offensive sweating. Can be thirsty, drinks a lot if fluids are there, but would not ask for them.

Baryta Carbonica

Often used as a throat remedy. Patient reports repeated attacks of throat infection, particularly after getting feet wet. Rawness or scraped feeling in throat with shooting pains on swallowing. Feeling of plug in throat. Chokes on solids and is much worse for empty swallowing. Swallows fluids easily. Hypersalivation. Small blisters on tongue. Hoarseness. Chronic enlargement of cervical glands and tonsils. Foul taste in mouth. Soft, chilly, pale, flabby, bloated patient. Has little stamina. Wants to be covered. Sometimes has swollen upper lip. Marked offensive foot sweat. Cracking noises in ears, worse for chewing and better for lying. Parotitis which is worse for cold. Accumulations of mucus in nose, throat, larynx and trachea. A useful remedy to follow these symptoms when first treated in their acute stage with Psorinum.

Baryta Muriatica

Throat remedy. Right-sided, or starts on right side. Burning pain with very enlarged tonsils. Feeling of lump in throat. Tongue white and mouth offensive. Salivation. Glands swollen. Marked thirst with dry lips. Aversion to all food. Pain worse on swallowing, referred to neck. Throat more dry than raw. Better sipping cold water. Works in fifty per cent of acute tonsillitis cases without definite symptoms. Recurring attacks with red face, dry lips and mouth. Throat red and congested with enlargement of superficial veins. Patient damp and warm to touch.

Belladonna

Congested face. Dilated pupils as a rule, although sometimes an extremely contracted pupil.

Throat. Heat. Redness. Burning. Violent heat everywhere. Very flushed face, which gets more flushed with swallowing and pain. Pupils dilated. Throat swollen, inflamed and darkish shiny red. Burning pains which tend to shoot to side of neck. Sense of blockage in throat, as if clutched. Spasm of throat on swallowing, or even when lying quite still, which lasts a few seconds and disappears. Worse on right side. Constant desire to swallow in spite of spasm. Fullness, congestion and throbbing in head. Marked thirst for lemon juice. Strawberry tongue. Neck tender to touch, and pain on speech, which is thick, and makes patient wince.

Acute Headache. Caused by exposure to sun, cold, emotional shock. Starts in early evening and lasts all night. Marked degree of mental excitement. Pain worse for cold draught blowing on head. Sensation as if whole forehead was bursting forward. Extreme pulsation in head. Pain worse for stooping, motion, lying down. Some relief from

(continued overleaf)

Belladonna, continued

bending head backward. Wants to lie with head high. Too many blankets on bed aggravates headache, and patient wants them off. Useful remedy in menstrual headaches. Headaches from washing hair and not drying it well. Intense photophobia much worse for stooping.

Eyes. Acute onset. Eyes burning hot with very acute pain that extends from eyes into back of head. Accompanied often with intense throbbing headache which is worse for lying down. Possibly the only eye remedy which has this symptom. In eye conditions the pupils are usually contracted. Sensation that eyes are bulging and pulsating. Burning sensation in eyes accompanied by dryness, followed by hot salty tears. Photophobia aggravated from movement. Bright red cheeks.

Berberis Vulgaris

Contradictory, changeable personalities. Mental dejection over their complaint. Difficulty in thinking. Aggravation time 4 p.m. until going to sleep at night. In twilight, dogs and people in the street appear much larger than they really are. Often feel their head is becoming larger. Feeling of having a cap on the head. Sickly expression with dry lips. Dry mouth with sticky frothy saliva, which looks like cotton wool or soapsuds. Appearances can be inconsistent. *Pains radiate from one spot*, commonly the right costal margin. Constant desire to defaecate, stools whitish, burning and sticky.

Renal Calculi. Burning pain in urethra, worse when passing urine and after stream has finished. This pain radiates. Pale yellow urine with transparent gelatinous sediment which floats in the urine, or clay-like mucus substance which settles. Acute pain in renal angle, worse for deep pressure.

Puffy swelling of left spermatic cord, worse on walking. Burning and soreness in vagina.

Stitching and shooting pains in neck and back with cold sensation which radiates. Pains in loin and back, without kidney trouble, which radiate across back to pelvis and thighs. Pain in any area which radiates with a feeling of weakness. Pains are worse for rest and better for standing or walking. Heaviness after pain. Pains in single joints.

Coldness, weakness and sweating before going to sleep. Feeling of heat in upper part of body. Chilly in morning, hot in afternoon. All sweating usually after midnight.

Bromium

Throats, always in hot weather. Worse left side. Prostration with deathly weakness. Face ashy-pale and grey. Surprisingly, no anxiety. Depressed and completely indifferent. Throat darkish with grey secretion. Complains of soreness rather than sharp pain. Aggravated by heat. Waves of heat over face, head and neck. Sweats on face. Sensation of cobweb on face, as though something had dried on the facial skin.

Bryonia

In acute illness, blotchy, bloated puffy face. Looks drugged. No fine features. Patient looks a dead weight. No life or vitality. Pretends to be asleep, is better left alone and undisturbed. Extremely irritable at interference. Worse for physical or mental effort. Drowsy during the day with evening aggravation around 9 p.m. Muttering delirium at night. If heavy sleep, is worse on wakening. Hot room aggravates and wants air. Lies still, feels nauseated and giddy on sitting up.

Worse for all movement. Does not want to be examined or questioned.

Constipation in children. Hard, dark, dry stools.

Rheumatism worse for dry cold and movement.

Chest. Hard dry cough with extreme pain on coughing. Holds on to side of chest. Lies on affected side. Mouth and lips dry. Very thirsty for long cold drinks. Cough worse at night, worse for movement and warm room. Pain better for any pressure or constriction which helps to keep still. Hyperpyrexia may be accompanied by bursting or stitching headache. Cough worse from 9 p.m. onwards and may be spasmodic. May follow second stage of Gelsemium cold or chill, mostly in cold dry weather.

Headache. Acute form often accompanies acute nasal catarrh, sneezing and coryza. May be due to overeating rather than overdrinking. Commonly occurs in Sepia patients. Dull congested face. Eyes look heavy and the patient keeps them closed. Dull aching frontal headache which often starts over nose and spreads to forehead and back of head. Better for pressure and worse for all movement.

Headache comes on in morning on opening eyes, and is worse for using the eyes. May be violent in type, with feeling that skull is being separated into two parts. Feeling of everything falling out of head on

(continued overleaf)

Bryonia, continued

stooping. Sudden vertigo on rising. In the acute neuralgic type of headache, pain is confined to left side of head and may radiate from left eye to left temple. This type of headache is also better for pressure and worse for movement, also better for cold applications. There is a feeling of heat in the head with coldness in the extremities, so that the patient wants to be covered with blankets. Headache may persist all day. Hair is sensitive to touch. Kind of headache one gets at the commencement of influenza.

Calcarea Arsenicosa

Epilepsy. Complains of rush of blood to head before fit. Headache begins in forehead and goes to back of head. May commence before fit. Cannot bear changes of diet. Pain in right eye with periodicity. A chilly remedy. Patient worse in cold weather. Irritable with mental and emotional strain. Irritable heart with extrasystoles which are more pronounced if angry.

Useful remedy in helping an alcoholic to abstain.

Calcarea Carbonica

Fat, flabby, lethargic and pale. Large head and rather large face. Especially a description of children who are charming, smiling and who take prizes at the baby show. They sit where they are put and do not wriggle about like other children. Slow walking, slow talking, slow teething. Face only fat, rest of body on thin side. Sweats profusely round head at night. Fatness without fitness, sweating without heat, bones without strength. Tissues 'plus quantity, minus quality'. Neck and body may be scraggy. Heads chilly and damp with boneless feeling. Calc. Carb. schoolchildren who are told by teachers that they are stupid go home bathed in tears, not loud or sobbing but just trickling down their faces. If not well they become particularly spineless. Very sensitive, and more so when they find they cannot keep up with other children at school. Must have their breakfast, when they have a craving for eggs. Adult hand is limp and feels boneless and clammy. Mentally and physically slow. Slow deliberate walk. Everything is in a minor key. Slow in speech, and pause to take in question before replying. Nasal polypi. Menses too early and too prolonged. Weakness in long bones and small of back. Conjunctivitis and congestion of right eye. Worse for alcohol. Often have pale mucous membranes. Occasional blue extremities. Soon chilled and have cold extremities. Sweating in cold room. Wear far too many clothes.

Mentals. Difficult to distinguish from Aurum. Melancholic. Heavy dull appearance, and sit staring in front of them telling their history, if they can be induced to speak. Full of self pity and hopelessness. Always telling of some recurring difficulty or worry. Harp on about these worries in the same old way and pattern. If you talk to them about their difficulties and worries they are apt to go to pieces and weep, tears trickle down. Bore their families and friends with the same old repetitive worries. Worry about friends, family and everything. Feel incapable of making any mental effort and have great disinclination to work. Weary of life and think they are failures. Despondent. 'Sitting solidly and bending pins' is a very good description. Do stupid finicky things. Can be dominated by someone else's personality. Can be roused to perform work only with difficulty. Brood over stupid things. Lack 'stuffing'. Think they are mentally below average. Very poor memories and are easily confused. Cannot remember dates of their illnesses and what they have recently read or written. Terribly sensitive, especially of criticism. Very upset if told to pull themselves together. Sensitive to cruelty or injustice. Lack courage and not likely to commit suicide, although they have a fear of becoming insane. Avoid people because of their mental confusion. Depression is very marked, fearful of the future. Can be peevish. Fear of dark. Intense anxiety at night and fear of cerebral haemorrhage. Uncertain sleepers and late in falling asleep. Awake in fright from alarming nightmares. Talk to themselves in bed.

Chronic Headaches. From exposure to heat or cold, or too much food or drink. Beating pain usually over right temple. Pain better for eyes closed, lying down and sleep. Worse for light, motion, stooping and walking.

Constipated, and feels better when constipated. They have useful appetites although not as good as you would expect from their fatness and flabbiness. May have gastric disturbances with marked eructations.

Dreams. Common dream remedy. People standing round the bed. Being killed or being very ill or dying. Constant dream of seeing corpses. Adults smell corpses.

Calcarea Fluorica
Chief use is in dispersion of bony growths. Useful in cataracts and opacities. Enamel deficiency. Bony growth of nasal septum. General modalities are worse for rest. Better for gentle movement, warmth, warm food and drinks, rubbing.

Calcarea Hypophosphorosa

Rheumatism in fingers, hand, thumb and wrist. Oppression and fullness round heart or in chest, often with dyspnoea.

Calcarea Iodata

Convulsions. Weight loss. Tiredness. Worry and anxiety. Gets angry over nothing. Dull and despairing. Important eye remedy. Conjunctivitis with inflammation and marked acute lacrimation. Burning pain in eye. Occasionally exophthalmos. Whatever the symptoms they are better for open air. Faints in a hot room.

Calcarea Phosphorica

Great adolescent remedy. Fair or dark, usually blue eyed with long eyelashes. Fairly active skin, not very fine, usually pale, almost sallow like suet pudding. Long legs rather than long back. Fat and flabby when very young. Damp hands and feet, face cold and clammy.

History of growing quickly. Children who are unable to stand. Cannot get up from seat. Lower limbs restless. Legs tired and weak. Cramp in calves on walking. *Many Calc. Phos. patients start as Calc. Carb. when a child, Calc. Phos. as an adolescent and go on to Phosphorus as an adult.*

Mentals. Difficult to differentiate between Calc. Phos. and Silica. Mentally tired, and when tired is irritable in a fretful way. Memory is weak and they are unable to concentrate. Have an indisposition to work and children get poor school reports. Do not work and do not want to try. Do not want to stop and talk to people and are soon aggravated by talking. Like to wander round and go where they like. Walk out of room when in company. Apt to get into a state of distress about anything. Resentful and discontented with their surroundings, place in life, in fact everything. Feel they are badly used by people and providence. Pick quarrels rather than rectify circumstances. Fears and dreads are worse in the evening. Easily disordered stomach. Choosy about food, particularly when anxious. Appetites vary but are usually good. Like salt but prefer it as salt bacon or salt meat. Stomach is worse for fruit or ice cream, especially if taken on a hot day. Cold milk may also upset them and may give them gastric pain or diarrhoea. Anxiety may produce stomach disorder and diarrhoea.

Adolescent Headache. Brought on by intense mental application, or exposure to cold, or tight hat, pressure or jar, and at night. Feels that ice is lying over back of occiput and at the same time has heat and smarting at the root of the hair. Feels there is a vice at the back of the head. Better for bathing head in cold water. In chest conditions there is a ticklish cough with abundant sour, offensive and purulent sputum. Head and neck sweat with cough. Dyspnoea is worse early evening until 10 p.m. Bronchospasm better when lying down and worse when getting up. Chest generally worse for cold, wet and wind. Cold damp feet. Chronic catarrhs are apt to get coryza in a cold room.

Calcarea Silicica

Deep-acting remedy. Patient pale and anaemic. Catarrh with thick greenish-yellow discharge. Sensitive to alcohol. Very chilly and sensitive to draughts. Feels worse at any time, especially after breakfast. Eating upsets them. They do not stand pain well and exaggerate it. Weak, fall down easily and sprain ankle. Most symptoms worse for motion. Numbness which is worse on the side lain on. Pains are burning in type. Can get excitable and angry although usually too weak or too indifferent. Symptoms are worse for anger. Main complaint is tiredness. Worry especially when going to sleep. Minimal sweating which disappears on change of atmosphere. Constipated.

Calcarea Sulphurica

An important remedy for acne vulgaris. Pale, fat, soft Calc. Carb. type with reddish unhealthy skin. Irritable and easily angered. Anxious about future and health. General weakness. Poor memory and stumbles over words. Lacks physical strength and meditates over possible misfortune. Indecisive. Periodical headaches morning, afternoon or evening which are better in open air and worse for noise and motion.

Throat. Whole mouth dry. Tongue dry and swollen, base yellow. Front of mouth clear. Back of throat red and swollen, with profuse yellow secretions which are difficult to get rid of. Pain on swallowing. Tendency to ulceration of tonsils. Neck glands soon involved. Sensation of choking. Hunger often marked. Thirst for cold drinks or fruit. Wants cool fresh air and is worse for heat to throat and worse for hot drinks.

Chest condition produces rattling choking cough with considerable hoarseness. Profuse phlegm. Better for throwing off clothing and in open air. Stitching pains in knees and legs which are worse for touch.

(*continued overleaf*)

Calcarea Sulphurica, continued

Sensitive to heat and cold. All pains are worse for heat. Headaches and cough worse for heat. Symptoms worse for walking fast and getting overheated. Worse for warmth of bed. Alarming and vivid imagination prevents sleep. *Has symptoms of Calc. Carb. and Sulphur.*

Cantharis

Follow-up to Causticum. Extreme anxiety with any acute condition. Screams. May lose consciousness. Extremely peevish, unpleasant and contradictory. Insolent. Refuses to listen to advice. Delirium. Violent. Unhappy sunken look. Says everything looks yellow. Disgust for food and has an urgent thirst. Cutting contracting pain in kidney region which is tender to palpation. Irritation of all urinary organs. Constant violent pain in bladder, with intolerable tenesmus. Urine passed in drops after haematuria. Pain before, during and after micturition. Great skin remedy. Erysipelas and burns. Blisters and vesicles. Skin cases may have accompanying anxiety. Patient always very ill. Burning inflammation which becomes rapidly worse and which may make patient excitable and difficult. Contracting pains from uterus down to urethra on desire to micturate. In men pain down to end of penis. Falling out of hair. *Afternoon aggravation.*

Capsicum

Throat. Constricted as if it will close. Worse when *not* swallowing. Smarting pain, with horrible mouth odour. Throat very red and looks as if it would bleed. Discoloured and purplish. Throat soreness drags on, no better or no worse.

Diarrhoea. In homesick children. With diarrhoea have difficulty in passing water. Stool frequent, small, dark slimy with mucus. Much colic and flatulence beforehand. If thirsty they get tenesmus.

Puffy lips which tend to crack. Face and nose red with cold nose. Old mastoid remedy.

Carbo Vegetabilis

Useful remedy in acute heart failure. Classical picture of collapse. Cold sweaty skin and mentally dull, rather foggy in outlook. Not sure where they are, or what will happen to them. Marked air hunger. Want air blowing on to them. Cannot bear bedclothes round neck. Better for cold air. Face pale, lips pale. Icy cold nose. Body cold and clammy and covered in sweat. Tired out mentally and physically. Attempts to eat or drink make them worse.

Causticum

Rather delicate-looking. Usually pale. Very marked distinctive greyish pallor. Fine hands and extremities. Fine features. Small warty growths round eyes and eyelids. Heavy-eyed drooping lids. Tendency to pimples or warts on nose. Timid patients. Worry. Fear that something awful is going to happen. If friends have an appointment and they are late the patient worries about dreadful happenings. Anxiety seeing boys climbing. Sympathetic to other people. General shyness – it is difficult to get going with them. Short answers to questions. Nervous laugh hides anxiety or true feelings. Can be reserved and almost refuse to answer questions. Weakness of memory in giving history, and may have written symptoms down. Irritable as a rule. Have good opinion of themselves. Likes things done at once and efficiently. If thwarted are apt to go into a violent temper and justify temper with excellent reasons. After bout of temper or when angry get unpleasant abdominal distension and heartburn. Neuralgic symptoms worse after anger. Can be melancholic, especially before sleep. Very bad sleepers, restless and uncomfortable in bed. Apprehensive in evening. Disinclined to work. Moodiness which is tiring and makes them unfit for work next day. Peevishness alternating with gaiety.

Flabby abdomen larger than one would expect in thin-faced, thin-necked patient. Great vertigo remedy. Falls forwards or sideways, never backwards. Vertigo is worse in bed and worse for lying and stooping. Better in afternoon. Feelings of giddiness 'all up and down'. Vertigo often accompanies menses.

Cystitis. Urgency with inability to pass urine, followed later by involuntary flow. Involuntary micturition on coughing or sneezing. Bladder weakness associated with coughing. Involuntary dribbling. Post-operative retention. Shooting pain in rectum on trying to pass water. Cystitis and leucorrhoea. There may be urinary symptoms after a chill. Cystitis remedy and not a renal remedy.

Great tendency to neuralgia, which is worse after temper. Muscular twitchings, jerkings and paralysis. Chorea after fright. *Bell's palsy.* Problems with jaw and mouth. Pains in teeth after exposure to cold winds. Many eye symptoms. Dryness of eyes in the morning and difficult to open lids. Burning, stinging photophobia. Feeling of sand in eyes. Itching and twitching of eyelids. Inclination to close eyes is typical. Inability to open eyes. Intense lacrimation worse for winds, in open air and cold rooms. Stiff neck sitting in draught. In influenza

(continued overleaf)

265

Causticum, continued

throat is dry, scraping and raw. Tickling cough with tough phlegm which cannot be expectorated. *Hoarseness.* Worse for cold and much better for rain. Laryngitis and coughs are better for rain. Rheumatism in one joint, usually the temporomandibular joint.

Cedron

Chronic headache with ocular disturbance beforehand. Dimness of vision. In some patients everything looks yellow or red. Pain in front of head which shoots from one temple to the other. Front part of head feels distended and pain is intense in this area. Associated with dizziness on standing or, not infrequently, tinnitus. Often starts at 11 a.m. and lasts all day and following night. More intense as evening wears on. Regular and recurring every two to three weeks. Starts at regular time for each individual patient.

Chelidonium

Livery patient. Despondent and hopeless – more hopeless than melancholic. Weepy. Awful feelings of anticipation. Cannot cope with life, and full of dreads for the future. Makes a specific worry the centre of their depression. Broody. Irritated by being talked to and worse if disturbed. Want to be left alone. Taciturn. Pain over liver or gall bladder extremely painful to palpation. *Anorexia.* Prolonged hiccough. Constipated in daytime. Mucus diarrhoea last thing at night. Unrefreshing sleep. Dreams about business problems, corpses, falling down and being killed or being buried alive.

Very much better for hot food or drink.

Chininum Arsenicosum

Chilly patient very sensitive to draughts. Anxiety. Marked weakness and marked restlessness. Irritable and tremulous. Very acute throat infections, verging on the diphtheric type, almost gangrenous. Back of throat very inflamed with putrid smell. Sensation of extreme contraction, and throat feels on fire. Exudate dark brownish. Extreme pain on swallowing. Tongue thick, yellow and slimy in early stages. Later on, dries and cracks. Gums swollen and may ulcerate and bleed. Very bitter taste, not putrid to the patient. Tendency to clear throat, but this is painful. Lips bluish and cracked. Thirst for cold drinks. General aggravation after sleep. Rapid irregular pulse.

Chininum Sulphuricum

Acute Headache. Associated with digestive disturbance. Pain starts at back of neck and extends to forehead. Violent aching pain associated with dampness and sweating about the head. With headache there is much flatulence which the patient is always trying to get up. Gets shaky with pain and looks sickly. Pain is better for pressing head against something cold, although patient himself is cold. Pain worse for turning head, using eyes and moving in open air. Intense hunger with appearance of feeling very sick. *Makes constant attempts to eructate with hunger.* Delicate chronic dyspeptic who feels hungry and is worse for eating food.

Chronic Headache. Gastric disturbance associated with nausea and vomiting. Pain is worse in both temples as if temporal arteries would burst. Hair tender to light touch. Relief from pressure over arteries. Better for keeping eyes open. Worse for lying or lounging. Better sitting up straight or standing. Tendency to sweat on head. Hypersensitive to cold, draught and open air. Night headache 1 a.m. to noon. Day headache beginning early morning and lasting till 2 p.m.–3 p.m.

Cinchona Officinalis (China)

Broken-down patient. Prolonged illness or worry. May have had severe loss of body fluids, e.g. haemorrhage, gastroenteritis. Has had prolonged spell of nursing. Hyperaesthetic. Hates noise. Depression due to physical exhaustion. Misery increases depression. Think people stop them doing things or prevent them getting better. Better for prolonged rest.

Clematis Erecta

Eruptions and urinary symptoms. Cannot bear being alone but also dreads company. Irritable, angry and fretful. Apprehension, weeping and homesickness. Weeps till exhausted. Small itching crusts in scalp. Pustular rash round loins, painful to touch. Small vesicles and pustules or ulcers on skin.

Swelling, inguinal glands which are more painful on walking.

Burning sensation before micturition. Pain in urethra long after passing urine. Feeling that urethra is closing up. Constriction. Very seldom does the bladder empty completely.

Toothache. Worse lying down at night. Better for cold air and cold drinks.

Cocculus

Acute headache from overwork or extreme nervous strain. Head feels empty when strain is over. Feels as if head would burst, and sensation at back of head as if opening and shutting. Pain worse after sleep, rough motion, using eyes and reading, stimulants – particularly coffee. Worse for tobacco smells and warm rooms. With pain in back of head there is aggravation from lying on back. Too tired to sleep after long hours of work. A near specific for travel sickness (in animals as well as humans).

Coffea Cruda

Insomnia from drinking coffee. To be effective, the patient must also fit the following picture: sensitive from any kind of emotion; overjoyed by pleasant surprise; sleeplessness in coffee drinkers after any ordeal.

Crotalus Horridus

Mentally depressed, weepy and fuddled, and with this cloudy state there is often a desire to escape.

In throat infections looks acutely ill. Congested lips, darkish in colour. Lips may feel numb. Tendency to yellowish tinge with cyanosis. Tongue smooth, fiery red as if polished. Blood-tinged salivation. Characteristic mouth odour – rather mouldy or almost sweetish. Complains of acute spasm in throat, worse on swallowing or even opening the mouth. Worse after sleep, wakes feeling suffocated. Easily develops epistaxis. Dark fluid blood that does not clot. Stomach easily out of order. Liable to dark offensive watery stools. Puffiness of extremities, particularly hands. Tendency to develop purpuric spots.

Croton Tiglium

Swollen brick-red hands. Look as if they would burst. Vesicles followed by pustules and then by crusts. Marked soreness. Hyperpyrexic. Debilitated. Sensation of emptiness.

Eyes when infected have swollen oedematous lids with little vesicles that may spread to cheeks. Left-sided. Early tendency to corneal ulcer.

Cuprum Metallicum

Principally a convulsive remedy. Characterised by violence, violent spasms, violent cramp, violent diarrhoea, violent cough. Pale and rather distressed-looking, or bluish with blue lips and extreme distress.

Jerkings, spasms and twitchings. Mentals vary. When ill they chatter incoherently and may be delirious. Cannot remember where they are.

Fretful and disinclined to work. On the other hand idleness is burdensome to them and they become bored and like to busy themselves. If not fretful can be amusing and show off with a kind of buffoonery. By and large they are fussy patients who are always on the move.

Vertigo. They fall forwards, or head feels as if it is falling forwards. Better for motion and better for lying down.

In acute illness they complain of metallic taste which is relieved by cold water. Dimness of vision. Rolling up of eyes. Itching lids.

Constriction of throat. Fast eaters. Prefer cold food and great thirst for cold water. Greedy without true appetite. Nausea and vomiting relieved by drinking cold water. Abdominal cramp and colic with sudden gushing stools relieved by drinking cold water.

Night cramp in legs.

Drosera Rotundifolia
Whooping cough. Rheumatism. Pain down legs, shinbone and arms. Drawing shooting pains worse in ankles. Bed too hard. Night sweating. Shivering when at rest.

Dulcamara
A red-faced Calc. Carb. Mentally a little confused. Cannot find the right word. Throat cases give a history of nasal catarrh. Worse in cold wet weather. Goes out and catches chill with onset of sore throat. Dry burning throat with stiff neck. Markedly red throat. Herpes around lips. Tongue dry and rough. Wants cold drinks. Early development of urticaria. Scratching relieves irritation but causes burning pains. Often accompanied by rheumatism. Hoarseness. May also develop lumbago with sore throat. Sore throat at time of menses.

Euphrasia
Acute catarrhal conjunctivitis with marked inflammation. Profuse irritating lacrimation. Lid margins look and feel very sore, bleed on touching. Eyes feel as if pepper had been put into them. Constant urge to rub eyes. Tiny septic pimples round eyelids, which may spread to cheeks. Feeling of dryness with sharp cutting pain behind the eyes. On examination the eyes and vessels of the eye look dark.

Ferrum Metallicum

Clear-skinned patient. Very unstable circulation. Pale, or else flushed up on stimulus of emotional excitement or exertion, food or drink. Fair skin with fair amount of colour round the cheek bones. Pale mucous membranes with definite anaemia. Easily tired, dyspnoeic and exhausted. Faint, giddy and chilly. Feels cold intensely. Cold extremities. Cramp in feet. Depressed and despondent. Weepy. Upset by opposition and advice. Very bad at standing and must sit down. Very irritable patient and markedly sensitive to noise. Sensitive to pain. Can be gentle and pleasant when feeling well. Depressed when constipated. Diarrhoea when eating. Children dislike eggs. Stomach upset by dry wines.

Ferrum Phosphoricum

Rheumatism of shoulder blades. Gets up in night to ease the pain. (The other two remedies which get up in the night and move about to relieve pain are Pulsatilla and Rhus. Tox.) Nice people but irritable. Worse for touch.

Gelsemium

Develops symptoms fairly slowly. Acutely flushed. Dusky. Element of fear in face. Blotchy-looking eruptions. Profuse or minimal sweating with a sticky feeling. Feeling of intense weariness. Eyes bright and glassy-looking, heavy-lidded and dull. Mentally dull. May look as if he cannot fix his attention because of pain. Dislikes any effort. Eyes may be congested with much lacrimation. Unpleasant occipital headache radiating to neck. Wants head to be supported and kept still. Tremulousness very typical, often with sense of instability. Feels he is falling out of bed. Wakes with a jerk. Has unstable circulation which is worse for draughts. Colds may come on days after exposure. History of getting chilled some three days before symptoms of illness appear. May not have noticed initial chill because he felt hot. Chilliness up and down spine in spite of being hot and sticky. Acute fluid coryza with marked sneezing, better sitting warm by fireside. Although body feels hot and sticky the extremities are cold.

Aching and soreness in muscles not very deep-seated. Feeling of heaviness. All symptoms may be intensified. May look heavy or sleepy but if excited by anything will have sleepless night. Mildly ill patient. He may be very sleepless, distressed and uncomfortable with restlessness which is the usual picture, or else he may be profoundly sleepy and emotional.

In throat infections there is pain, swelling and redness of throat with some slight ulceration. Spasm of throat on swallowing. There is generalised aching. Patient is better for hot fluids and worse for cold drinks. Very often thirstless. Swallows frequently to relieve throat pain. Sometimes nausea. May complain of chilliness with urinary frequency or occasional incontinence.

Palpitation with irregular heart beat. Empty feeling in chest or down to stomach *not* associated with hunger. No appetite.

May have a yellowish appearance. In acute headache patient is slightly flushed and has besotted appearance. Some ocular disturbance before headache starts. Blindness, partial blindness or diplopia. Pain worse over right eye in one type of patient. Another type may have frontal headache. Sensation of coldness in occiput which starts in forenoon and is present until patient goes to bed, associated with feeling of faintness and intense sleepiness. Pain worse on initially lying but passes off if perfectly still. Worse for light and better for sleep. In recurring headache secretion of urine is increased as pain subsides. Acute type comes on with acute coryza or exposure to cold. Pain is relieved by vomiting. When ill, may develop fear of death. Anxiety more marked with sore throat than is usual in Gelsemium patient, possibly because of accompanying head, neck and ear pains.

Glonoinum

Very acute headache, like Belladonna with even more intense pain. Follows exposure to sun or very bright light. Intense dusky redness of face. Hot face and head with a good deal of sweating. Pain may be all over, or on one or other side of head and is then associated with ocular disturbance. Disturbance in colour on looking at objects. Bursting pain and head feels expanded. Pain is worse for motion, stooping and jarring. Better sitting holding head to keep it still and better for ice bag. Definite pulsations on painful side. Starts at sunrise, is worse at midday and tends to go at sunset – an important clue.

Graphites

Large heads and faces. Fattish features, heavy and not very distinct. Pale mucous membranes. Pale extremities. Mauvish powdered appearance. Drooping eyelids after a bad night's sleep. May have styes on lower lids.

Can be very depressed. More sad than depressed. Sit down and think how soon they are going to die, or how soon their illness is going

(continued overleaf)

Graphites, continued

to kill them. Worry about if they will go to heaven when they die. Marked indecision when depressed. *Indecision runs through this remedy.* Any problem makes them waver and hesitate. Mental work excites and worries them; they fret about it but carry on. Weeping and foreboding of trouble ahead. Like to criticise rather than being sensitive to criticism themselves. Sensation of blood flowing from feet. Very sensitive to music, which makes them weep and increases their depression.

They suffer from photophobia in sunlight and often have crusted eye lashes. Offensive sweating. Any discharge is offensive. Wetness behind ears, side of nose and occipital hair line.

Stomach pains are better for eating. Patients are always better after taking food, which they usually like. Marked aversion to fish, salt meat and sweets. Better for warm milk. Flatulence better for belching but they get painful incarcerated wind. They are always better in the evening and better for warmth. They sleep well but get uncomfortably hot. Overheated by exertion. Worse on wakening. Constipation may be a feature in their history. *Painless* swollen cervical glands. Chilly patients who feel better in a draught but must be covered. Feeling of cobweb over face.

Guaiacum

Mentally dull. Depressed. Lazy and indolent. Forgetful and absent-minded. Congested swollen red face in early stage of throat infections. Usually has dilated pupils. Severe pain in throat which feels full and swollen. Pain on outside of neck better for holding neck and putting something round it. May have occipital pain. Some joint pains which are worse for heat. Very thirsty for cold water. Definite aversion to milk. Slight desire for sour things such as hot lemon juice.

Hepar Sulphuris

Thin, nervous and fair. Discontented. Look as if unwell for some time. Possibly sweating. Look tired. Give the impression they have come to see you against their will. Resentful when you start asking questions. Sink into chair as if physically tired. Give impression they are up against things. Dissatisfied with conditions. More fed up than fearful. Sensitive beyond bounds of reason. They live in the wrong place, have the wrong friends and the wrong job. They have had bad luck. Nobody is nice to them, and nobody backs them up.

Sensitiveness to personal atmosphere. Ungoverned temper. Quarrelsome and impulsive. More irritable than anxious. Impulsiveness is suicidal. Annoyance may give impulse to kill. Children lose temper, hit and kick and do damage. Mother looking after child will turn round and hit it with anything to hand. Wishes he could change his job, which he feels is unhealthy. If he changes his surroundings he improves, then reverts back again. Goes over his past continually.

Tendency to suppuration. Catarrhal state of mucous membranes. Hoarse from being out in cold wind. Marked cutaneous hyperaesthesia, especially to touch and draught. Extremely sensitive to cold. The most chilly patient who feels the slightest draught. Hand out of bed, even warm draught in summer makes him worse, and aggravates any condition from which he is suffering. Worse particularly in cold dry weather. Better in damp weather. Hands very cold and clammy.

Worse morning and evening, no definite hour although morning aggravation on waking. Respiratory, laryngeal and nasal symptoms worse in evening, 6 p.m. or 7 p.m. to midnight, during which time there is marked cough aggravation. Cough is dry and teasing with tearing sore chest. Very hot but cannot move or uncover without feeling chilly. Suffocative croupy cough. Sweats without relief.

Common to find patients with aversion to fats, although they may want them. Always wants something with strong taste, pickles, herring etc. Deep desire for sour things. Likes wine dry. Better after eating.

Throat. Recurring infection. Feeling of needle or fish bone in throat. Early formation of pus. Old quinsy medicine. Ulceration at corner of lips, crack in centre of lips, which is very painful. Offensive mouth and breath. Throat sensitive to swallowing, even opening mouth and putting out the tongue. Better for warmth applied to neck. Very sensitive to pain. Sour-smelling sweat. Better for warmth applied to neck. Tongue dry, slightly coated, sore round margins and very sensitive.

Eyes. History of weak eyes. Eye conditions intensely painful with early ulceration. Corneal ulcers. Early development of oozing pus. Complains of blunt stick feeling pressing into eyes. Intense photophobia. Conjunctivae puffy, swollen and oedematous. Muddy cornea. Feeling that a string is pulling eyes into back of head. Eye pain worse for examination.

Hepar Sulph. pain is stabbing, stitching – jabbing of sharp sticks whatever part of body is involved.

273

Hydrastis
Broken-down chronic bronchitic. Thick ropey yellow mucus which is profuse in open air and stops when in the house. Nose full of pus. Often an association between bronchitis and ulceration of the legs. Autumn and a winter aggravation, with patients complaining of the onset of both symptoms at the same time. The bronchitis is productive and the areas of ulceration have firm edges and are painful at night. General weakness and easily discouraged.

Iris Versicolor
Acute headache remedy. Symptoms caused by eating sweets. Usually right-sided. Blindness or disturbance of vision beforehand. *Pain is worse keeping still or on vigorous exertion.* Better in fresh air and moving about quietly. Worse in really cold air. Vomits.

Kali Bichromicum
Fair, fat and somewhat sluggish individual. Face puffy. Generalised puffiness. Unhealthy skin, and a majority have definite tendency to acne vulgaris. Rather a muddy appearance of eyes with yellowish tinge to conjunctivae. Impression of weak eyes. Rather above average height, muscularly strong, easily tired, almost lazy. One group of these patients may not be so fat and heavy, and may have more colour in their cheeks and darker hair. This group usually complain of rheumatism. Commonest complaints are 'catarrhal dyspepsia' and bronchitis with asthma. Acute respiratory conditions tend to be worse in spring and autumn. Capillary bronchitis shows cough with marked tendency to choking. Abundant stringy difficult muco-pus on waking, and early morning aggravation between 2 a.m. and 5 a.m. Chests are better in open air if not too cold or damp, and better for warmth of bed.

Catarrh is troublesome in wet cold damp weather. Nose and sinuses choke up with stringy yellow mucus. The more chronic the condition the more white the mucus. The more acute the condition the more yellow it becomes. Early involvement of accessory sinuses. Boring pain as if a blunt plug were being forced into the affected area, frontal sinus commonest. General headache with pain over antra and eyes. Back of throat deeply congested with strips of mucus hanging from posterior nares. Oedematous appearance of uvula and soft palate.

When catarrh involves stomach there is typical acute gastritis or even ulcer. Anorexia. Flatulence. Sudden onset of nausea and vomiting. Distressing sense of weight in stomach after taking food. Marked dislike of meat. Bad taste in mouth, and water tastes unpleasant. Develops dislike of fats. Craves sour things. Has a marked longing for beer. The chronic beer drinker is a typical Kali Bich. They have a definite coffee aggravation, also a beer aggravation which sets up vomiting or diarrhoea. Stringy yellow watery sour vomitus with heaviness in right hypochondrium.

Eyes. Deep sharply-defined corneal ulcer tending to perforate with sharp clear cut margins. Eye looks painful, patient says it is not painful at all. Thick stringy discharge. Acute iritis in rheumatoid conditions with associated conjunctivitis. Intense heat in the eye. Marked photophobia. Granulated lids at margins.

Chronic Headache. Dimming or loss of vision before headache. Interval between eye disturbances and headache varies from a few minutes to half an hour. Comes on in early morning, gets worse during day and fades towards evening. As a rule left-sided. Worse for light and noise and motion, especially stooping. As a rule better for lying, but pain worse if lying on painful side. Otherwise amelioration of pain from pressure. Pain may be confined to small area on temporal side. Better for open air and food, particularly hot soup.

Rheumatism. Pains migrate from joint to joint. Acute pain of sudden onset, which goes quickly. Comes on in summer and is worse for cold and movement. Better for warmth but a little worse from too much heat. Better for rest. May have sciatica in hot weather, which is better for applied heat and flexing leg. The sciatica is better for movement and the rheumatism is worse for movement. Very sensitive to weather changes. Most Kali Bich. patients are definitely worse in summer if the weather is hot. When ill, Kali Bich. are chilly and feel the cold and are worse from damp cold weather. They are worse in open air and feel shivery. In all Kali salts you get a definite early morning aggravation between 2 a.m. to 5 a.m. – Kali Bich. is earlier than Kali Carb. They have aggravation and less energy after food.

There is definite alternation of symptoms, rheumatism will clear up followed by digestive or bowel trouble.

Boils over tibia. Ulcers of leg with dirty white discharge. Feeling of coldness below the knee.

Liable to 'catarrh' of bladder with yellowish white stringy mucus in urine. *Pain in coccyx during micturition.*

Kali Bromatum

Fair, fat and lethargic. Rather depressed. Heavy, dull adolescents. Restlessness of feet, twitching. Tendency to fall asleep if not exerting themselves. Numbness of hands, legs and feet. Discomfort of limbs with trembling feelings. There are three pathological conditions in which this medicine is useful: (i) choreic symptoms after shock, (ii) uraemic convulsions, (iii) infantile diarrhoea with meningeal irritation.

Epilepsy. More frequent before or during a period. Definite relationship between periods and fits. Extreme headache. Prodromal sensation of swelling, associated with excitement *which must be present*. Aggravation time around 2 a.m.

Acne vulgaris which is worse pre-menstrually. Prolonged periods in adolescent. Hot-blooded. Worse for heat, summer and hot rooms.

Kali Carbonicum

Pale, fat, flabby, soft, sweating patients. Slow and easily tired out. General weakness, and when tired get backache. Slack joints, broad pelvis. Puffy ankles – more oedema than fat. Tend to flat feet. In colouring more dark than fair. General appearance of puffiness, especially upper eyelids. Rather muddled mentally. Give impression of confusion and have fears during confusion of poverty, future and death, even though life to them may not be worth living. Easily mentally confused and become forgetful. Inability to get things done. Use wrong words and say the wrong things. Complain of lack of physical and mental energy. Constantly misplacing things. If accused unjustly they make no effort to defend themselves. Jealous and possessive, have hoarding instinct. Hang on to their husbands when they positively loathe them. Hang on to their money. Miserly. Feeling of failure. Annoyed at their mental state. Irritable. Dislike being touched. Sensitive to noise. Mentally muddled after food. Fear of being alone. Timidity.

Catarrh. Yellow tenacious mucus when overheated in hot room, or following exertion. Worse for weather change. Nasal discharge may be profuse after a temporal headache. May be brought on by chilling in cold air. May develop sore painful, hot throat at late stages with white-yellow mucus. Enlarged cervical glands painful and worse for cold.

Dry hacking spasmodic cough worse from 2 a.m. to 4 a.m. Stabbing pain in chest, better for sitting propped up and leaning forwards. Right lower lobe most often affected in chest conditions. Pain is worse for lying on affected side. In respiratory conditions do not confuse with Hepar Sulph., which has a time aggravation from 7 a.m. to 9 a.m., does not have a puffy face, is much thinner, more depressed and anxious-looking.

Nearly always have tendency to digestive troubles. Marked flatulence and distension after food, involving whole abdomen. Feeling of emptiness with internal chilliness. Take food with no improvement.

Dental caries. Rarely seen with sound set of teeth. Unhealthy mouths with pale, flabby fattish tongue.

Cholecystitis with marked colic. Painful haemorrhoids with tendency to thrombose. Constipation.

Love of sweets and sugar. Thirst for sour liquids. With physical weakness they have sugar hunger. Aversion to meat and a liking for starchy foods. Usually worse for eating, which gives them a drowsy kind of distension.

Haemorrhagic tendency. Periods too frequent and too profuse, flooding. *Intensely chilly* – as cold as any remedy in the materia medica. Sensitive to draughts and any cold air. Complaints aggravated by mental or physical exertion and damp weather. Yet there are apparent contradictions – the patient is worse for warm drinks and eating warm food. Pains better for heat, worse for pressure and movement. When ill worse if uncovered, *internal* coldness. Sweat on slightest exertion.

Sacral backache a common symptom, sharp, cutting and burning. Worse for exertion, walking and standing. Better lying on hard surface.

Tendency to polyps and fibroids.

An aggravation common to all Kali salts occurs after sexual intercourse. Undue excitement with absolute prostration afterwards.

Dangerous to use Kali Carb. in tuberculosis as it may disseminate the infection. *Valuable in intestinal and gallbladder colic, but if Kali Carb. is the constitutional remedy an aggravation can be expected. Kali Carb. patients with colic, especially gallbladder colic, can be well treated with Aconite.*

Kali Iodatum
Fall into two groups – acute and chronic.

Acute Type. Fatter than you would expect them to be. More flushed and deeper red than the chronic type. Heavier-featured, rather cyanotic, and heavy lipped. Bad at giving history in acute attack of illness.

Chronic Type. Pale, delicate-looking with unstable vaso-motor system. Flush easily. Usually fair skinned with fair hair. Both types depressed and easily discouraged. Definite disgust of life. Bad-tempered, irritable and abusive if annoyed. Restless, more marked if annoyed. Agitated and weepy.

There is a 2 a.m. to 5 a.m. aggravation of all symptoms. Headache, dry throat and general depression on waking.
Hot-blooded and worse for heat. Better in open air.
Hungry patients worse for cold food, cold milk and ice cream. This in spite of general feeling of aggravation from heat. They have moderate thirsts.
Tendency to urticaria which is worse at the seaside. Slight asthma in some cases, also worse at the seaside.
Inflamed hip joints with tenderness above and below joint. Affected part must be uncovered. Better for cold applications and continued movement. Sciatica with one spot on nerve which is exquisitely painful and tender to touch. This is worse lying on affected side, sitting and standing. Better moving.
In rheumatism there is tenderness over joint and diffuse pain above and below. Give Kali Iod. in a hot-blooded patient with tinnitus.

Eye. Very purulent inflammation. Pus under lids which are swollen and red inside and out, worse under upper lid. Pain and tenderness very marked. Intensive conjunctivitis with blepharospasm. Conjunctivae oedematous with thick greenish-yellow discharge. Peri-orbital bone tenderness. Intense burning. Early tendency to corneal ulcer. Marked headache. Better for warmth, worse for cold and damp.

Inflammation of Accessory Nasal Sinuses. Puffiness of forehead spreading to eyes. Bursting pain at root of nose extending into skull. Acrid watery coryza. Burning in eyes with intense lacrimation. Nose sore and raw. Upper lip swollen. Small ulcers at tip of tongue. *Intense pain at root of tongue on trying to put tongue out.*

Kali Phosphoricum

Thin, pale-skinned and mostly dark-featured. All other Kali salts tend to be fat. Curious people, extremely exhausted mentally and physically. Irritable and tend to flare up. Irritability comes in spasms, especially when they are annoyed. Emotional excitement leaves them trembling. Sporadic irritability leaves them in a tremulous state and physically weak. Shy and nervous of friends and strangers. May have a fear of meeting people. Tremble in crowds of people. Although stressful when talking to people they have a definite fear of solitude. Conscious inability to cope with things, break down and cry and get into state of exhaustion and exasperation. Want someone to hold on to them, either to save their reason or help them to control themselves. Fear of strange surroundings, especially of open spaces. Averse to going away from home. Neurasthenic type of anxiety. If left alone tend to develop their many fears. In spite of nervous and physical weakness they often become restless and easily startled. Obstinate and difficult to handle, especially when being advised about their health. They have a dislike of life, they loathe it yet have a fear of death. Never the sort of people to commit suicide. When excited they have a malar flush. Faint in a crowd. Tendency to stagger, too tired to walk straight or cannot be bothered to try. May have vertigo due to weakness of legs.

Main complaint is one of general weakness, numbness, tremor, fleeting generalised pains mostly confined to extremities. These are better for warmth and gentle movement, and immediately better if the patient eats. Strenous exercise or exertion makes them much worse. Appetite is quickly satisfied and they become uncomfortable. Often crave ice cold water. Like sweet and sour things, sometimes crave vinegar. Kali Phos. is the only Kali salt that does not take too much starch. In general they are usually worse for food, and eating may aggravate their condition. Practically all suffer from digestive disturbance.

There is a peculiar apparent contradiction regarding appetite. They have a feeling of hunger which disappears on taking food, and they immediately feel full, as if the whole abdomen was swollen out. There is much flatulence, and within a few minutes of stopping eating they have a feeling of emptiness. Flatulence often gives rise to colic. Dislike bread and meat. They have an acute gnawing hunger pain around 5 a.m. which is better for nibbling biscuits. Tendency to sweating after eating. Headache which is worse for working late. Comes on in night during the usual time aggravation and on waking. Better for getting up

(*continued overleaf*)

Kali Phosphoricum, continued

and gentle movement. It is worse for cold and very sensitive to noise. They have tender scalps and wrap up head to keep warm. They are particularly sensitive to cold and most reactions are aggravated by it. Better for warmth. Pre-menstrual aggravation, better when menses start.

Peculiar pain at 7th cervical vertebrae which involves whole dorsal area of spine – a common complaint of Kali Phos., worse when tired, lying, sitting. Weak feeling in back which is worse for touching.

Headache in student after intensive study. Has usual modalities.

Hypotension. Toneless heart muscle.

Old people with dysuria which continues after flow has ceased.

Diabetes (provers develop glycosuria).

Violent dreams and nightmares.

Kali Sulphuricum

A cross between Sulphur and Pulsatilla. Appearance of heaviness, weariness and sluggishness, as if they could not be bothered to move. Coarse skin and high colour. Rather fat and slow. Complain of tiredness, which is due to laziness. Aversion to physical and mental work. Extremely anxious and sorry for themselves. Depressed and lack confidence. Timid, impatient and changeable mood, lively one moment and depressed the next. Gloomy view of life and show anger in response to optimistic advice. Anxiety without reason. Very obstinate. Symptoms are worse in the evening and on early wakening. Itching skin all over body, anywhere and everywhere. Itchiness is a useful peg on which to hang their symptoms.

Always catarrhal. Crusted eyelids with violent itching. Worse in warm room. Crusts are yellowish and any discharges are yellow. All Kali Sulph. discharges are thick, yellowish or greenish-yellow. Nasal discharge causes intense itching of nose.

Congestive headaches. Feeling of fullness, heaviness and heat in head. May complain of giddiness. Face very hot. Headache starts over eyes and forehead and spreads over head. Marked on the right side. Worse on waking, evening, warmth, after food, sudden movement, menses. Better for open air, cold applications, pressure and lying down.

Respiratory Conditions. Face bright red. Chest usually worse on right side. Tongue has yellow coating with insipid taste. Sputum typically yellowy-greenish. Some tracheitis. Râles. Cough is worse for eating. Better for cold drinks and cold air.

Rheumatism. Migrating pains with marked sweating. Very cold hands and feet. Pains worse in summer and worse in heat. Better for gentle motion in cold air.

Haemorrhoids with peri-anal itching. Skin dry, scaly and itching. All symptoms are worse indoors, especially when it is warm. Exertion makes symptoms worse, which produces sweating. Sensitive to noise. Dream of ghosts and robbers. Struggle and fight in their sleep.

Kalmia Latifolia
Wandering pains in children, commencing in shoulders and referred to arms and hands. Top of leg to ankle. Pain always moved downwards. Rapid onset and rapid disappearance.

Kreosotum
Bronchitis during teething or summer diarrhoea. Blotchy discoloured red faces. Cough worse for heat and better for cold drinks. Subjective smell of creosote at back of nose. Brown-coated tongue. Excoriation of lips and nares. Feeling of pulsation over body when excited. Extremely sensitive to music.

Lac Caninum
Fair, gentle sort of people. Weep easily and get very despondent and irritable. Fear of loneliness and darkness.

Throats. Alternating sides. Tongue white silvery coating with similar coloured exudate on tonsils. Throat very painful. Sensitive to touch and on swallowing pain radiated to ear. *Aversion to milk very marked.* If girl gets sore throat at menses the remedy is likely to be Lac Caninum or Dulcamara. Saliva thick and difficult to get up. Worse when swallowing saliva than semisolid or solid food. Hunger in spite of sensitive throat. Sensation of floating on air. Distressing and persistent dreams of snakes. No aggravation from warmth.

Lac Defloratum

Chronic headache with ocular disturbance. Complete loss of vision before pain. Starts in forehead and passes to occiput. Throbbing with intense nausea. Better for pressure and binding up the head. Worse for noise, light and motion. Often worse during menses. Increased secretion of pale urine during headache without any relief of pain.

Lachesis

High colour. Venous engorgement. Bluish face. Hands red, puffy and tremulous. Restless. Cannot keep to point of conversation. *Loquacity. Jealous.* Mix up time of day. Self-conscious with a 'weird conceit'. Narrow religious outlook. *Suspicious.* Irritable and malicious. Worse for heat and after sleep. Intolerance of tight clothing.

Headache. During menopause or at menses. From exposure to heat of any kind, sun, hot room, stove, light, fright, shock or emotional upset. If caused by grief there is uncontrolled weeping.

Feeling of rush of blood to head, with throbbing, bursting, pulsating, burning pain. Felt all over head, especially on vertex. Sensation of weight pressing on top of head, as if head was expanding. Often acute pulsations in temples. Flushed face with marked excitement. Generalised coldness with shivering. Any movement makes feeling of fullness worse yet pain is worse for pressure, lying down, stooping and after sleep, emotional excitement. Feeling of tiredness in neck which is worse for constriction. Sensitive to stimulants. May go to bed with slight headache and wakes with it blazing. Apt to get flooding at menopause, which relieves headache at once. Headaches are often right-sided and are ameliorated by eating.

Throat. Tends to be left-sided. Feels swollen and closed up. Pain acute and referred to ear on swallowing. Throat looks dark and purplish. Ropey, stringy saliva at back of throat. Tongue reddish, feels raw and burning. Mouth offensive. Swelling inside and outside throat. Restless, nervous, tremulous, hot, sweaty and irritable. Aggravation from anything tight, and worse after sleep. Pain worse for hot applications and drinks, warm food. Worse during sleep, and feels choked on waking. Sometimes acute headache in association with throat infection.

Cardiac Conditions. Cannot stand pressure of bedclothes. Feeling of constriction around chest. Cyanosed. Face, lips and fingers cyanosed. Tremor of tongue and hands. Numbness of left arm and hand. Worse lying left side and worse for heat.

282

Laurocerasus

Marked cyanosis. Pain in precordium. Apex beat slow and irregular. Intense dyspnoea after exertion.

Ledum

Penetrating wounds. Foot and leg on injured side cold. Local heat with cold feeling on touch. Muscle twitching round injury. Local hyperaesthesia.

Lilium Tigrinum

Mostly a female remedy. Appearance difficult to place. Compact and set in stature. Full-blooded. Fair rather than dark. Fat rather than thin. Lips darkish in cold and rather full. All grades of blueness of lips. Definitely hot-blooded. Irritable, snappy and impossible to please. Exacting and want things to centre round themselves. Depression, which may take form of a religious melancholia. Tormented about future and especially salvation. Sense of own importance and great sense of responsibility. Feel they have important duties to perform and are unable to do them. Blame everyone around for feelings of failure. Feel they should be the ones who are giving advice. Bad-tempered when they are being helped and when given consolation. Offended at slightest thing and take advice as criticism. Strange idea that they have done something they should not have done and that people are therefore against them. Can be difficult patients and can be violent. Indifferent to loved ones and to surroundings, become depressed and weep. Idea of undiagnosed fatal disease. Fear of insanity when stressful. Aimless hurry, full of rush and torment. Cannot achieve what they set out to do. Heat aggravation in every form. Intolerance of warm stuffy rooms. Better in open air, cool air and moving out of doors. Often have physical disturbance, worse at night especially when in bed. Push off bedclothes. Headache and dyspnoea in stuffy room.

Dragging-down feeling in pelvic organs, wants to support perineum and lower abdomen. Anteverted uterus with marked bowel irritation. Urgency to stool and micturition. Sensation of lump in lower abdomen with urgent desire for bowel movement. Pelvic congestion. Sexual excitement marked. Scanty menses.

Epigastric pressure makes patient feel sick. Hungry and remains so after a big meal. No satisfaction from eating. Desire for meat. Dislike coffee and bread. May be some discomfort in right iliac fossa.

Frontal headaches associated with mental muddle, cannot think. Ocular disturbance. Pain referred to occiput. Better for fresh air.

Lycopodium

Spare, sallow wrinkled people from the time they are small babies. A Lycopodium baby who is ill has nothing but lines on his face, frown on forehead, very poor colour and abdominal pain at some time of the day. As they get older they grow above average height and develop a stoop. A long narrow patient who looks as though he has gone in the middle. Always has a worried expression, even as a schoolboy. At school he is a very good worker, ambitious and wants to succeed in life. He appears reticent, even distrustful and has a reputation of being haughty with his school friends, but this attitude really hides a feeling of insecurity. He does not get on well with other boys and probably has only one friend with whom he is really expansive. The younger Lycopodium child dreads going to school, cannot eat breakfast and clings to mother until at the school gate, then easily persuaded to enter school. A reasonable youngster who will listen to persuasion. Never wants to play games or attend parties. Comes home from school and reads a book, stating that he sees his friends at school all day and wants to be alone. Apprehensive before examinations but settles down once they have started.

Hard workers. Very slow getting to sleep and often go over their lessons and recite poetry in bed and complain that mind is too active to sleep. Do not like the feeling of being quite alone and often will not go to bed until someone else goes at the same time (does not want to talk to them but likes to know there is somebody nearby).

Nearly all have digestive difficulties. Cannot go beyond his time for a meal, he has to sit down and feels awful. Says he is ravenously hungry and after a few mouthfuls will feel full and push his plate away, although he may feel hungry again soon after. Frequently has a craving for sweet things and likes hot food. A cold meal may upset him. Feels blown out after his meal. He often makes a better meal of jam than of savouries. Can always eat sweet foods. Does not like tepid food much, and prefers hot food and drink.

Lacks stamina, easily tires mentally and physically, and by the end of the afternoon feels quite exhausted. *A great remedy for mental fatigue.* The businessman who is slow off the mark in the morning. Better if he eats his breakfast but usually does not. Tendency to morning depression. An intellectual who distrusts his own competence. Haughty and headstrong. Looks lean and livery. Difficult to get symptoms from him. Never really wants to give anything away even if they know you well. Always likes to keep something up his sleeve. No true Lycopodium patient is expansive. When unwell fears that business may fail and then apt to get careful with money matters, fear he will not have enough to live on. Narrow in outlook. May take up eccentric causes. When depressed he sits around, does not want to be disturbed and becomes irritable, fretful and peevish. Cannot bear contradiction. If left alone for long he wanders round and wants to get in touch with someone, cannot bear being left alone. Moods vary, always with an element of anxiety. Uses wrong words and is confused about everyday things.

Better for sympathy and worse for cold. Worse for tight clothing round abdomen. Tight hat gives them a headache, which is better for head uncovered and for fresh air. Headache is usually right-sided. Very sensitive to noise and smells.

Dry hot hands and feet. Sweating, especially when apprehensive as in making a speech. Delivers it well once he has started. *An important remedy for sleeplessness.* Sleeping remedy for ambitious boys. They have many dreams but can never remember them. Wide awake at 4 a.m. If dreams are between 4 a.m. and breakfast they can remember them. Dreams are often of wild animals and things they are afraid of. May have vertigo on rising. All symptoms have a time aggravation between 4 p.m. and 8 p.m. and often between 4 a.m. and 8 a.m.

These patients are very faithful. They never say 'Thank you'. It is all in a firm handshake.

Throats. Tend to be right-sided. Tongue dry and often swollen. Dirty throat comes on early. Sour taste. Sharp stitching pain worse on swallowing. Worse after sleep. Aggravation 4 p.m. to 8 p.m. Better for cold drinks, as a rule. Pale, worried and anxious. Flatulence and eructations. If mouth is infected can have tootache.

In virus infections Lycopodium comes in as a late remedy about the third day. With chest infections the patient is not usually flushed. Face pale, almost yellow. Very distressed-looking, wrinkled face and forehead. Looks ill. Pinched nose, flapping nostrils not synchronous with heart beat or respiration. Possible twitching of facial muscles. Nothing pleases them and they are very difficult to nurse. Want their own way. Resentful, peevish and irritable. Characteristic tongue, sore and stiff when extruded, with extremely painful vesicles which spread to lips. Dislikes being left alone, someone must be near but does not want to be disturbed. Short dry cough with little expectoration. If there is sputum at all it is saltish or bitter. Marked lack of thirst. Better for hot drinks and worse for cold drinks. Minimal sweating. Likes to be propped up. Wakes up in state of fright.

Lycopus Virginicus

Aortic and mitral valvular disease. Cardiac degeneration. Irregular pulse. Pale rather than cyanosed. Cough with throbbing in head and neck. Intense feeling of activity in the chest. Worse lying on right side. Great desire for food and smell of food.

Magnesia Phosphorica

Well-developed bony framework, although rather emaciated. Sallow greyish complexion with dark rings under eyes.

Headaches.
(i) Acute superficial neuralgic type with pains along superficial nerves. Due to exposure to cold, general nervous strain or excitement. Shooting pains worse on right side. May settle over right eye.
(ii) Deep headache starting at back of head and spreading all over. Found always in tired broken-down patient in poor health. Tendency to recurrence.

Both types sensitive to touch but better for firm pressure. Always very sensitive to cold. Have dread of uncovering head. Better for warm applications.

Medorrhinum

Rheumatism. Starts in several joints but settles in only one. There is often sciatica with other joint pains. Pain in ball of foot. Sleeps with feet out of bed. Pain worse for all movement.

Medusa

Between picture of Sepia and Natrum Mur. Slightly greasy hair and skin. Skin is rather sallow or brownish. Often dark rings under eyes. Tired-looking. *Useful in adolescents.* In looking at Medusa one must consider the two types of Sepia: (i) rather bright patients who go off at the deep end at the slightest provocation and are exceedingly irritable, and (ii) rather stupid and tired out.

Medusa is neither of these but fits somewhere in between. They can be silent and do not want to talk, they never give their history in one go and do not want to answer questions. They always think of something else to add to their history. Rather resent their friends and people. Do not sleep well although better for sleep, better for movement and taking food. Must have some sleep or they feel useless. Nearly always have dull headache. Do not like a lot of changes and prefer pleasant routine.

Mercurius Cyanatus

Pale, soft, flabby sweating patient. Malar flush. Mentally dull and slow to reply. Suspicious and distrustful. Difficulty in finding the correct words. Speech indistinct due to difficulty in forming words. Large tremulous tongue and in general tremulous.

Typical 'Vincent throat'. Dark red and very swollen throat with early superficial ulceration. Usually right-sided and offensive. Tongue yellow and slimy. Feeling of lump in throat with dysphagia. Pain referred to neck and to lesser extent the ear. Nightly aggravation of pain. Hot sweating with increase of discomfort. Very marked thirst for cold drinks. Early tendency to pus. Greasy slimy saliva.

Mercurius Solubilis

Pneumonia. Patient deadly ill. Profuse sweating. Marked tremor, more so in hands. Too hot or too cold, clothes on and off. Tongue pale, flabby and swollen and teeth marked, greasy to touch and profuse salivation. Never lie on right side. Marked thirst for cold water. Characteristic chatter, talks at a terrific rate. Restless. Generalised muscle twitching. Feels as if chest is going to burst. Cough is paroxysmal until sputum comes up, and this is always offensive.

Mercurius Sulphuricus

Eyes. Due to exposure to cold, usually in a rheumatic subject. Acute inflammation, red and swollen eye. Photophobia marked. Irritation. Tears irritate skin of face. Worse for heat or warm applications. Useful in burns near the eye. Marked sweating. Pain much worse in evenings.

Natrum Arsenicosum

Pale bluish pallor, blue rings round the eyes. Dry cracked lips. Nervous and frightened with physical restlessness. Twitching of shoulder or face. Outwardly tired. Shy and walks with a shy gait. Fears of disease, evil and impending disaster. Overconscientious, and exerts much effort. Feeling of working against time. Mental effort very tiring. Physical and mental weariness. Trembles after anger.

Definitely chilly and must have warmth. Slight mental amelioration in open air. Much worse in winter and damp cold. Symptoms aggravated by mental or physical exertion. Feels worse after food, especially milk, rich foods, fatty foods and starch. Has intolerance of fruit, and alcohol produces aggravation. Likes sweets and has craving

(continued overleaf)

Materia Medica

Natrum Arsenicosum, continued

for bread. Thirst for cold drinks. May desire cold food, which upsets him. Definite aggravation on waking and around midnight.

Discharges are sticky, thinnish, offensive and yellow. Tongue flabby, toneless with viscid mucus. Bitter taste.

In gastric trouble has burning pain with feeling of emptiness *without* feeling hungry. Food may produce nausea and vomiting, which is more sour than acid. Likes small drinks and hypersensitive to hot drinks.

Bright yellow evening diarrhoea after evening meal.

Natrum Carbonicum

Fleshy, pale, doughy features. Flushes when talking, blotchy redness. Tired with a tired gait and often puffy ankles. Slouches in chair, marked reaction to sudden noise. Acutely irritable. Mentalities nearly correspond to Natrum Mur. Hypersensitivity more marked, reacts with irritability or palpitation. Dislike of people for no reason, particularly strangers. Feels cut off from friends whom they ultimately antagonise by criticism.

They are chilly patients, much worse for cold and much better for heat, with one exception – they cannot stand hot sun on their heads, which produces headache. Marked aggravation from thunder. There is a 5 a.m. aggravation in gastric symptoms, better for getting up and eating. General aggravation arund 5 p.m.

Outstanding feature of gastric disturbance is flatulence, loud and heavy eructations, heartburn and waterbrash. Abdominal pains are better for eating. Desire for food every two hours and have hunger period early morning and late evening. Stomach is aggravated by milk, which produces sour vomit if taken during gastric upset. May also produce diarrhoea. Rich foods, fatty foods, sweets, fruit and starches cause aggravation. Thirst for cold drinks. Likes sweets and heavy farinaceous foods. Loathes coffee, fat and milk.

Mucous membranes feel dry. Any discharges are yellow, watery, sticky and offensive. May be white and not so watery in some cases, and then comes away in lumps and pieces. May have glossitis with tendency to blisters on edge of tongue. Constipation may be a constant feature.

Natrum Muriaticum

Persons of definite character. Not generally thin except as children. Usually fairly well covered and tend to be rather broad. Tend to be scraggy around neck and sometimes thin-faced. Colouring anything from sandy to actually dark, not as a rule dark-haired. Skin at rest is always sallow, but if excited or hurried come in with a malar flush, so alive and flushed that one does not at first notice the pallor.

In waiting-room picks up parcels with a hand tremor, almost scared. Comes in with air of apparent assurance and shakes hands firmly. Short rapid definite movements, walks across floor meaning to get to other side. Sits down as if everything has been a strain. Carotid pulsations. Tends to oily greasy look, worse in a hot room. Greasy hair.

If patient has a cold there is a tendency to herpes on lips. Have rather red lips with rough crack in centre of lower lip. May have ulcers on tip of tongue or lips. Mapped tongue. Many are contrary to textbook pictures. Although thin around face and neck from the waist down they are well covered and have quite fat thighs with rather thick ankles and feet. Tend to be anaemic with pale mucous membranes and low haemoglobin.

Mental. Mental instability, either up or down and never on an even keel. Either melancholy and miserable or overexcited. Never in either mood for long. A weird mixture of contradictions. Laugh without a sense of humour, or have a twisted sense of humour. Sense of fun totally absent. Can laugh and weep, but it is never a pure and simple act. A slightly embarrassed patient; self-conscious and you have to break through before you get their confidence. Have a marvellous capacity for remembering every slight or insult since they were born, and brood over past events. Resentful if they do not get attention, which they crave, yet when given it they can become nasty in return. They make themselves the centre of attention. They do not like their depression ignored and demand extra attention.

They develop a passionate friendship and then suddenly terminate it. They are said to have absolute intolerance of consolation, but really crave consolation and appreciation from the right people. Their symptoms are aggravated if consolation and sympathy are given by the wrong people, especially when depressed, and they will then break down and weep, which makes them better.

They are hypersensitive to noise, surroundings, music, thunder and
(continued overleaf)

289

Natrum Muriaticum, continued

people. They have a strange susceptibility to music, although are not necessarily musical people. They wallow and weep over sentimental music. Their hypersensitivity often runs to extremes – they may be over-conscientious or may lose all interest. They may be afraid, or they will get into a state where they will set themselves against fear. One day they will tackle anything; another day they will need support. They are nice to know but not nice to live with.

Temperature. Temperature reactions are like their mentality – hot-blooded. Intolerance of hot stuffiness more than warmth and of a stuffy room crowded with people. Cannot stand exposure to sun or getting hot from exertion. On the other hand cannot stand draughts or cold. Suffer from cold extremities in extreme cold. Mental symptoms better in fresh air. Develop greasy face from emotional stress, physical effort, strain of seeing doctor and hot rooms. Worse in summer and intense heat and do not stand heat well. Sun aggravation worse at noon and tails off early evening. Any symptoms that the patient has are worse mid-morning between 10.30 a.m. and 11.30 a.m. Must have coffee and a bun.

Gastrointestinal. Very hungry mid morning, when they get an empty sinking feeling. There are apparent contradictions in desires for food and their aggravations. All Sodiums have a definite bread and starch aggravation. Some have a definite desire for bread, which is marked in Natrum Mur. All have more or less marked desire for salt, although some may have an aversion to salt, including Natrum Mur. All Sodium salts have an aggravation from milk. There is a definite desire for soups. Thirsty for cold drinks and like sweets. They like bitter foods.

Sluggish and acidic. Uncomfortable after a meal due to slow digestion. Digestion always worse for eating. In acute upset is always better for vomiting. Aversion to coffee in upset period. Cold drinks relieve indigestion, temporarily. There is flatulence and abdominal distension which is intolerant of pressure. May have hepatic and splenic enlargement. Definite and obstinate constipation, worse at the seaside.

Acute Headache. Wakes with it in the morning. Lasts well into next night. Associated with menses before or afterwards. Another form of headache comes on 10 a.m. to 11 a.m. and is worse around midday, eases off between 3 p.m. and 4 p.m. This is usually in summer and is related to the intensity of the sun's heat. Eyes tired and smarting with photophobia. Headache worse for using eyes. Aggravated by tobacco, thunder and sour wine.

Chronic Headache. Pre-menstrual, heat of sun, rail journey, eye strain, mental exertion or excitement. Starts in occiput and spreads all over head. Is splitting in character and worse on left side, worse for motion, using eyes and warmth. Extreme photophobia and sensitive to noise. Aggravated by lying with head low. Rather better in open air. Scalp and hair particularly sensitive to touch, which produces pain. Sweating just before relief of pain over face and head. May be zigzag vision prior to headache. Restless, fidgety and keyed up. Worse at seaside. When attempting to relax they may fall off to sleep and are liable to sudden muscular twitchings.

Menses are like their mentality, irregular. They develop backache which is worse on waking and better for moving about, pressure and lying on something hard. Mucous membranes always feel dry and any discharges are like white of egg. Skin complaints are urticarial or vesicular in type. *Possibly the greatest shock remedy.*

Natrum Phosphoricum
Thin, underweight, tall and scraggy. Skin pale but flushes under stress. Most are past middle life. Rather untidy.

Loss of keenness and sparkle. Difficulty in remembering details of ailment. Hopeless about their condition, do not think they can be helped and have come to see you by compulsion. Impatient of friendly advice. Delay seeking advice because of fear of illness. Restless and fidgety in spite of weariness. They criticise people who are not present.

Children present with stiffness and tightness in muscles. Feel as though the tendons in their legs are shortened. Limbs weak and heavy, worse in right wrist and elbow. Tend to be worse on right side. Pain in shoulder moving to wrist and palm of hand.

Chilly and most sensitive to draughts. Much worse for cold and change in weather, bath and damp.

Digestive troubles are worse after a bath. Better for eating and taking food. Aggravated by milk, rich food, fatty foods, fruits, starches, sour and acid foods and alcohol. Thirst for cold drinks. Desire for cold food, although this produces an aggravation. Desire for eggs, fried fish and highly seasoned foods. Feeling of emptiness which is worse after bowels move. Sour eructations.

(*continued overleaf*)

Natrum Phosphoricum, continued

Tendency to greenish watery diarrhoea with much flatus and marked urgency, and feeling of weakness in rectum.

Discharges are yellow and pussy, acrid and excoriating with sourish smell.

Prostrated by sexual intercourse.

Natrum Sulphuricum

Fat and undersized. Florid with underlying yellowness. May get jaundice in acute conditions. Tendency to greasy skin with eruptions. Miserable and discontented. May be bad-tempered and depressed with feeling of hopelessness. Looks sluggish and liverish. Converse appearance, exophthalmos with thyroid enlargement (which is always definite). Fat necks. Thoughts of suicide. Dislike of people. Suspicious. Sullen with apprehension and anxiety. Worse when people are about. Definite fear of crowds and fear of evil.

Hot-blooded. Worse in warm weather. Sensitive to lack of air, warm and stuffy room. Sensitive to damp, wet, hot, muggy days. In spite of aggravation from heat they are particularly sensitive to night air if it is misty. They have a spring aggravation.

Worse in morning on waking. Singularly unpleasant before breakfast and better for bowel movement. Nausea after breakfast.

Aggravation from milk and rich food, particularly fatty foods, starchy foods and fruit, and vegetables of all kinds, especially greens. Potatoes may aggravate, and coffee certainly does affect them. They have a thirst for cold drinks and a craving for ice cream. They rather like boiled milk even though they have a loathing for milk.

Sluggish, liverish patient. Full tender stomach with a feeling of weight in right costal margin. Dragging sensation in liver area. They have a congested stagnant colon with a full caecum and tendency to chronic appendicitis. Urging to stool produces massive amounts of flatus. Tendency to diarrhoea after rising from bed in morning. Aggravation time for abdominal conditions is 4 p.m. to 8 p.m. Frequent bleeding piles.

All discharges are greeny-yellow, profuse and offensive. Tongue has a thick dirty brown coating with much mucus. Blisters on cheek and inside lips. A slimy taste is present with loss of taste.

Rheumatism presents as stiffness in left side of leg and left forearm with a feeling of compressed band around elbow. Markedly left-sided remedy.

Nitricum Acidum

Dark. Vital. Usually thin. Flushing followed by pallor. Dark rings under eyes. Pigmentation (as freckles) enhanced in appearance. Brown, dark brown, black eyes. Mentally active. Not sure that they have a definite illness. Despair about health and have a fear that they are going to die. Feel ill but do not specify any special illness. Irritable to a point of anger, and can be very obstinate. Very sensitive to pain and touch and any physical disturbance. Pain upsets them out of all reason. Pain may make them angry and vindictive. They are hard-working people who become upset if they do not get a regular quota of sleep. Chilly and worse in cold weather, be it dry or wet. May get sudden intolerance of heat. Perspire profusely at night.

Desire fat, which makes their symptoms worse. Liking for savouries and food with definite bite, e.g. pickles and curries. Aversion to bread, milk, meat and sweets. Complain of sweet taste in mouth. Symptoms are definitely worse after taking food. Dysphagia with choking, sticking pain which distorts the face and causes pain in ear.

Chronic Headache. After travel, especially a rail journey. Pain presses all over the head, with flushings of heat in head and neck. Pain better for taking off hat, cold air and lying down. Worse for noise, particularly voices. Generalised pains – stabbing, stitching and splinter-like. One of the 'fishbone in throat' remedies. Pain worse for cold.

Throats. All fevers are worse at night. Throat extremely sensitive to touch, and the pain is worse if one tries to examine throat. Pains tend to come and go, and radiate to ear. Oedematous throat. Mouth and sweat smell putrid. Stringy salivation. *Always thirstless.* Yellowish coating on tongue and small white patches on tonsils. Ulcers at corner of mouth which tend to crack. Very offensive urine. Irritable and hyperaesthesic.

Nux Vomica

Two types: (i) Fair to dark. Any colouring. Weary-looking as if he has sat up all night reading. Slouches with abdomen sticking out. Slow and studious-looking. (ii) Spruce, well-groomed and full of life.

Both get a bit excited when talking and flush up – a dusky flush rather than a bright red. Dark under eyes. Sallow, rather wrinkled skin, lined faces. Tend to be underweight.

Peevish and morose, they are fault finders. Very much strung up and will fly into rage at anything. Very hard to please in business and at home. Conditions are never quite right for them. Cannot tolerate contradiction. Never quite contented, and anxiety is usually associated with things outside themselves, work, friends, financial future rather than ill health. Apt to be silent and rather sullen, and hate to be spoken to. This type needs Nux Vomica, but you have to follow up with Sepia. Anger from consolation. Nerves always on edge, and if startled will turn round and curse you. Very impatient, cannot wait for things to be done for them. If doing anything themselves they will not persevere. Soon throw things in. Thought of doing anything exhausts them, even when feeling well.

The chronic case is the one who has been overdoing it steadily, not only in diet but in very hard work with undue stress and constant anxiety. He does not sleep well, and reads late to become sleepy. Wakes between 3 a.m. and 4 a.m. with active brain. May work then and go back to sleep around 7 a.m. Has a peaceful good sleep and then is difficult to rouse for breakfast. Wakes up with terrible taste and headache, and generally feels off colour.

Gastric. Attacks of gastric upset after dietary indiscretion. Too large and rich a dinner with alcohol intake. If heavy meal is taken in a hot room he will at times go dusky, with marked flatulence and feeling of faintness. Must loosen clothes. Likes fat and digests it well. Definite meat and milk aggravation. Particularly susceptible to coffee, which will give him a sleepless night. Upset by stimulants, tea and tobacco. Taking of cold food may give an attack of abdominal pain. Definitely better for small amounts of food and will often only want a little meal. If they overeat they feel full and heavy in stomach with much yawning. Sensation of stone in stomach one hour after a meal. They may have disturbances in power of swallowing, gets food down a good way and then feel uncomfortable, as though a large mass had stuck a long way down oesophagus. There is then regurgitation as if peristaltic action had gone wrong. This is not connected with pain. They have a

294

particular craving for 'pick-me-ups' and frequent the cocktail bar, and are apt to taste everything at the bar. They are much improved in chronic and acute gastric disturbance if they can vomit. Vomiting is very difficult – they strain and retch and finally vomit sour, bitter, scalding material. Worry adds to digestion difficulties. There may be upper abdominal distension, and liver may be affected by repeated rich diets. A useful remedy in hepatic colic. Constipation with a feeling that rectum is full after a bowel movement, which is accompanied by much straining. Some have troublesome diarrhoea, but even with urgency to stool have difficulty in evacuation.

Pains are typically spasmodic, and cramping wherever they are. Cutaneous sensitivity with a tendency to twitching, irritated by cold, touch or noise. Pains are worse for movement, better for heat and worse for pressure. Backache is worse for lying or trying to rotate in bed. Oversensitive to external impressions – visual, auditory, olfactory and tactile.

They are worse in cold dry weather and better in damp weather. They sweat easily and the least current of air causes coryza and headache.

There is a tendency to jaundice in all febrile conditions.

Alcoholic 'morning after' headache is worse before getting out of bed. Pain is better for keeping still and is accompanied by feeling of nausea. Worse for stooping, working and mental effort. Heaviness and congestion are characteristic. There may be amelioration when walking in open air.

Chills and colds are of rapid onset. The patient stays wrapped up to keep warm, then uncovers to cool. Better for warm drinks. Often a useful remedy in influenza. If cough is present he cannot move without a cough starting, sore retching, spasmodic and tickling in larynx. Feels that something is torn loose in chest. Great rheumatic remedy, especially single joints. Cold dry weather aggravates. Very chilly, better for warmth, hot drinks and rainy weather.

Tendency for actions to be turned in opposite directions, acute peristalsis in constipation, the more he strains the more difficult it is to pass. Urine dribbles but stops on straining.

Opium

Shock in cerebral haemorrhage: (i) Violent delirium. Staring eyes, bright red face, delusions. Has great strength and courage in himself. Apprehension and fear of death. (ii) Stupor. Looks intoxicated, eyes open, very red face. Inert. Sad and solemn with some degree of mental activity. Later is disinclined to work. There may be a phase of complete insensitivity and apoplectic freezing. Extreme constipation.

Phosphorus

Two types: dark-haired or fair-haired. One common feature is a reddish glint in hair. Well-proportioned. Slender hands. Skin always fine and tends to vary in colour very quickly, but skin is never damp. They flush up quickly, which may be due to nervousness. They never perspire except for a reason, mental or physical exertion.

An alert, bright and intelligent patient. Nice to know. Tires quickly and is often tense with restlessness. When overworked or overtired they develop a kind of mental apprehension and think they are going to be ill, and wonder what kind of illness they will have. Get tense about business. Are efficient but worry about accidents at work. They are always watching you. They have a dislike of talking to people and are terrified in a crowded room. They cannot talk in a crowd and cannot think of anything to say. Crave the company and sympathy of others. When tired become apathetic and indifferent. Fly into a passion when opposed and then are very ashamed. Experience strange feelings on meeting other people whom they do not really know. Easily exhausted by talking even to one or two people. A silent crowd may sap their strength. Sensitive to atmospheres and external impressions. Indifferent to the family when they are ill. May have anxious forebodings and maniacal attacks with violence. They fear the dark, twilight, loneliness, thunder and death. They have premonitions waking or sleeping. In fright they may have involuntary stool or micturition.

Food. They are hungry at night and always go to bed with something to eat. Food peculiarities similar to Calc. Phos. Like highly seasoned foods. Desire refreshing things, and salt rather than salted foods. Like spicy foods and sour foods (wines). Dislike sweets, or may like them until ill and then cannot bear them. Phosphorus is the thirstiest of remedies. When ill the patient will drink volumes of cold water and then vomit. Loves ice cream. May have an aversion to tea and meat.

Dislikes beer. Coffee may constipate. Child dislikes milk and milk puddings.

Headaches. Congestion and throbbing in head, better for cold air and rest. Worse if lying low and must be propped up with pillows, which is a typical Phosphorus posture. Pain is better for pressure. Artificial appetite precedes headache with unusual hunger. Sensation of extreme coldness at base of brain, relieved by heat.

Pneumonia. Clear pale skin with reddish flush, initially dry and hot and later sweaty. Scared stiff and responds to reassurance. Fear of death and of being alone. Must have light. Very thirsty for iced water and sour cold drinks. Dry tongue, dry lips and a dry cough which is hacking and sounds painful. More commonly right-sided. Bright red sputum. Marked chest pain worse for lying on unaffected side. Lies or sits propped up in typical position. Cough worse for talking, laughing, eating.

Phytolacca
Throat remedy. Acute onset. Darkish red throat with whitish grey exudate, worse on right side. Oedema of uvula. Patient feels very ill, hopeless and is indifferent. Pain is burning in character and is worse for hot drinks. Pain at root of tongue, referred to ear on putting out tongue. Complete inability to swallow. Tongue feels raw and scalded, with yellow streak down centre or definite yellow coating. Mouth offensive with much stringy saliva. Aching in joints and often an acute backache. Tremor of hands and feeling of exhaustion. Sweating of face with cobweb sensation as though something had dried on the face.

Platina
Very characteristic depression. Unpleasantly arrogant. Excessive self-esteem. Warped. Pay undue attention to stupid footling little things, or minor disagreements which they magnify and brood over. Reasoning is taken as an argument. Restless, and very worked up by excitement. With their marked feeling of self-esteem they have a feeling of failure. Prevaricate. Cannot stand opposition – weep if opposed and this brings out all their worst characteristics. They feel much larger than anyone else – a very queer symptom – other people are seen as being smaller. Always think they are going to die. Mr Dombie in *Dombie and Son* is a perfect Platina.

Psorinum

Unshaven miserable tramps. They have no self respect, or tell you so. However much they wash they never look clean – always dirty-looking. Depressed and even melancholic, and feel quite hopeless. Absolutely joyless and despair of themselves. No energy, the slightest effort does them in, want to lie down and do absolutely nothing. Fearful of death. Rough dry skins. Extremely chilly. Apt to lie flat in bed with arms by their sides.

May have chronic headache associated with dimness of vision or flickering sparks in front of eyes. Intense hunger coming on before headache starts, persisting throughout headache. Acute stabs of pain running through head. Better on bathing head (in contrast to general Psorinum symptoms). Worse for cold and fresh air. Wraps up head, pain eased if head begins to sweat. Throat infections are like those of Baryta Carb. When they recur they require Psorinum. Sweaty skin which is greasy to touch. Scalded feeling in throat. Tough and offensive salivation. Throat worse for cold. Generalised aching pains. With any rise of temperature there is a marked skin irritation. Children get peevish towards night and are sleepless.

Plumbum Metallicum

Pale people with skin of dingy hue. Sallow. Yellow sclerotics. Expression of anxiety. Very dilated pupils. Indolent and very disinclined to work. Melancholic and slow of perception. Answer slowly and give wrong names and words. Apathy. Insomnia with restless sleep. Talk to themselves. Inclination to cheat and deceive. Feeling of tight band round leg. Constipation. Abdominal colic with pain drawing to back of spine, which may give them paroxysms of screaming.

Pulsatilla Nigricans

The best picture is shown in the teenage girl. Patient is like an April day. Fair-skinned and usually well covered. Pleasant and affectionate and must have fuss and attention. Described as taking everything and giving nothing. (I do not entirely agree – some of the finest characters I know have been Pulsatilla when unwell.) As a rule sweet-natured, yielding and very loving. Under stress, mental or physical or as a result of infection, the patient may become the April day, everything about her is changeable. Smiling and apparently happy one minute and in tears the next minute, and these tears are perhaps the most characteristic thing about Pulsatilla. Easily depressed, particularly in the evening and hates to be alone, but if someone is cross and irritable with her she will burst into tears. At this stage a little attention and the feeling that someone wants to help her dries those tears quickly, but they will recur at any other upset. When depressed they feel they are under somebody's thumb. Extremely capricious and satisfied at nothing. Extremely ill-humoured, cannot concentrate and her thoughts wander. Easily takes offence and bursts into a stormy kind of weeping.

Feels the heat and wilts in hot summer, can never sit in the sun, Pulsatilla babies left in the sun are upset and miserable. Upset in airless hot room. They are always better moving gently in open air.

Tongue moist but feels dry to the patient, who is usually thirstless. Loathes fat and fatty foods, which cause nausea, vertigo and headache. This acute headache is worse on stooping or pressure and better in cool and air and for gentle movement.

Sleeps in characteristic position, on back with arms above head. Slow in getting off to sleep. If the bedroom is warm, sleeplessness may be prevented if allowed to move around before going to bed, and a cool drink makes them feel better before going to sleep. May look purplish if they are very sleepless. Overeating will wake them up. They may be slow going to sleep if they have a worry on their mind and will go over it again and again, but once asleep can be difficult to wake in the morning.

Complains of pains anywhere, but like her general personality they are changeable, going from one place to another. Pulsatilla pain patterns are a pain coming on suddenly and going off gradually. Single-joint rheumatism, especially the knee joint, which is painful, swollen and distressing. The pain is worse for a hot bath or heat from pressure of bandage, and better for gentle movement.

Eyes. Acute catarrhal conjunctivitis nearly always with a history of styes. Pustular irritation around lids with profuse yellow or yellowish discharge which is bland. Irritating and much scratching. One contradiction is that they like their eyes bathed with hot water.

Nose. In the cold weather the nose runs and then becomes stuffed up in a warm room. Discharge usually thick and yellow, but never excoriates.

Throat. Pain comes on in spasms, suddenly and then gradually subsides. Throat gives feeling of fullness and choking. Tongue is coated thick yellow and feels greasy as do the lips, which are cracked

(continued overleaf)

299

Pulsatilla Nigricans, continued

and swollen. The patients are thirstless. During throat pain they become chilly and are much worse if you make them warm.

Pneumonia. Chest infections in autumn and early spring. Patient mild, gentle and yielding with congested appearance. Tight chest which feels raw. Pain in chest wanders from place to place and is sharp in character. Patient propped up and worse for heat, or lying down. Dry, teasing irritating cough difficult to expectorate, and may vomit. Sputum is tough and yellow. Thirstless with dry mouth, better for sucking a lemon. Better for lying on unaffected side. Worse for hot bed, clothing and room. Great anxiety at night, especially if hot. Tremulous with the anxiety, which may wake them up.

Chronic Headache. Caused by digestive disturbance, often from eating rich foods. Pain in temples, usually of throbbing character, more marked on one or the other side. One-sided flush on painful side. Photophobia usually present. Pain is worse for close stuffy atmosphere, lying down, stooping and in the evening. Better for walking in open air and pressure.

May be the indicated remedy in leucorrhoea which is yellowish and not excoriating. Useful in menstrual troubles, menopause and morning sickness for this type of patient.

Radium Bromatum

Lumbo-sacral pain radiating to one or both hips. Not relieved by pressure or heat.

Rhododendron

Needed in early summer when the flowers are out. Rheumatism which is worse for cold wind and rain at beginning of June. Pains shift about and are inclined to go from above downwards.

Rhus Toxicodendron

Cold wet-weather rheumatism. Tearing pain round joints, worse for initial movement and better for continued movement and warm dry applications. The patient has insomnia from the pain and gets up during night, drinks tea and walks about. Pains worse from keeping still.

In acute febrile conditions is extremely restless and moves around in bed. Marked fears. Metallic taste with coated tongue and red streaks

300

down sides, fiery red tip. Intense thirst for cold drinks. Generalised aching with nightly aggravation of all symptoms. Better for continued movement and heat. Worse keeping still, cold and damp.

Inflammation of perineal or peri-anal areas.

Eyes. All eye conditions quickly spread to cheeks. Lids sore and raw with herpetic eruption from corner of each eye. Marked pain and scalding tears. Patient cries when trying to open eyelids. Bulging swelling of eye. Intense photophobia. Worse for cold bathing.

Rumex Crispus
Looks miserable because of cough, which is barking and irritable. Irritation just below larynx. Feeling of rawness, worse if breathing cold air. Cough worse from any change of atmosphere, particularly going into cold air. Copious catarrh from nose, initially watery and later thick and ropey. Places blanket over head when coughing to avoid breathing or inhaling cold air. Cough is worse for moving about.

Ruta Graveolens
Eye injuries with bruising of surrounding tissues. Virtually the specific remedy for sprains and strains, particularly for ligamentous tissue.

Sabal Serrulata
Confused. Strange and unusual feelings. Cannot remember anything. Must have time to think, and concentrates on complaint. Depressed, despondent and irritable. Furiously angry at sympathy.

Enlarged prostate. Painful micturition. Bladder feels full with initial pain on starting flow. Feeling of blockage in urethra. Testicles feel drawn up and painful. With the enlarged prostate there is constipation. Dysuria in the female is associated with ovarian pain. Pains are better for sleep.

Headaches are generalised and referred to temples, worse on right side. Pain often starts at root of nose and goes up into head. Pain at base of brain, which refers to mid cervical area. Headache often accompanied by vertigo.

Afraid to go to sleep, fearing unknown danger if they do.

Eczematous patches on hands and face.

Sanguinaria

Haggard face. Pale with inclination to vomit. Dry lips. Circumscribed redness of cheeks. Tongue feels burnt with dry feeling in throat. Dysphagia. Dry throat may be accompanied by tickling cough, better for sitting up and passing flatus or producing eructations. There may be a crawling feeling under sternum. Sputum tough, bloodstained and purulent. Cough may produce fetid breath, patient is dyspnoeic and unable to inspire deeply.

Vertigo on rising, with dull heavy feeling in stomach. Dares not turn quickly or will fall. Faintness on turning head quickly or on rising from stooping position. Worse in mornings. Dullness in temples, worse on right side with feeling of blood rushing to head and whirring in ears. Head is painful to touch. May complain of paroxysmal frontal headache with nausea and vomiting and chilliness. Pain is worse rising from seat or from taking exercise. There may be burning dryness in the eyes.

Acute headache of sudden onset. Very like Gelsemium pain in character. Starts in morning and gets worse as day goes on. Begins in occiput, spreads over head and settles in right eye. No increase in amount of urine secreted as headache subsides, and this is often the only distinguishing feature from Gelsemium headache. Pains in nape of neck, shoulders and arms, especially right side. May wake with pain under clavicle and scapula.

Tired and languid on waking. Feels faint with some sweating and feeling of nausea. Pulse irregular and with reduced force. Sudden nausea with excessive salivation and spitting. Dull heavy feeling in stomach as if there is a hard mass. Vomiting bitter material is more usual when headache is present.

Bowels loose with spluttering flatus.

Burning heat alternates with shivering. Heat goes from head to stomach. Neuralgic pains in face and upper jaw, starting in morning and lasting all day. Will clear with sleep and is better for dark room and quietness. Pain in ball of thumb.

Symptoms may have a seven-day periodicity.

Sarsaparilla

Looks ill, old and wrinkled. A bladder remedy rather than a kidney remedy. Urging and inability to pass urine. Dysuria which stops flow, resulting in discharge of elongated flakes of mucus. Urine turbid like clay water, accompanied by tenesmus of bladder – this is a prescribing point. There may be gravel in urine. Patient may be incontinent during the day, when urine is highly coloured. Very little urine may be passed or else frequent pale urine may be a feature in some patients.

May have temporal headache with sinking sensation, better for rest and worse for motion. Most symptoms are worse for walking and going up and down stairs. Pains make them impatient and mentally depressed.

They have poor appetites. Food tastes bitter, sweetish or metallic. Sinking empty feeling after food. Distress after little food. Better for cold diet and worse for warm food. Thirst for water.

Rash on eyelids with swelling of eyes and nose. There may be blockage of one nostril. Scabs on face like crusted milk.

This remedy is characterised by skin eruptions and urinary complaints.

Senega

Pneumonia of intense onset. Cannot bear to be examined. Percussion hurts them. Sensitive chest wall. Senega has the most tough and gluey sputum of all remedies. Generally better for very gentle movement in bed. Very sensitive to cold air. More commonly right-sided than left. Worse lying on right side. Emphysematous and drowsy.

Sepia

Tend to be fair rather than dark. Sullen expression. Definitely stupid-looking. Stupid appearance may be due either to overtiredness or to slow-acting brain, and these aspects form the two types of Sepia. As a rule both types are tallish with long backs. Faces are fatter than you would expect from the rest of their appearance, which is one of tall thinness. They have a sallow yellow colour which you will not find in any other remedy. Under-eye shadow which looks to be halfway down their cheeks, brownish and often extending across nose and out to cheek bones. Often have warty growths on face and neck which are deeply pigmented, especially after age of forty. Pale lips.

Slumps into chair and looks absolutely depressed and physically weary. Has some effort in supporting long back. Comes into room without pleasant greeting, has not come to see you of own accord, will not accept fact that she is ill. They have a resentment against their fate, and feel that they have had a poor deal. People are not fair to them. Tired-out mentally and physically, feel beaten and cannot go on. If you break through their defences they weep and feel better for it. When depression is marked they do not want to be helped. It is a

(continued overleaf)

Sepia, continued

mistake to try and cheer them up, for they become resentful, obstinate and disagreeable. In this state they feel like martyrs. This induces more weeping, which is profuse and of the despairing type. They are much worse from consolation. Independent usually and hate to be helped when they are ill.

Apt to become melancholic and then are taciturn, although excitable if stressed. Overworked mother who is looking after children becomes worried and excited and very restless. Fear of something dreadful if children are ill. Feels that daily routine is going to be too much. Fear of poverty, that husband will be unable to work. Has dread of asking for help rather than of actual poverty. Envious of others and may be spiteful in remarks. Has indifference to friends, work and relatives. May shut herself in room and reject family. Talking may make her snappish, nervous and apprehensive. Avoids company yet dreads to be alone.

A chilly patient, although worse standing in a warm room and could faint. Often faints in church. Cold clammy extremities as a rule, with offensive foot sweat. Does not stand cold well in any form, and sensitive to weather change. Stuffiness tends to upset them, rather than heat. Worse for cold damp or for change from cold dry to warm and dry wet weather.

Morning aggravation. Must have sleep and is better for a good night's sleep. If she only has a short sleep she wakes up feeling she is going to die. Has headache which gets worse as day goes on and then often terminates in evening with sickness. It is better for applied heat, worse for a warm room and light or noise. Tight pressure to head will ameliorate.

Hypersensitive to smells and smell of cooking, which may cause sickness. Likewise to smell of tobacco, to which they have a marked intolerance. Likes spicy pungent foods and may crave stimulants, wine etc. Desire for vinegar.

Often retroverted uterus. Feeling that pelvic organs are going to fall out, more marked when depressed. Sense of something bulging into rectum, no tenesmus or urging to defaecate. Acute dysmenorrhoea and scanty periods. Sacral pain spreading to flanks. Spinal hyperaesthesia. Backache which is better for support and for walking, and quick movement, such as dancing.

Palpitation as if heart would force its way through chest wall. Comes on with extreme attacks of anger. Better for walking a long distance and walking fast. General relief from movement, food and sleep.

Chronic headache starts in occiput and spreads over head. Pain very intense and associated with menses. May come on after theatre, concert, or shopping when tired. Bursting pain all over head, which is worse for motion and mental exertion. Definite amelioration from taking exercise, not just walking about. If you can make the patient walk fast for half an hour it will go. Headache may be better after a meal, also better for dancing. Useful remedy for falling hair, especially with itching scalp. *Of value in sterility.*

Silicea

Usually small and undersized, especially as children, although they may grow very tall eventually. They have small hands and feet, well proportioned. Rather mouse-coloured hair with clean skin and good colour; face may be dead white. May have sore patches round eyes and nose, and cracked corners to mouth and nose. Pleasant yielding gentle people on the whole. Give the impression that they would give up easily, but this is entirely false. Have enormous courage and capacity for work. Weakness is in their physique, which at times makes them give up. This leads to a lack of self confidence, and they worry that they may not be able to perform even the smallest duties. They dread being asked to do a job, but when they do it they will do it well, to a point of overconscientiousness.

Gentle and polite up to a point, but if you push them they can be obstinate, peevish and irritable and as difficult as anyone can be. They are very persistent – if they think a thing strongly it is difficult to get it out of their heads. The children are lively and pleasant and can be great fun, but if they are mismanaged they are obnoxious, resentful and fiendish. On the other hand, they can also be the most miserable of children, delicate and cold. Their feet are always cold, and they cannot get them warm.

They cannot sleep, and sweat profusely round the head with soaking pillows. Offensive foot sweat. Sweating is characteristic. Wake up at night because hands have 'gone to sleep'. The adults are sleepless when under mental or physical strain. Fall asleep for an hour or two, wake up and mull over their work and go to sleep again when it is time to get up. After half an hour's sleep in the morning they wake up and wonder what they were worrying about all night.

Headache. Recurring. Bilious. Starts in occiput and spreads down spine, then spreads over the head and settles over right eye. Persistent

(continued overleaf)

305

Silicea, continued

pain to outer side of eye. The whole head aches and throbs, going on to feeling of nausea and then vomiting. Keeps head up and lies on hot bottle. Worse for cold draught, pressure of tight hat, movement and exertion (especially shopping).

Another type of headache is brought on by mental concentration or sudden mental effort. It is frontal over the forehead and may go from one side to the other. The whole frontal area is tender and painful. Patient may have chronic headaches usually due to fatigue or overexposure to sun or cold, particularly draught of cold air. Associated with vertical half blindness, and there may be an interval between this and the onset of headache. Interval associated with some sensory disturbance such as anaesthesia of one limb or some part of body. Headache starts over one eye, usually right, and radiates from this spot. May vomit, and is better for this. Better for soft shawl wrapped round head. Subsides with increase in urinary output. Worse for pressure over painful area.

A chilly patient who likes ice cream and cold foods. Definite dislike of warm food and drink, which if taken upsets them. Flushes and sweats from hot drinks. Violent flushes from drinking hot tea, especially at the menopause. Acute indigestion from taking milk in quantity.

Bronchitis and bronchial asthma. Coarse rattling chest with much mucus. Chest conditions worse for cold draughts and cold thundery weather. Asthma may develop from suppressed sweating. Best remedy for a chest that does not clear up, as well as in a broken-down patient with bronchitis or unresolved pneumonia after antibiotics. Skin tends to be damp, especially hands and feet. Fingers and toes go dead in winter, better for immersing in hot water.

Cuts and skin lesions go septic. Cracks and fissures round finger-nails. Sore throat with enlarged cervical glands. Sweating hands and feet, neck and forehead. Tinnitus.

Boils which do not resolve. *Of value in the extrusion of foreign bodies, but only effective when suppuration has begun.*

Spigelia

Typical nervous headache which starts in occiput and spreads over the head to left eye or temple. Pain throbbing and shooting. Left eye feels too big for socket. Comes on in late morning and subsides by evening. Pain worse for using eyes, reading and sewing, noise, jarring and motion. Head sensitive to touch and better lying on right side. Likes head and shoulders propped up. Emotional upset causes pain. Angina pectoris with fibrillation. Apex pain goes through to left shoulder and down left arm. Numbness. Better propped up to one side.

Spongia Tosta

Angina pectoris. Heart feels that it is getting bigger, that it is swollen in chest and spreading up to neck. Marked aggravation lying down. Extremely chilly. Draught increases pain. Numbness in fingers which may spread to lower extremities.

Squid

Menopausal patients. Bright, quick and intelligent. Interested in other people and not self-centred. Energetic women who have irregular and scanty periods. Possible mastitis before period. Chilly. Mildly depressed without irritability.

Sting Ray

Sallow and usually dark. Looks tired with rings round eyes. Very chilly but cannot stand stuffy room. Sensitive to all weather changes and cannot stand real heat. Must have sleep. Wakes with morning headache which is better towards evening, worse for noise and jarring. Faints if stands too long. Low backache better for walking. Tired-out patients who in general are better for movement and better for taking food.

Sulphur

Stooping, untidy, unwashed. Often underweight, sometimes to a point of emaciation, in spite of good appetite. They look much older than they are. Dry scaly and spotted skin, very unhealthy-looking. Hair is dirty-looking, stiff and brittle. Lazy, slow-moving and always tired.

Peevish, irritable, depressed and tired of life. Philosophizes and dreams. Selfish, with little regard for other people. Has delusions of grandeur, thinks he is wealthy and sees beauty in rags. May have religious melancholia. Forgetful and has difficulty in remembering simple things and names.

Prone to skin infections. Normal Sulphur skin burns and itches and is worse for scratching and washing. Scratching causes burning sensation. Redness, burning and irritation of orifices with offensive

(continued overleaf)

Sulphur, continued

perspiration. Marked intertrigo. Itching is worse for warmth, especially warmth of bed, soles of feet burning, sticks feet out of bed.

In acute illness they sweat and have intense burning feelings. May feel faint. Worse after sleep and very thirsty for cold water. Hot hands and feet, cold body. Sweat is offensive.

Morning aggravation at 11 a.m., when they feel hungry with epigastric discomfort. Aggravations may show periodicity. Worse on standing, washing and bathing. Better for dry warm weather.

Terebinthina

Have a half-intoxicated look. Queer people – full of pressure in the head and a fear of getting epilepsy. Burning is a constant feature in their symptomatology. Dull headache with great tendency to sleep. Feeling of tight band round the head. Voice sounds unnatural to them – they think there is something queer about their voice. Tinkling in the ears and unable to determine direction of sounds.

Red smooth tongue with no papillae showing. When ill very hungry, and very thirsty. Tight feeling in upper abdomen. Chronic liver complaints. Much distension, gurgling and tenderness in abdomen. All better for movement.

Pains go from left to right side of body.

Constipation with urinary symptoms which are worse for sitting.

Pressure on kidneys when sitting down. Better for movement. Frequency and dysuria with diminished secretion. Occasional profuse flow and then deposit of mucus. Urine thick and muddy-looking with some haematuria.

Clammy sweating in bed at night. Drowsiness even during conversation. Three special symptoms: (i) smooth glossy tongue, (ii) tinkling in the ears, (iii) drowsiness.

Theridion

Headache of puberty, sometimes menopause. Spreading pain at back of eyes, spreading deep into brain. Definite and intense giddiness, worse for closing eyes. May be accompanied by nausea. A distinctive point in this remedy is that the patient does not want to keep his eyes closed with the headache. Abnormal hyperaesthesia to noise which can make them sick. Headache better for lying down in silent room.

Thuja Occidentalis
Fair haired and fine skinned. Appearance associated with TB diathesis. Singularly well-mannered, sensitive, polite and grateful. Some impatience, and may be depressed. Mental fogginess. Dislike strangers. Shy. Hate to be touched. Scrupulously truthful. Sensitive. Anger about minor irritations. Weep profusely at music.

Profuse sweating on uncovered parts, especially on neck. Sweat oily and offensive. Eruptions on covered parts, better for scratching.

Persistently sleepless. Restless and gets out of bed. When they sleep they dream of dead people. Marked insomnia after vaccination. When they sleep after vaccination they dream of corpses and the smell of them, of falling from a great height and of body being in a vice. On waking may have a headache which is better for bending head back.

May complain that they feel thin and that their legs are delicate, as if made of glass. People who hurry, and hurry you along with them. Very chilly people – often called the cold Pulsatilla.

Tuberculinum Bovinum
Appearance can be all kinds of colourings but fairly constant are their blue sclerotics and long eyelashes. Hairy backs. Marked family history of TB. Mental restlessness and a state of dissatisfaction with everything. Desire to move about which is desire for change. Always want to do something else from what that are doing, and *long to travel*. Whatever their complaint they are better for movement. A good-tempered patient who changes to a disagreeable and easily upset adolescent. Bursts into tears continually and get very angry. Dislike of mental work and makes excuses for not working. Aversion to people. In adolescence a good remedy for headaches. Hypersensitive to thunder, storms, damp and dogs. Nearly always musical and very sensitive to it. Weeps. Queer kind of rheumatism worse in damp cold and damp heat, or change from hot to cold or cold to hot. Much worse for standing.

Repertory

CONSTITUTIONAL PRESCRIBING – APPEARANCE

Abdomen: flabby, Causticum

Acne vulgaris: pale, fat, soft, Calc. Sulph.

Adolescent remedy: blue-eyed, Calc. Phos.; dark, Calc. Phos.; fair, Calc. Phos.; long eyelashes, Calc. Phos.

Adult hand: boneless, clammy, Calc. Carb.

Adult: speech slow, Calc. Carb.

Alive: fidgety, Arsenicum Alb.; rapid walkers, Arsenicum Alb.

Ankles: puffy, Natrum Carb.; thick, Natrum Mur.

Appearance: mauvish powdered, Graphites

Asleep: tending to fall, Kali Brom.

Bends forward: Aurum Met.

Bloated: Baryta Carb.

Blotchy: bloated, Bryonia; puffy face (in acute illness), Bryonia; redness, Natrum Carb.

Bright-eyed: Apis

Children: do not play, Antimonium Crud.; lower limbs restless, Calc. Phos.; slow talking, Calc. Carb.; slow walking, Calc. Carb.; tears trickling down face, Calc. Carb.; unable to stand, Calc. Phos.

Collapsed: pale child, dusky, twitching, Aethusa

Colour: high, Lachesis

Cracks: around nose, thick-coated white tongue, Antimonium Crud.

Cyanotic: (acute type), Kali Iod.; in old men, Aesculus

Damp: and warm to touch, Baryta Mur.; face cold, Calc. Phos.; feet, Calc. Phos.; hands, Calc. Phos.; sweating of head, Apis

Dark: Nux Vom.; brown pigmentation, Nitric Acid.; fair-haired, reddish tint, Phosphorus; fine skin, Phosphorus; rings round eyes, Nitric Acid; tender hands, Phosphorus; thin, Nitric Acid

Delicate-looking: greyish colour, Causticum; pale, Causticum; warty growths round eyes, Causticum

Drowsiness: Terebinthina

Dull: heavy eyes, sullen face, Baptisia

Expression: melancholic, Plumbum Met.; of anxiety, Plumbum Met.; sickly, Berberis; fine, Causticum; pale, Graphites

Eyelids: drooping, Graphites

Eyes: rings round, Antimonium Crud.

Face: ashy, Bromium; depressed, Bromium; large, Calc. Carb., Graphites; pale grey, Bromium; red, Baryta Mur.; sallow lined, Nux

Vom.; fair, Kali Brom.

Fair-haired: Thuja

Fair-skinned: well covered, Pulsatilla; with sweating on uncovered parts, Thuja

Fair: Kali Bich, Nux Vom.

Falls: forward, Causticum; sideways, Causticum

Fat: Kali Bich, Natrum Sulph.; flabby, Calc. Carb.; in old men, Aesculus

Fatter than one would expect: Kali Iod.

Feet: hot, Sulphur; irritation of, Aloes; thick, Natrum Mur.

Flabby: Antimonium Crud.

Fleshy: Natrum Carb.

Flush, malar, when excited: Natrum Mur.

Flushed: Kali Iod.; puffy face, Apis

Footsweat: offensive, Aconite, Silicea

Hair: darker, Kali Bich.; falling out, Cantharis; fine, Arsenicum Alb.; greasy, Medusa; greasy-looking, Natrum Mur.; mouse-coloured, Silicea

Hands: fine, Causticum; hot, Sulphur; red, Lachesis; tremulous, Lachesis

Height above average: Kali Bich.

Large: with fattish features, Graphites; head, Calc. Carb.; head, Graphites

Lethargic: Calc. Carb., Kali Brom.

Limbs: weak, Natrum Phos.; worse right side, Natrum Phos.

Lips: dry, Baryta Mur., Berberis

Livery patient: Chelidonium

Looks: drugged, Bryonia; half-intoxicated, Terebinthina; older than they are, Sulphur; unhappy and sunken, Cantharis; unhealthy, Sulphur

Mouth symptoms: Baryta Mur.

Muscularly strong: Kali Bich.

Pains: from left to right, Terebinthina; radiate from one spot, Berberis

Pale: Baryta Carb., Calc. Carb., Natrum Carb.; bluish pallor, Antimonium Crud.; delicate-looking, Antimonium Crud.; flabby, Antimonium Crud.; mucous membranes, Graphites; sunken face, Arsenicum Alb.; unhealthy skin, Calc. Sulph.

Perspire: do not, Phosphorus

Physical strength, lacks: Calc. Sulph.

Physical weakness: Natrum Ars.

Prostration with weakness: Bromium

Puffiness: generalised, Kali Bich.

Pupils: dilated, Plumbum Met.

Restless: Aconite

Restlessness: of feet, Kali Brom.

311

Saliva: frothy and sticky, Berberis
Sclerotics, blue: hairy hands, long eyelashes, Tub. Bov.
Sclerotics, yellow: Plumbum Met.
Short-necked: in old men, Aesculus
Skin: brownish, Medusa; clammy, Baptisia; coarse, with cracks,
    Arsenicum Alb.; dingy hue, Plumbum Met.; dusky, Aloes; eruptions,
    Natrum Sulph.; fine, with tendency to sweat, Arsenicum Alb.; florid,
    Natrum Sulph.; greasy, Natrum Sulph.; hot, Baptisia; hot dry, Aloes;
    moist, Baptisia; pale greyish tint, Aluminium Met.; sallow, Medusa,
    Natrum Mur., Plumbum Met.; scaly, Sulphur; unhealthy-looking,
    Sulphur
Sluggish: Kali Bich.
Soft-looking: Baryta Carb.
Spruce: Nux Vom.
Stagger: tendency to, Kali Phos.
Stooping: Sulphur
Sweat: offensive, Baryta Carb., Sulphur; tendency to, Arsenicum Alb.
Sweating: occipital hairline, Graphites; offensive (in acute illness),
    Baptisia; on face, Bromium; on side of nose, Graphites; round head at
    night, Calc. Carb.; usually after midnight, Berberis; wetness behind
    ears, Graphites; without heat, Calc. Carb.
Taciturn: wants to be alone, Chelidonium
Thighs, fat: Natrum Mur.
Thin build: Arsenicum Alb.
Thin: pale-skinned, Kali Phos.
Tongue: bright red, Sulphur; smooth glossy, Terebinthina
Tremulousness: Aconite
Undersized: Natrum Sulph., Silicea
Underweight: Sulphur
Untidy: Sulphur
Venous engorgement: Lachesis
Weakness in physique: Silicea
Weary-looking: Nux Vom.

CONSTITUTIONAL PRESCRIBING – MIND

Affectionate: Pulsatilla
Alone: does not like being left, Lycopodium; hates to be, Pulsatilla
Annoyance: may have urge to kill, Hepar Sulph.
Anticipation: Chelidonium
Anxiety: neurasthenic, Kali Phos.; with acute condition, Cantharis; with
    restlessness, suicidal thoughts, Arsenicum Alb.

Anxious: Kali Sulph.

Apprehension before examinations: Lycopodium

Atmosphere: sensitive to, Phosphorus

Attention, must have loving: Pulsatilla

Case-history, never gives in one go: Medusa

Changeable: Pulsatilla

Changed surroundings give temporary relief: Hepar Sulph.

Children: kick, do damage, Hepar Sulph.; peevish, whining, Aluminium Ox.

Confused, may easily become: Aluminium Ox.

Contented, alert, confident: Aluminium Ox.

Contradiction, cannot bear: Lycopodium

Contradictory, changeable, dejection: Berberis

Courageous: Opium; with great capacity for work, Silicea

Criticises people not present: Natrum Phos.

Cry, finds it difficult to: Aurum Met.

Depressed: Aesculus; Kali Sulph.; when constipated, Ferrum Met.

Depression: due to exertion, China; without irritability, Squid

Despairs about health: Nitric Acid

Difficulty in thinking: Berberis

Dislike: of life, Kali Phos.; of people, Natrum Mur.; of strangers, of being touched, Thuja

Disorientated: Hepar Sulph.

Dissatisfaction with everything: Tub. Bov.

Distressed about everything: Calc. Phos.

Dull, mentally: Merc. Cy.

Evil, fears: Natrum Ars.

Exacting, sense of own importance: Lilium Tig.

Fastidious: Arsenicum Alb.

Fatigue, mental: Lycopodium

Fault, easily finds: Arsenicum Alb.

Fear: of death, Arsenicum Alb., Kali Carb., Opium; of disasters, impending, Natrum Ars.; of future, Kali Carb.; of outside, open spaces, Kali Phos.; of poverty, Kali Carb.

Feelings, unusual: Sabal Serr.

Friendship, can suddenly terminate: Natrum Mur.

Grandeur, delusions of: Sulphur

Head: feeling of cap on, Berberis; feeling of tight band around, Terebinthina

Heat: dislikes, Pulsatilla; on upper part of body, Berberis

Hopeless: Natrum Phos.

Hopeless rather than melancholic: Chelidonium

Hyperaesthetic: China
Indecision, mental work excites: Graphites
Indifferent: dreads to be alone, Sepia; to family when ill, Phosphorus; to loved ones, Lilium Tig.
Insanity, fears of: Lilium Tig.
Insolent: Cantharis
Instability: Natrum Mur.
Insult, capacity for remembering: Natrum Mur.
Intelligent: Arsenicum Alb.
Irritable: Calc. Phos., Nitric Acid; can react with palpitation, Natrum Mur.; when annoyed becomes tremulous, Kali Phos.
Jealous: Kali Carb., Lachesis
Lacks 'stuffing': Calc. Carb.
Laughs without sense of humour: Natrum Mur.
Legs feel as if made of glass: Thuja
Loquacity: Lachesis
Malicious: Lachesis
Melancholia: Natrum Mur.; brooding, Aurum Met.; self-pity, Calc. Carb.; tears dribble down, Calc. Carb.
Memory, poor: Calc. Carb.
Menopausal patients: Squid
Mental effort, incapable of: Calc. Carb.
Miserly: Kali Carb.
Muddle-headed after eating: Aesculus
Music: sensitive to, Tub. Bov.; weeps profusely at, Thuja
Nervous: restless, twitching of shoulders, face, Natrum Ars.
Noise, sensitive to: Kali Carb.
Obstinate: Nitric Acid
Overconscientious: Natrum Ars.
Overexcitable: Natrum Mur.
Oversensitive: Arsenicum Alb.
Pain, sensitive to: Nitric Acid
Peevish: conditions never right, flies into rage, Nux Vom.
Peevishness alternating with gaiety: Causticum
Pelvic organs feel as if going to fall out: Sepia
Remembering, difficulty with: Sulphur
Resentful: against fate, Sepia; if not getting attention, Natrum Mur.
Resents friends: Medusa
Restless: Natrum Phos.
School: dreads going to, Lycopodium; reticent as schoolboy, Lycopodium
Secretive: Hepar Sulph.
Selfish: Sulphur

Sensitive: to criticism, cruelty, injustice, Calc. Carb.; to noise, Ferrum Met.

Sleep, late in falling to: Calc. Carb.

Stupor, eyes open, red face: Opium

Suspicious: Lachesis, Merc. Cy.; that people stop them doing things, China

Sympathetic: good opinion of themselves, Causticum; nervous laugh, Causticum

Sympathy, angry at: Sabal Serr.

Talk, must have time to: Sabal Serr.

Talks at terrific rate: Merc. Sol.

Tearful: Pulsatilla

Temper bad, when helped: Lilium Tig.

Terrified in crowded room: Phosphorus

Thunderstorms, hypersensitive to: Tub. Bov.

Timid: Kali Sulph.; fears something is going to happen, Causticum

Tinkling in ears: Terebinthina

Tired: craves company when, Phosphorus; mentally, Calc. Phos.; of life, Sulphur; weeps and feels better, Sepia

Tiredness, anxious with: Kali Sulph.

Travel, longs to: Tub. Bov.

Tremulous: Merc. Cy.

Voice, thinks something is queer about it: Terebinthina

Weepy: unstable, upset by advice, Ferrum Met.

Worries: about imaginary diseases, Arsenicum Alb.; repetitive, Calc. Carb.; sensitive to music, Graphites; with feeling of cobweb over face, Graphites

Worry, concentrates on one particular: Chelidonium

Yellow, everything looks: Cantharis

EMERGENCY REMEDIES

Appendix: Arnica, Crotalus Horr., Rhus Tox.

Boils: Calc. Sulph., constitutional remedy, Hepar Sulph., Kali Bich., Pyrogen, Silicea, Tuberculinum

Bruises: Arnica

Carbuncle: Anthracinum, Arsenicum Alb., Rhus Tox., Tarentula

Cellulitis: Pyrogen, Rhus Tox., Snake venoms

Cerebrovascular accident: Opium

Empyema: Pyrogen

Fractures: Arnica, Hypericum, Rhus Tox.; comminuted, Hypericum

Gallbladder, pre- or post-operative: Phosphorus

Gastroenterostomy: Carbo Veg.
Glandular tissue: Bellis Per., Conium
Ileus, paralytic: Carbo Veg.
Injuries: to head, Arnica, Calendula, Cicuta, Helleborus Nig.,
    Hypericum, Natrum Sulph., Opium, Pyrogen; to joint, Bryonia,
    Strontium Carb.; round coccyx, Hypericum
Mastoid infection: Capsicum
Pre- and post-operative: Aconite, Argentum Nit., Ignatia
Sensitive tissue damage: Hypericum
Shock: Aconite, Natrum Mur.
Sprains: Arnica, Hypericum, Rhus Tox.
Tetanus: prophylactic for, Hypericum
Tonsil: operation, Arnica, Merc. Sol., Rhus Tox.
Ulceration: Calendula, Carbo Veg., Kali Bich., Lycopodium, Merc. Sol.
Weakness: Calc. Carb., constitutional remedy, Rhus Tox.
Wounds: lacerated, Calendula; penetrating, Ledum

DEPRESSION – GENERAL

Anger: attacks of, Sepia
Annoyance: causes, Lilium Tig.
Anxiety: at night, Pulsatilla
Appearance: heavy and dull, Calc. Carb.
Apprehension: Natrum Ars.
Arrogant: Platina
Broken-down person: Cinchona
Broods: Aurum Met.; over stupid things, Calc. Carb.
Changeable: Pulsatilla
Cold: sensitive to, Ferrum Met.
Colour: dusky, Aurum Met.
Concentrate, cannot: Pulsatilla
Confidence: lack of, Kali Sulph.
Consolation: bad-tempered when given, Lilium Tig.
Cry easily: Pulsatilla
Depressed: Aesculus, Antimonium Crud., Guaiacum, Kali Sulph.,
    Crotalus Horr.
Depression: Lilium Tig.; acute, Calc. Carb.; concentrates on worry,
    Chelidonium; misery increases, Cinchona; no real substance behind,
    Ferrum Met.
Despondent: Chelidonium
Die: think they are going to, Platina
Disturbed, cannot bear being: Chelidonium

316

Envious: Sepia
Exertion: overheated by, Graphites
Expressing themselves, difficulty in: Calc. Carb.
Falls: to left side, Aurum Met.
Fear: of death, Arsenicum Alb.; of failure, Platinum; of going insane, Calc. Carb.; of poverty, Psorinum, Sepia
Fears: full of, Platinum
Fears worst is going to happen: Sepia
Fuddled: Crotalus Horr.
Helpless: Chelidonium
Hopeless: Psorinum
Hopelessness: Calc. Carb.
Ignored: hates being, Natrum salts
Ill-humoured: Pulsatilla
Illness: thinks it will kill him, Graphites
Indecision: runs through remedy, Graphites
Interest: makes himself centre of, Natrum salts
Irritable: Ferrum Met., Lilium Tig., Pulsatilla
Life: cannot cope with, Chelidonium; disgust of, Aurum Met.
Melancholia: Aurum Met., Calc. Carb.
Mental dejection: Berberis
Mental effort: incapable of making, Calc. Carb.
Mind: cannot make up, Graphites
Opposition: upset by, Ferrum Met.
Overtired: Sepia
Pain: gallbladder, Chelidonium; over liver, Chelidonium
Relied upon, likes to feel: Lilium Tig.
Resents: job, Sepia
Responsibility: sense of, Sepia
Restless: Platina
Restlessness associated with depression: Arsenicum Alb.
Sad: more than depressed, Graphites
Self-esteem: excessive, Platina
Self-respect: lack of, Psorinum
Sense of humour: absent, Natrum salts
Sensitive to: music, Natrum Carb.
Silence: wants absolute, Aurum Met.
Spiteful: Sepia
Suicidal: Aurum Met.
Suicide: not likely to commit, Calc. Carb.
Sweats: profusely in cold room, Calc. Carb.
Sympathy: does not want, Natrum Mur.

Tears: drip silently, Calc. Carb.
Tremulous: Pulsatilla
Upset: if told to pull themselves together, Calc. Carb.
Vertigo: bouts of, Aurum Met.; turning head suddenly <, Calc. Carb.
Violence (in acute condition): Arsenicum Alb.
Wakes: after being asleep for a short time, Pulsatilla
Weep: tends to, Chelidonium
Weepy: Crotalus Horr.
Work: dread of having to, Cinchona
Worry: from prolonged illness, Cinchona

DEPRESSION – AGGRAVATION

Aggravation: Lilium Tig.
Evening: Lilium Tig.
Heat: Lilium Tig.
Midnight to 1 a.m.: Arsenicum Alb.
Music: Graphites
Night: Lilium Tig.
Noise: Sepia

DEPRESSION – AMELIORATION

Evening: Graphites
Food: Graphites
Warmth: Graphites

HEADACHE, ACUTE – GENERAL

Aching: dull frontal, Bryonia
Adolescent: Calc. Phos.
Bad as you can get: Sanguinaria
Bilious: Silicea
Congestion: Apis
Constipated: Nux Vom.
Coryza: Bryonia
Dampness: on forehead, Apis; of head, Chininum Sulph.
Deep: Mag. Phos.
Excitement: associated with emotion, Apis
Eyes: does not want to keep closed, Theridion; pain on opening, Bryonia; tired, Natrum Mur.
Flatulence: Chininum Sulph.

Giddiness: < closing eyes, Theridion
Hair: sensitive to touch, Bryonia
Head: dampness around, Apis; pulsation in, Belladonna; wants to keep high, Belladonna; whole is sore, Apis
Headache: dull frontal, Bryonia; extends over occiput, Bryonia
Hypersensitive: to noise, which can make sick, Theridion
Menopause: Theridion
Menses: accompanies suppressed, Apis; after, Natrum Mur.; before, Natrum Mur.
Menstrual: Belladonna
Nasal: catarrh, Bryonia
Nausea: Silicea
Neuralgia: along superficial nerves, Mag. Phos.
Ocular disturbances: Gelsemium
Pain: boring over right eye, Gelsemium; goes on throbbing, Apis; stabbing, Apis; stabbing of sudden onset, Apis
Periodic: Gelsemium
Photophobia: Natrum Mur.; < stooping, Belladonna
Puberty: Theridion
Pulsating: Belladonna
Recurring: Gelsemium; Silicea
Scalp: tender, Apis
Skull: feels tight, Apis
Sneezing: Bryonia
Tenderness: over forehead < motion, Bryonia; over forehead > pressure, Bryonia; over forehead when cold, Bryonia; over head, Bryonia
Throbbing: Belladonna
Urine: increased quantity (with relief), Gelsemium; secretion pale during (no relief), Lac Def.
Vertigo: on rising, Bryonia
Vision: disturbed beforehand, Iris; sees colours, Glonoinum
Vomiting: Arsenicum Alb.; Silica

HEADACHE, ACUTE – AGGRAVATION

Blankets: too many on bed, Belladonna
Cold: Mag. Phos.; windy, Iris
Draught: Silicea
Eating: sweet things, Iris
Everything: Cocculus
Excitement: Apis
Exertion, vigorous: Iris, Silicea

Eyes: using, Natrum Mur.
Head: turning, Chininum Sulph.
Heat: Apis; followed by cold wind, Belladonna
Hyperaesthesia: Apis
Keeping still: Iris
Light: Gelsemium
Lying down, when first: Gelsemium
Menses: Natrum Mur.
Mental excitement: Nux Vom.
Motion: Gelsemium; jarring, Glonoinum; stooping, Glonoinum
Movement: Apis, Silicea; head low, Belladonna; in open air, Chininum Sulph.; of eyes, Belladonna, Chininum Sulph.; stooping, Belladonna
Neuralgic type: movement, Bryonia
Pressure: Silicea
Thunder: Natrum Mur.
Tobacco: Natrum Mur.
Wine, sour: Natrum Mur.
Work: Nux Vom.

HEADACHE, ACUTE – AMELIORATION

Cold air: Glonoinum
Cold applications: Bryonia, Glonoinum
Cold water: bathing in, Calc. Phos.
Cold: Chininum Sulph.
Fresh air: Iris
Leaning back: Belladonna
Lying down: Kali Sulph.; in silent room, Theridion
Moving about: Iris
Open air: Kali Sulph.
Pressure: Apis, Kali Sulph.; over arteries, Chininum Sulph.; firm, Mag. Phos.
Sitting holding head: Glonoinum
Sitting up: Chininum Sulph.
Sleep: Gelsemium, Glonoinum
Standing: Chininum Sulph.
Sunset: Glonoinum
Vomiting: Gelsemium
Walking about gently in open air: Iris
Warmth: Mag. Phos.

HEADACHE, ACUTE – APPEARANCE

Complexion: greyish, Mag. Phos.

Congested: Apis
Eyes: rings under, Mag. Phos.
Face: hot, Kali Sulph.; intense dusky redness, Glonoinum
Head: keeps up, Silicea
Heavy appearance: Gelsemium
Lies on hot bottle: Silicea
Puffy: Apis
Sick: looks as if could be, Chininum Sulph.
Sits holding head so that it will not move: Glonoinum
Slightly flushed: Gelsemium
Swollen: Apis
Tired broken-down patient, Mag. Phos.
Vessels pulsate on affected site: Glonoinum

HEADACHE, ACUTE – CAUSATION

Acute illness: Gelsemium
Alcoholic: Nux Vomica
Cold: Belladonna, Calc. Carb., Calc. Phos., Mag. Phos.
Coryza, acute: Bryonia
Dietary over-indulgence: Pulsatilla
Digestive: Chininum Sulph., Pulsatilla
Eating sweets: Argentum Nit.
Emotional cause: Belladonna
Excitement: Argentum Nit., Natrum Mur.
Eyestrain: Natrum Mur.
Hair: not drying, Belladonna; washing, Belladonna
Heat: Calc. Carb., Sepia
Influenza: Gelsemium
Jar: Calc. Phos.
Journey, after: Argentum Nit.
Menstrual period: irregular, Apis; suppressed, Apis
Mental application: Calc. Phos.
Mental exertion: Natrum Mur.
Nervous strain: Cocculus, Mag. Phos.
Overwork: Argentum Nit., Cocculus
Railway journey: Natrum Mur.
Shock: Belladonna
Sun: Aurum Met., Belladonna, Glonoinum, Natrum Mur.
Theatre: Natrum Mur.
Tight hat: Calc. Phos.

HEADACHE, ACUTE – SENSATIONS AS IF

Extremities: coldness in, Bryonia
Hair: smarting at root of, Calc. Phos.
Head: everything falling out on stooping, Bryonia; heat in, Bryonia; vice at back, Calc. Phos.
Heat: Calc. Phos.
Occiput, ice lying over back of: Calc. Phos.

HEADACHE, ACUTE – SITE

Back: Mag. Phos.
Eye: right, Silicea
Eyes: back of, spreading deep into brain, Theridion; over, Kali Sulph.
Frontal: Silicea
Head: Silicea; spreading all over, Mag. Phos.; spreads over, < right side, Kali Sulph.
Neck: back of, to forehead, Chininum Sulph.
Occiput: Silicea; begins in, spreads over head, settles in right eye, Sanguinaria
Right-sided: Iris
Spine: down, Silicea

HEADACHE, ACUTE – TIME

10 a.m.–midday <, 3–4 p.m.: Natrum Mur.
Afternoon: Belladonna
Early in day until going to bed: Gelsemium
Lasts all day: Bryonia
Lasts all night: Belladonna
Morning: Bryonia; < as day goes on, Sanguinaria
Wakes up with it in the morning: Natrum Mur.

HEADACHE, CHRONIC – GENERAL

Burning: Arsenicum Alb.
Cold extremities: Lachesis
Comes on gradually: Argentum Nit.
Congestion: Psorinum
Constipation: accompanied by, Aluminum Met.; associated with, Aurum Met.
Gastric association: Calc. Carb.
Giddiness: on standing, Cedron

Hair: tender to touch, Chininum Sulph.
Head: stiffness at back of, Argentum Nit.
Heavy: Aluminium Met.
Hunger: intense, Psorinum
Nausea: Argentum Nit.; Lac Def.
Pain: comes on gradually, Argentum Nit.; starts with feeling of tension, Argentum Nit.; suddenly goes off, Argentum Nit.
Periodicity, marked: Arsenicum Alb.
Photophobia: Natrum Mur.; marked, Pulsatilla
Pulsating: Lachesis
Recurring: Aluminium Met.; regularly, Cedron; whenever constipated, Aluminium Met.
Scalp, superficial tenderness of: Argentum Nit.
Sensory disturbance: vertical half-blindness, Silicea
Soreness: Argentum Nit.
Suddenly gone: Argentum Nit.
Throbbing: Aluminium Met., Lachesis; intense, Arsenicum Alb.
Urine, pale during headache (no relief of pain): Lac Def.
Vomiting: Arsenicum Alb.

HEADACHE, CHRONIC – AGGRAVATION

Alcohol: Calc. Carb.
Cold: draught in open air, Chininum Sulph.; fresh air, Psorinum
Exertion: Argentum Nit.
Funny (unpleasant) sounds: Aurum Met.
Light: Calc. Carb.; Kali Bich.; Lac Def.
Lying: down, Pulsatilla; lounging, Chininum Sulph.
Lying: with head low, Natrum Mur.
Mental concentration: Silicea
Motion: Argentum Nit., Calc. Carb., Cocculus, Lac Def., Lachesis, Natrum Mur.; using eyes, Natrum Mur.; walking far in open air, Calc. Carb.
Noise: Aurum Met., Kali Bich., Lac Def., Nitric Acid.
Pressure: Silicea; soreness on surface of cranium, Aurum Met.
Seaside: Natrum Mur.
Sleep: Cocculus, Lachesis
Smell: of cooking, of food, of tobacco, Arsenicum Alb.
Smells: Aurum Met.
Stimulants: particularly coffee, Cocculus
Stooping: Calc. Carb., Lachesis, Pulsatilla
Stuffy atmosphere: Pulsatilla

Talking, effort of: Argentum Nit.
Touch: Aurum Met.; pressure, Arsenicum Alb.
Using eyes: Argentum Nit., Cocculus, Natrum Mur.
Walking: Calc. Carb.
Warmth: Natrum Mur.

HEADACHE, CHRONIC – AMELIORATION

Cold application (early in attack): Arsenicum Alb.
Drinks, hot: Kali Bich.
Evening: Kali Bich.
Eyes: closed, Calc. Carb.; keeping open, Chininum Sulph.
Food: Lachesis
Fresh air: Argentum Nit.
Icy cold applications: Aluminium Ox.
Lying down: Aluminium Ox., Calc. Carb., Kali Bich.
Open air: Natrum Mur.
Pressure: Argentum Nit., Kali Bich., Lac Def., Pulsatilla; over arteries, Chininum Sulph.
Sitting up: Chininum Sulph.
Sleep: Calc. Carb.
Standing: Chininum Sulph.
Walking: Pulsatilla; in open air, Aluminium Ox.
Warmth: Mag. Phos.

HEADACHE, CHRONIC – APPEARANCE

Bloated: Lachesis
Dull: Aurum Met.
Eyes: sits with them shut, Calc. Carb.
Flush: on cheek, same side, Pulsatilla
Flushed: Aurum Met.
Gloomy: Aurum Met.

HEADACHE, CHRONIC – CAUSATION

Cold: Silicea
Excitement: Argentum Nit.
Fatigue: Silicea
Food/drink, too much: Calc. Carb.
Gastric disturbance: Chininum Sulph.
Heat/cold, exposure to: Calc. Carb.

Menopausal: Lachesis
Menstruation, associated with: Sepia
Mental overwork: Argentum Nit.
Nausea: Chininum Sulph.
Sun: Silicea
Vomiting: Chininum Sulph.

HEADACHE, CHRONIC – DESIRES

Somebody to talk to: Argentum Nit.
Sweets: Argentum Nit.

HEADACHE, CHRONIC – SENSATIONS AS IF

Brain, soreness in: Argentum Nit.
Cranium, soreness on surface: Aurum Met.
Eyes, sand in, with lacrimation: Aurum Met.
Head is drawn back: Argentum Nit.
Temporal arteries would burst: Chininum Sulph.
Tension, stiffness: soreness at back of head, soreness at back of neck, Argentum Nit.

HEADACHE, CHRONIC – SITE

All over: Lachesis
Forehead: Arsenicum Alb.; shoots from one temple to other, Cedron
Head: Arsenicum Alb.
Left side: Bryonia
Nose: root of, Arsenicum Alb.
Occiput: all over head, Natrum Mur.; spreads over head, Sepia
Temple: pain beating over right, Calc. Carb.; spreads all over but becomes localised left, Argentum Nit.
Temples: Chininum Sulph.; pain with headache all over, Pulsatilla

HEADACHE, CHRONIC – TIME

1–2 a.m./p.m.: Arsenicum Alb.
9–11 a.m./4–8 p.m. <: Mag. Sulph.
11 a.m.–all day and night, into following night: Cedron
3–4 p.m.: Natrum Mur.
Day: Kali Bich.
Early morning till 2-3 p.m.: Chininum Sulph.

Early morning: Kali Bich.
Evening: Kali Bich.
Night, 1 a.m. to noon: Chininum Sulph.
Noon: Argentum Nit.
Summer: midday, Glonoinum

HEADACHE, CHRONIC – VISION

Disturbance: eye, flickering, specks in front of, Psorinum; ocular, Cedron
Eyes: agglutinated in morning, Aurum Met.; zigzag in front of, Natrum Mur.
Sight: distortion of, Aurum Met.
Vision: dimness of, Kali Bich., Psorinum; disturbance of, before headache, Kali Bich.; loss of, Kali Bich., before pain, Lac Def.; upper half of, impaired, Aurum Met.

EYES

Blindness: Gelsemium
Burning sensation accompanied by dryness: Belladonna
Cheeks, condition spreads into: Rhus Tox.
Cold: < bathing, Rhus Tox.; sensitive to air, Aconite; water, Apis
Colour, disturbance in: Glonoinum
Conjunctivae, puffy: Hepar Sulph.
Conjunctivitis: catarrhal, Euphrasia, Pulsatilla; congestion of right eye, Calc. Carb.; with blepharospasm, Kali Iod.
Cornea, muddy: Hepar Sulph.
Corneal ulcer, sharply defined: Kali Bich.
Diplopia: Gelsemium
Discharge: greenish-yellow, Kali Iod.; stringy, Kali Bich.; yellow, Kali Sulph.; yellow, bland, Pulsatilla
Draughts, sensitive to: Aconite
Dryness in morning: Causticum
Eruption, herpetic from cornea to eye: Rhus Tox.
Evenings: Merc. Sulph.
Eye: looks painful but not to patient, Kali Bich.; symptoms start right side, Apis
Eyelids: crusted with itching, warm room, Kali Sulph.; difficult to open, Causticum; granulated at margins, Kali Bich.; margins bleed on touching, Euphrasia; mucuous membranes like raw beef, Apis; rash with swelling, Sarsaparilla; redness round margins, Allium Cepa; swollen, Apis; swollen and red, < under upper lid, Kali Iod.

Feeling of string pulling into head: Hepar Sulph.
Grit, feeling of: Aconite
Head, pain extends into back of: Belladonna
Heat <: Merc. Sulph.
Inflammation: acute, Apis; purulent, Kali Iod.
Irritation: burning, Allium Cepa; pustular lids, Pulsatilla
Lacrimation: < burning, Apis; irritating, Euphrasia; winds, Causticum
Lashes crusted: Graphites
Onset acute: Belladonna
Open air: Allium Cepa
Pain: < evenings, < heat, Merc. Sulph.
Painful conditions: Hepar Sulph.
Pains, sudden stabbing: Apis
Photophobia: Graphites, Hepar Sulph., Kali Bich., Merc. Sulph.; < cold bathing, Rhus Tox.; < movement, Belladonna; < warmth, Argentum Nit.; inclined to close eyes, Causticum
Pupils: contracted, Belladonna; dilated, Aconite
Pus, development of: Hepar Sulph.
Swelling, red: Merc. Sulph.
Tears: irritate facial skin, Merc. Sulph.; scalding pain, Rhus Tox.
Tenderness, periorbital: Kali Iod.
Ulceration, early: Hepar Sulph.
Urge to rub: Euphrasia
Vessels: congested bright red, Apis; look dark, Euphrasia

THROATS & INFLUENZAS – GENERAL

Aching: generalised, Gelsemium, Phytolacca; in part lain on, Baptisia
Acute: almost gangrenous, Chininum Ars.; onset, Phytolacca
Anxious: Aconite, Arsenicum Alb., Psorinum
Aversion: to milk, Guaiacum
Awake: muttering until morning, Baptisia
Burning (including mouth): Apis
Cervical glands: chronic enlargement, Baryta Carb.; swollen, Apis; tender, Apis
Chilly shivering: Apis; wants to be covered up, Baryta Carb.
Cold drinks, wants: Dulcamara
Confused: Dulcamara
Coughing, paroxysm of: Causticum
Dark: Merc. Sol.
Darkish red: Phytolacca
Depressed: Guaiacum

Desire: for cold drinks, Dulcamara; for sour things, Guaiacum

Diarrhoea: collapse, Baptisia; dark, Crotalus Horr.; violent, Baptisia; vomiting, Baptisia; watery, Crotalus Horr.

Dirty: Lycopodium

Dreams of: snakes, Lac Caninum

Dry: Apis

Dryness: at back of throat, Causticum

Ear: pain radiates to, Lachesis, Nitric Acid.

Earache: Dulcamara

Ears: cracking in, eating, Baryta Carb.; cracking in, lying down, Baryta Carb.; eruptions, Lachesis

Epistaxis: Crotalus Horr.

Extremities, puffy: Crotalus Horr.

Exudate: right side, darkish red, Phytolacca; right side, whitish grey, Phytolacca; brownish, Chininum Ars.; dark, Chininum Ars.; tenacious, Dulcamara; thick yellow, Merc. Cy.; yellowish, Dulcamara

Faint on sitting up: Aconite

Fear, acute of death: Gelsemium

Feels: hopeless, very ill, Phytolacca

Feet, icy cold: Dulcamara

Fever, high: Aconite

Flushed: face, Belladonna; when lying down, Aconite

Foot sweat, offensive: Baryta Carb.

Fuddled: Crotalus Horr.

Glands: involvement of, Calc. Sulph.; swollen, Baryta Mur., Phytolacca; swollen, chronically enlarged, Baryta Carb.

Glistening and oedematous: Apis

Gums, swelling: Chininum Ars.

Heat: general burning, Dulcamara; violent, everywhere, Belladonna

Hoarseness talking: Causticum

Hot weather, always in: Bromium

Hot: Lachesis

Hypersalivation: Baryta Carb.

Hypersensitive people: Hepar Sulph.

Illest of all: Phytolacca

Illness: acute, Baptisia

Indifferent: Phytolacca

Inflamed: Lachesis; darkish red, Belladonna

Inflammation, acute: Apis

Irritable: Chininum Ars.; Lachesis; towards evening (children), Psorinum

Melancholy: Psorinum

Move about, has to: Phytolacca

Mucus: glairy and offensive, Baptisia; in larynx, in nose, in throat, in trachea, Baryta Carb.

Muddled: Merc. Sol.

Nasal discharge, excoriating watery: Arsenicum Alb.

Neck: glands involved, Calc. Sulph.; sensitive to touch, Belladonna

Nervous: Crotalus Horr.

Oedema of uvula: Phytolacca

Oedematous: Nitric Acid.

Offensive: Merc. Cy., Merc. Sol.; mouth, Baptisia, Hepar Sulph.; urine, Nitric Acid.

Pain: acute, referred to ear, Lachesis; back of neck, Guaiacum; burning, with enlarged tonsils, Baryta Mur.; ears, Gelsemium; excrutiating, Merc. Cy., Nitric Acid.; extending into neck, Phytolacca; in spasms, Lachesis; neck, Gelsemium; on swallowing, Calc. Sulph.; outside neck, holding it, Guaiacum; radiates round neck, Merc. Sol.; radiates to ear, Nitric Acid.; redness, Gelsemium; sensitive to, Hepar Sulph.; stabbing on swallowing, Calc. Sulph.; stinging on swallowing, Apis; stitching, Lycopodium; swelling, Gelsemium; ulceration, Gelsemium; with every period, Dulcamara, Lac Caninum

Painful: congested burning, Aconite

Painless ulcers: Baptisia

Pains: come and go, Nitric Acid; shooting, on swallowing, Baryta Carb.

Patient very ill: Baptisia

Peevish: Psorinum

Perspiration smells unpleasant: Nitric Acid.

Prostration – deathly weakness: Bromium

Pulse: irregular, Chininum Sulph.; rapid, Chininum Sulph.

Purplish: Lachesis

Pus: early formation of, Hepar Sulph.; early tendency to, Merc. Sol.

Quinsy: Calc. Sulph., Hepar Sulph.; recurring, Psorinum

Recurring: infection, Hepar Sulph.

Red: Dulcamara, Merc. Sol.; bright, Apis; congested, Baryta Mur.; glistening, Apis

Redness: Psorinum

Restless: Aconite, Arsenicum Alb., Chininum Ars., Lachesis

Saliva: blood-tinged, Crotalus Horr.; greasy, Merc. Sol.; offensive, Psorinum; slimy, Merc. Sol.; stringy, Lachesis; thick, Lac Caninum; tough, Psorinum

Secretion: darkish-grey, Bromium

Shivery: Apis

Skin: dry, rough, 'nutmeg-grater', Psorinum

Snappy: Hepar Sulph.

329

Solids, difficulty in swallowing: Baptisia
Sore throat: recurrent, Baryta Carb.; at menses, Lac Caninum
Soreness over whole body: Apis
Sour taste: Lycopodium
Spasm: on swallowing, Belladonna, Gelsemium
Speech: indistinct, Merc. Cy.; makes patient wince, Belladonna; thick, Belladonna
Sputum: putrid, Arsenicum Alb.
Sudden (acute): Guaiacum
Superficial ulceration: dark red, Merc. Cy.; swollen, Merc. Cy.
Swallow: constant desire to, Belladonna; desire to, Belladonna; difficult to, Merc. Sol.; fluids with great difficulty, Baptisia
Swallows frequently: Gelsemium
Sweating: Lachesis; on face, Bromium; on face, cobweb sensation, Phytolacca
Swollen: Lachesis, Merc. Sol.; closed up, Lachesis; inside and outside, Lachesis
Taste: bitter, Chininum Ars.; horrible, Gelsemium
Thirst: for cold drinks, Chininum Ars., Merc. Sol.; and fruit, Calc. Sulph.; for lemon juice, Belladonna; for water, Guaiacum; intense, Aconite; with aversion for food, Baryta Mur.; with dry lips, Baryta Mur.
Thirstless: Gelsemium, Pulsatilla; always, Nitric Acid.; throat, purplish swollen, Baptisia
Tight: cannot bear anything, Apis, Lachesis
Tongue: blisters, Baryta Carb.; bright, fiery red, Crotalus Horr.; coated, Hepar Sulph.; coated, putty-coloured, Lycopodium; coated, yellow, Nitric Acid.; dry, Aconite, Hepar Sulph., Lycopodium; dry, red streak down centre, Baryta Carb.; dry, swollen, Pulsatilla; dry, swollen base, Calc. Sulph.; greasy, Pulsatilla; mouth offensive, Merc. Cy.; red, Aconite; salivation, Baryta Carb.; slimy, Merc. Cy.; strawberry, Belladonna; swollen, Lycopodium; thick, yellow, slimy, Chininum Ars.; white, Merc. Cy.; yellow, Calc. Sulph., Merc. Cy., Pulsatilla; yellow streak down centre, Phytolacca
Tremulous: Lachesis
Trying to clear: Chininum Ars.
Ulceration: corner of lips, Hepar Sulph.; crack in centre of lips, Hepar Sulph.
Ulceration: tonsils, Calc. Sulph.
Urticaria: Dulcamara; marked, Apis
Weak: Chininum Ars.
Yellowish coating: Nitric Acid.
Yellowish: Crotalus Horr.

THROATS & INFLUENZAS – AGGRAVATION

Applications, hot: Lachesis
Chewing: Baryta Carb.
Cold: Causticum, Psorinum; drinks, Gelsemium, Lycopodium; food, Lycopodium
Draughts: Arsenicum Alb.
Empty swallowing: Baryta Carb.
Fevers at night: Nitric Acid
Food: liquid, Lachesis; solid, Apis
Heat: Bromium, Phytolacca; to throat, Calc. Sulph.; applications, drinks, Lachesis, Phytolacca; room, Apis; things, Calc. Sulph.
Movement: Aconite, Nitric Acid.
Pain: nightly, Merc. Cy.
Seat: Merc. Sol.
Sleep: Chininum Ars., Crotalus Horr., Lachesis, Lycopodium
Swallowing: Aconite, Apis, Baptisia, Lac Caninum; pain referred to neck, Baryta Mur.
Tight: anything, Lachesis
Warm food: Lachesis
Warmth (patient): Pulsatilla
Weather, changes in: Arsenicum Alb.

THROATS & INFLUENZAS – AMELIORATION

Cold: fluids, Lycopodium; water, Baryta Mur.
Hot fluids: Gelsemium
Lying: Baryta Carb.
Moving about: Dulcamara
Rain: Hepar Sulph.
Sitting up: Apis
Warmth applied to neck: Hepar Sulph.

THROATS & INFLUENZAS – APPEARANCE

Acutely ill, yellow tinge with cyanosis: Crotalus Horr.
Anxious: Gelsemium, Lycopodium
Befogged look: Baptisia
Bluish: Gelsemium
Dull: Baptisia, Gelsemium
Dusky: Baptisia
Face: ashy-pale, Bromium; congested, Belladonna, Guaiacum; grey, Bromium; pale, Apis; puffy, Apis; red, Apis, Baptisia, Guaiacum; swollen, Guaiacum

Fair: Lac Caninum
Fat: Calc. Sulph.
Feet got wet: Baryta Carb.
Flabby: Merc. Cy.
Gentle: Lac Caninum
Hands, tremor of: Phytolacca
Heavy-looking: Gelsemium
Ill – bluish: Crotalus Horr.
Pale: Calc. Sulph., Lycopodium, Merc. Cy.
Pupils, dilated: Belladonna
Soft: Calc. Sulph.
Sweating: Merc. Cy.
Worried: Lycopodium

THROATS & INFLUENZAS – CAUSATION

Catarrh, chronic postnasal: Dulcamara
Cold: spell, Hepar Sulph.; wind, Aconite
Provocation, any: Hepar Sulph.
Walked in open, got feet wet: Baryta Carb.

THROATS & INFLUENZAS – SENSATIONS AS IF

Choked: Belladonna
Choking: Calc. Sulph.
Contraction, extreme: Chininum Ars.
Eye, black: Belladonna
Face: cobweb over, Bromium, Phytolacca
Floating on air: Lac Can.
Full: Guaiacum
Fullness: Calc. Sulph.
Have to move about: Phytolacca
Lump in throat: Baryta Mur.
Numb: Gelsemium
Part of them lost: Baptisia
Plug – cannot swallow without pain: Baryta Carb.
Shut in against will: Crotalus Horr.
Spasm, going into: Crotalus Horr.
Swollen: Guaiacum, Lachesis
Throat: fishbone in, Hepar Sulph.; is closing, Aconite; on fire, Chininum Ars.
Tongue, raw, swollen: Phytolacca

Veins: boiling water flowing through, Arsenicum Alb.; ice water flowing through, Arsenicum Alb.

THROATS & INFLUENZAS – SITE

Alternating sides: Baryta Mur.
Left-sided: acute, Lachesis
Right-sided: Baryta Mur., Lycopodium, Merc. Cy.

THROATS & INFLUENZAS – TIME MODALITY

Afternoon, middle of, <: Apis

PNEUMONIA – GENERAL

Air hunger, marked: Pulsatilla
Anxious: Phosphorus
Appearance: collapsed, Sulphur; dusky, Sulphur
Breathing: difficult, Rhus Tox.; rapid, Rhus Tox.; shallow, Rhus Tox.
Cannot bear to be examined: Senega
Chest, burning pain in: Sulphur
Cough: aggravated by draught, Senega; dry, Phosphorus, Pulsatilla; irritating, Pulsatilla; short, Phosphorus; teasing, Pulsatilla
Delirium: Rhus Tox.; talks incessantly, Merc. Sol.; talks rapidly, Merc. Sol.
Delusion – going to do important work: Rhus Tox.
Either too hot or too cold: Merc. Sol.
Face: distressed-looking, Lycopodium; nose pinched, Lycopodium; pale, Lycopodium; wrinkled, Lycopodium
Faint, feels as if going to: Sulphur
Fear of thunder: Phosphorus
Head up, a little bit back on pillow: Phosphorus
Hot rawness in chest, feeling of: Pulsatilla
Illness, intense: Senega
Inspiration, catching, painful, short: Phosphorus
Lack of reaction: Sulphur
Look: chilly, collapsed, pale, Sulphur
Mouth, intense dryness: Pulsatilla
Pneumonia, viral: Pulsatilla, Rhus Tox.
Râles, unilateral, commonly right-sided: Senega
Relief from moving about: Rhus Tox.
Salivation: Merc. Sol.
Scared: Phosphorus

Sensitive: to cold air, Senega; to noise, Lycopodium
Skin: clear, dry, hot: Phosphorus; reddish flush, Phosphorus
Sleep, restless: Lycopodium
Sputum: blood-streaked, Lycopodium, Pulsatilla; bright red, Phosphorus; glairy, Senega; offensive, Merc. Sol.; purulent, Lycopodium; tough, Pulsatilla, Senega; yellow, Pulsatilla
Sweat: soaking with, Merc. Sol.; in virus infection, Lycopodium
Talk – does not want to be talked to: Lycopodium
Taste, unpleasant metallic: Rhus Tox.
Temperature, swinging: Merc. Sol.
Thirst, intense, for cold drinks: Rhus Tox.
Thirstlessness: Pulsatilla
Tightness, feeling of: Pulsatilla
Tongue: coated, Rhus Tox.; fiery red tip, Rhus Tox.; red streaks down sides, Rhus Tox.; sore, Lycopodium; white coating to, Pulsatilla
Tremor, general: Phosphorus
Wants to keep perfectly still: Senega

PNEUMONIA – AGGRAVATION

After sleep: Sulphur
Heat: Pulsatilla
Lying down, on right side: Senega

PNEUMONIA – AMELIORATION

Lying on unaffected side: Senega
Movement, gentle: Senega

PNEUMONIA – TIME MODALITIES

4–8 a.m./p.m. <: Lycopodium
Nightly <: Rhus Tox.

RESPIRATORY CONDITIONS – GENERAL

Asthma: Silicea
Autumn remedy: Rumex
Bronchitis: Silicea; summer diarrhoea, teething, Kreosotum
Bronchospasm, > lying: Calc. Phos.
Chest: much mucus, rattling, Silicea; something torn loose in, Nux Vom.; sore, Hepar Sulph.

Chills of rapid onset: Nux Vom.

Cough: barking, Rumex; choking, Calc. Sulph.; dry, Hepar Sulph., Kali Carb., Lycopodium; hacking, Kali Carb.; irritable, Rumex; little expectoration, Lycopodium; rattling, Calc. Sulph.; sporadic, Kali Carb.; suffocative, Hepar Sulph.; tickling, Causticum

Coughing (Sept.–Dec.): M.A.P.

Discharges, excoriating: Kreosotum

Dislikes being left alone: Lycopodium

Dyspnoea: < early evening, Calc. Phos.; stuffy room, Lilium Tig.

Emphysematous: Senega

Feeling of pulsation when excited: Kali Sulph.

Fingers go dead: Silicea

Hands: clammy, cold, Hepar Sulph.

Headache: fullness, Aesculus; motion, Aesculus; tension, < coughing, Aesculus

Hoarseness: Calc. Sulph., Causticum

Hot, cannot uncover without feeling chilly: Hepar Sulph.

Irritable: Lycopodium

Larynx: irritation below, Rumex; tickling in, Nux Vom.

Lips, excoriation of: Kreosotum

Lobe, right lower affected: Kali Carb.

Move, cannot without coughing: Nux Vom.

Muco-pus on waking: Kali Bich.

Music, sensitive to: Kreosotum

Nares, excoriation of: Kreosotum

Pain: in arms and legs, Hydrastis; stabbing, in chest, Kali Carb.

Patient, broken-down: Silicea

Peevish: Aesculus, Lycopodium

Phlegm: profuse, Calc. Sulph.; tough, Causticum

Râles: Kali Sulph.

Rawness, sensation of, < cold air: Rumex

Resentful: Lycopodium

Retching: Nux Vom.

Skin: damp feet, hands, Silicea

Soreness, spasmodic: Nux Vom.

Sputum: bitter, Lycopodium; offensive, Calc. Phos.; profuse on exposure to air, Hydrastis; purulent, Calc. Phos.; ropey, Hydrastis; saltish, Lycopodium; sour, Calc. Phos.; stringy, Kali Bich.; thick, Hydrastis; yellow-greenish, Kali Sulph.

Sweating at night: Drosera

Sweats without relief: Hepar Sulph.

Thirst, marked lack of: Lycopodium

Toes go dead: Silicea
Tongue: bitter taste, Kali Sulph.; brown, coated, Kreosotum; painful
vesicles which spread to lips, sore, Lycopodium; stiff, Kreosotum;
yellow, Kali Sulph.
Wheezing (Sept.–Dec.): M.A.P.
Whooping cough: Drosera

RESPIRATORY CONDITIONS – AGGRAVATION

After meal: Aesculus
Aggravation: 2–4 a.m., Kali Carb.; 2–5 a.m., Kali Bich.; 6 p.m., Hepar
Sulph.; 7 p.m.–midnight, Hepar Sulph.
Anger: Calc. Sil.
Autumn (acute conditions): Kali Bich.
Change of atmosphere: Rumex
Cold: Causticum; draughts, Silicea; drinks, Lycopodium; dry weather,
Hepar Sulph.; thundery weather, Silicea
Coughing: Rumex
Eating: Kali Sulph.
Heat: Kreosotum
Hot drinks: Kreosotum
Lying on affected side: Kali Carb.
Movement: Rumex
Right side: Kali Sulph.
Spring: Kali Bich.
Stuffy room: Aesculus

RESPIRATORY CONDITIONS – AMELIORATION

Cold: air, Kali Sulph.; draught of air, Aesculus; drinks, Kali Sulph.,
Kreosotum
Damp weather: Hepar Sulph.
Leaning forward: Kali Carb.
Open air: Kali Bich.
Rain: Causticum
Sitting up: Kali Carb.
Warm drinks: Nux Vom.
Warmth of bed: Kali Bich.

RESPIRATORY CONDITIONS – APPEARANCE

Broken-down chronic bronchitics: Hydrastis

Face: blotchy, Kreosotum; bright red, Kali Sulph.; cyanotic, Aesculus; discoloured, Kreosotum; distressed-looking, Lycopodium; fat, red, Aesculus; red, Kreosotum; wrinkled forehead; Lycopodium
Fair: Hepar Sulph.
Flushed, not usually: Lycopodium
Looks ill: Lycopodium
Miserable because of cough: Rumex
Nervous: Hepar Sulph.
Nostrils: flapping, not synchronous with heartbeat, not synchronous with respiration, Lycopodium
Pale and anaemic: Calc. Sil.
Thin: Hepar Sulph.

ASTHMA – ADULTS WITH FAMILY HISTORY

Better alone: Carbo Veg.
Chest: distended, full, Kali Sulph.
Chilly: Carbo Veg.
Hoarse: Carbo Veg.; after attacks, Kali Sulph.
Irritable: Carbo Veg.
Phlegm: sticky, thick, Kali Sulph.
Rhonchi: Kali Sulph.

ASTHMA – ADULTS WITH NO FAMILY HISTORY

Breathless, bluish-grey: Phosphorus
Chilly: Cactus
Cough, paroxysmal: Phosphorus
Fears, full of: Cactus
Irritable: Cactus
Salt, desires: Phosphorus
Skin, clear: Phosphorus
Thin: Cactus, Phosphorus
Thirsty: Phosphorus
Withered-looking: Cactus

ASTHMA – AGGRAVATION

1–3 a.m.: Cactus
Early morning: Kali Sulph.
Talking: Phosphorus

ASTHMA – IN CHILDREN

Appearance, exhausted: Tub. Bov.
Appetite, poor: Thuja
Attacks: bad, nightly, Sambucus; midnight, Tub. Bov.
Chilly: Thuja
Dyspnoea at sunset, going on into night: Thuja
Fair: Thuja
Fat: Sambucus; dislikes, Thuja
Feels heat: Tub. Bov.
Flabby: Sambucus
Following every cold: Thuja
Fond: of meat, salt, Thuja
Frightened: Thuja; easily, Sambucus
Lung, marked signs in left: Natrum Sulph.
Nasal, yellow discharge: Thuja
Pale: Sambucus, Tub. Bov.
Pink-skinned: Thuja
Râles: Tub. Bov.
Reserved: Tub. Bov.
Salt, desire for: Natrum Sulph.
Scared: Tub. Bov.
Sweat: over chest, head, Tub. Bov.
Thin: Tub. Bov.
Thirsty, seldom: Tub. Bov.
Tuberculosis on mother's side: Tub. Bov.
Warm patient: Natrum Sulph.
Weep, inclined to: Tub. Bov.

CATARRH – GENERAL

Accessory sinuses, inflammation of: Kali Iod.
Acrid watery: Kali Iod.
Copious: Rumex
Forehead, puffiness of: Kali Iod.
Headache: general, Kali Bich.
Lacrimation, intense burning: Kali Iod.
Mucus, tenacious: following exertion, Kali Carb.; yellow, < in overheated room, Kali Carb.
Nose: intense itching of, Kali Sulph.; raw, sore, Kali Iod.
Pain: boring in affected area, Kali Bich.; intense at root of tongue, Kali Bich.; very trying to the patient, Kali Bich.
Pus: Hydrastis; stringy yellow, Kali Bich.; thick, yellowish, greenish-yellow, Kali Sulph.

Tongue, ulcers at tip of: Kali Iod.
Watery, initially but later thick: Rumex
Weather, troublesome in cold and damp: Kali Bich.

CATARRH – AGGRAVATION

Weather change: Kali Carb.

CORYZA – GENERAL

Acrid: Allium Cepa, Kali Iod.
Acute, bluish: Gelsemium
Body, hot and sticky: Gelsemium
Circulation, unstable, < draughts: Gelsemium
Clear: Allium Cepa
Comes on days after exposure: Gelsemium
Conjunctivitis, acute localised: Allium Cepa
Current of air, caused by: Nux Vom.
Discharge, bland, thick, yellow: Pulsatilla
Excoriation, external nares, upper lips: Allium Cepa
Extremities, cold: Gelsemium
Eyes, as if being torn out: Allium Cepa
Headache: Nux Vom.
Lacrimation, bland, excessive: Allium Cepa
Lips, tendency to herpes on: Gelsemium
Onset, rapid: Nux Vom.
Sneezing, > warm: Gelsemium
Spine, chilliness up and down: Gelsemium
Stuffed up in warm room: Pulsatilla
Sweats easily: Nux Vom.
Watery: Kali Iod.

CORYZA – AGGRAVATION

Cold dry weather: Nux Vom.

CORYZA – AMELIORATION

Damp weather: Nux Vom.
Open air: Allium Cepa
Warm drinks: Allium Cepa

CIRCULATORY SYSTEM – AGGRAVATION

Draught: Spigelia
Drink, attempting to: Antimonium Tart., Carbo Veg.
Eat, attempting to: Carbo Veg.
Heat: Lachesis
Lying: down, Spongia; left side, Lachesis; right side, Lycopus
Movement: Spigelia
Stuffy room: Antimonium Tart.

CIRCULATORY SYSTEM – AMELIORATION

Propped up on one side: Spigelia

CIRCULATORY SYSTEM – ANGINA

Chest, tightening of: Arsenicum Alb.
Chilly: Arsenicum Alb., Spongia
Congested: Spongia
Death, afraid of: Cactus
Distress, accompanied by tremulousness: Aconite
Distressed: Arsenicum Alb.
Constriction, feeling of: Arsenicum Alb.
Fibrillation: Spigelia
Frightened: Arsenicum Alb.
Heart: feels as if getting bigger, Spongia; sensation of squeezing travels laterally, Cactus
Hot – wants air: Lilium Tig.
Irritable: Lilium Tig.
Left-sided remedy: Spongia
Lies propped up: Spigelia
Numbness: Spigelia; in fingers, Spongia
Pain: at apex to left shoulder, Spigelia; chronic, Latrodectus; down left arm, Latrodectus, Spigelia; stabbing, Spigelia; through to left axilla, Latrodectus
Pains: burning, Arsenicum Alb.
Palpitation: Spigelia
Patient, broken-down: Arsenicum Alb.
Relief in first attack: Aconite
Restless: Aconite
Terrified: Aconite
Unreasonable: Lilium Tig.
Waxy: Arsenicum Alb.
Weak: Lilium Tig.

Woman's remedy: Lilium Tig.
Wrinkled: Arsenicum Alb.

CIRCULATORY SYSTEM – CARDIAC FAILURE, ACUTE

Air hunger, acute: Carbo Veg.
Air, feels cannot get enough into lungs: Arsenicum Alb.
Anxiety: Arsenicum Alb.
Appearance, dusky, sooty, sunken: Antimonium Tart.
Bed, wants to spring out of: Arsenicum Alb.
Clammy: Carbo Veg.
Cold: Carbo Veg.
Face, pale: Carbo Veg.
Fear: Arsenicum Alb.
Feeling: cold, Arsenicum Alb.; of chest contraction, chest oppression, Arsenicum Alb.; of fullness in chest, Antimonium Tart.
Fingernails, bluish: Antimonium Tart.
Hopeless: Antimonium Tart.
Keeps deathly still: Antimonium Tart.
Lips: pale, Carbo Veg.; pinched, wrinkled and grey, Arsenicum Alb.
Lungs, oedema of: Antimonium Tart.
Mental distress: Arsenicum Alb.
Mentally worn out: Carbo Veg.
Miserable: Antimonium Tart.
Nose, icy cold: Carbo Veg.
Physically worn out: Carbo Veg.
Râles, marked: Antimonium Tart.
Restlessness: Arsenicum Alb.
Sweating: Arsenicum Alb.
Tongue, coated white, thick: Antimonium Tart.
Water, constant thirst for small sips of: Arsenicum Alb.

CIRCULATORY SYSTEM – CARDIAC FAILURE OF SLOW ONSET

Blue: Laurocerasus
Breathless, intensely: Laurocerasus
Chest: feeling of intense activity in, Lycopus; sense of constriction in, Lachesis
Cough, with throbbing in head, neck: Lycopus
Disease, aortic, mitral: Lycopus
Dyspnoea after exertion: Laurocerasus
Food, desire for: Lycopus
Hands, swelling of: Naja

341

Head, throbbing in: Lycopus
Heart irregular, slow: Laurocerasus
Heat, cannot stand: Lachesis
Neck, throbbing in: Lycopus
Numbness: Laurocerasus; in left arm, Lachesis
Pain: in precordium, Laurocerasus; stabbing to scapula, Naja
Pale: Lycopus
Patient, purplish-coloured: Lachesis
Pressure, cannot stand: Lachesis
Pulse, irregular: Lycopus
Suspicious: Lachesis

INTESTINAL TRACT – GENERAL

Alone, fear of being: Kali Carb.
Blown out, feels after meal: Lycopodium
Chilly, intensely: Kali Carb.
Colic: gallbladder, Kali Carb.; hepatic, Nux Vom.; intestinal, Kali Carb.
Colon, congested, stagnant: Natrum Sulph.
Cooking, loathes smell of: Arsenicum Alb.
Digestive: difficulties, Lycopodium; disturbance, Kali Phos.
Dysphagia: catarrhal, Kali Bich.; choking, Nitricum Acid.; sticking pain, Nitricum Acid.
Eater, fast: Cuprum Met.
Epigastric discomfort: Sulphur
Feeling: of emptiness, Kali Carb.; of emptiness after defaecation, Natrum Phos.; of emptiness without hunger, Natrum Ars.; of fullness after a few mouthfuls, Lycopodium; of weight in right costal margin, Natrum Sulph.; of weight in stomach after food, Kali Bich.
Flatulence: Chininum Sulph., Kali Bich.; in bowels, Natrum Carb.; distention after food, Kali Carb.; marked eructations, Argentum Nit.; much, Kali Phos.
Food, distress after: Sarsaparilla
Fruit, intolerance of: Natrum Ars.
Gastric: trouble, Natrum Ars.; upset, Nux Vom.
Gastritis – acute ulcer: Kali Bich.
Greedy without appetite: Cuprum Met.
Hungry: Sulphur; empty sinking feeling mid-morning, Natrum Mur.
Hypersensitive: cooking, Sepia; hot drinks, Natrum Ars.; tobacco, Sepia
Indecision runs through remedy: Graphites
Intercourse, prostration after: Kali Carb.
Internal chilliness: Kali Carb.
Liver area, dragging sensation in: Natrum Sulph.

342

Mealtime, cannot go beyond: Lycopodium

Milk, intolerance of: Aethusa

Nausea: intense, Antimonium Crud.; vomiting, Kali Bich.; vomiting, > cold water, Cuprum Met.; without vomiting, Argentum Nit.

Pain: burning, Natrum Ars.

Regurgitation, in oesophagus: Nux Vom.

Secretions, acrid: Arsenicum Alb.

Sensation: blood flowing from feet, Graphites; stone in stomach after meal, Nux Vom.

Sickness, intense: Aethusa

Stomach, tender: Natrum Sulph.

Swallowing, disturbance in power of: Nux Vom.

Sweat, offensive: Graphites

Sweating after eating: Kali Phos.

Taste: horrible, Aconite; metallic, > cold water, Cuprum Met.; sweet, Nitric Acid.

Thirst: for cold drinks, Natrum Ars., Natrum Carb., Natrum Sulph.; for cold water, Cuprum Met.; for sour liquids, Kali Carb.; great, Cuprum Met.

Thirstiest of remedies: Phosphorus

Tongue, dry: Aconite

Uncomfortable after meal: Natrum Mur.

Upset: fatty greasy food, Arsenicum Alb.; juicy fruits, Arsenicum Alb.; melons, Arsenicum Alb.; tea, Nux Vom.; tobacco, Nux Vom.

Vomiting: bile, Aconite; bitter, Antimonium Crud.; difficult, Nux Vom.; mucous, Aconite; violent, Antimonium Crud.

Vomitus: stringy, watery, yellow, Kali Bich.

INTESTINAL TRACT – AGGRAVATION

5 a.m. : Natrum Carb.

11 a.m.: Sulphur

4–8 p.m.: Lycopodium, Natrum Sulph.

Alcohol: Natrum Phos.

Bread: Natrum Mur.

Coffee: Arsenicum Alb., Natrum Sulph., Nux Vom.

Drink: Antimonium Crud.

Eating: Kali Carb.

Fat: Arsenicum Alb., Nitric Acid.

Food: Antimonium Crud., Arsenicum Alb., Nitric Acid.; cold, Natrum Phos., Sarsaparilla; rich, Natrum Sulph.; rich, fatty, Natrum Carb., Natrum Phos.; sour, acid, Natrum Phos.

Fruits: Natrum Phos.

Meat: Nux Vom.
Milk: Natrum Mur., Natrum Phos., Natrum Sulph., Nux Vom.
Starches: Natrum Carb., Natrum Mur., Natrum Phos.
Sweets: Natrum Carb., Nitric Acid.

INTESTINAL TRACT – AMELIORATION

Cold: diet, Sarsaparilla; drinks, Natrum Mur.
Eating: Natrum Carb., Natrum Phos.
Food, small amounts of: Nux Vom.
Vomiting: Natrum Mur.

INTESTINAL TRACT – APPEARANCE

Alert: Phosphorus
Anxious: Arsenicum Alb.
Bluish: Cuprum Met.
Bright: Phosphorus
Compact in stature: Lilium Tig.
Dark: Nitric Acid
Depressed: Antimonium Crud.
Distress: extreme, Cuprum Met.; tremulousness, Aconite
Dusky: Aethusa, Nux Vom.
Exophthalmos – thyroid enlarged: Natrum Sulph.
Face: pale sunken, Arsenicum Alb.; puffy, Kali Bich.
Faintness, feeling of: Nux Vom.
Fair: Kali Bich., Lac Can.
Fat: Kali Bich., Natrum Sulph.
Fattish features, mauvish-powdered: Graphites
Flatulence, marked: Nux Vom.
Florid: Natrum Sulph.
Fretful: Arsenicum Alb.
Gentle people: Lac Can.
Hair, reddish tint in: Phosphorus
Ill: Sarsaparilla
Intelligent: Phosphorus
Lips darkish in cold: Lilium Tig.
Mental anxiety: Arsenicum Alb.
Mucous membranes pale: Graphites
Old, looks: Sarsaparilla
Pale: collapsed child, Aethusa; distressed-looking, Cuprum Met.; flabby, Antimonium Crud.
Sadness: Arsenicum Alb.

Sallow: Lycopodium
Sluggish: Kali Bich.
Spare: Lycopodium
Tall, scraggy: Phosphorus
Thin: in build, Arsenicum Alb.; underweight, Phosphorus; usually, Nitric
  Acid.; wrinkled child, Argentum Nit.
Twitching: Aethusa
Undersized: Natrum Sulph.
Vital: Nitric Acid.
Well covered: Natrum Mur.
Worried: Arsenicum Alb.
Wrinkled: Lycopodium, Sarsaparilla

INTESTINAL TRACT – AVERSIONS

Bread: Kali Phos., Lilium Tig., Nitric Acid.
Coffee: Lilium Tig., Natrum Carb., Natrum Mur.
Fat: Arsenicum Alb., Natrum Carb.
Fish: Graphites
Meat: Graphites, Kali Phos., Nitric Acid.; (marked), Kali Bich.
Milk: Natrum Carb., Nitric Acid.; (in a child), Phosphorus; (marked),
  Lac Can.
Salt: Graphites, Natrum Mur.
Sweets: Graphites, Nitric Acid., Phosphorus

INTESTINAL TRACT – CAUSATION

Children, recently weaned: Argentum Nit.
Chill: Antimonium Crud.
Cold drinks, excessive: Antimonium Crud.
Dietary indiscretion: Nux Vom.
Hot weather: Arsenicum Alb.
Iced foods: Arsenicum Alb.

INTESTINAL TRACT – DESIRES

Beer: Kali Bich.
Bread: Natrum Ars., Natrum Mur.
Drinks: Lycopodium; small, Natrum Ars.
Eggs: Natrum Phos.
Farinaceous foods: Natrum Carb.
Fat: Nitric Acid, Nux Vom.

Fish: fresh, Natrum Phos.
Food: cold, Natrum Phos.; hot, Lycopodium; seasoned, Natrum Phos., Phosphorus; starchy, Kali Carb.; two-hourly, Natrum Carb.
Ice-cream: Phosphorus
Meat: Lilium Tig.
Pick-me-ups (particularly): Nux Vom.
Refreshing things: Phosphorus
Salt: Natrum Mur., Phosphorus
Sour things: Kali Bich., Kali Phos.
Sugar: Kali Carb.
Sweet things: Lycopodium
Sweets: Kali Carb., Natrum Ars., Natrum Carb.

CONSTIPATION

Brooding: Aurum Met.
Colour, dusky: Aurum Met.
Constipation: Aurum Met., Calc. Sil., Graphites, Kali Carb., Natrum Carb., Nux Vom.; extreme, Opium
Delirium: Opium
Face: feeling of cobweb over, Graphites; large, Graphites
Faeces, small balls of: Plumbum Met.
Features, fattish: Graphites
Feeling, rectum full: Nux Vom.
Feels better when constipated: Calc. Carb.
Flabby: Kali Carb.
Fleshy: Natrum Carb.
Haemorrhoids, painful: Kali Carb.
Head, large: Graphites
Melancholic: Aurum Met.
Pain: drawing to back of spine, Plumbum Met.; umbilical, Plumbum Met.
Pale: Kali Carb.; anaemic, Calc. Sil.; doughy features, Natrum Carb.
Peristalsis, acute: Nux Vom.
Spruce: Nux Vom.
Stupor: Opium
Sweating: Kali Carb.
Weary-looking: Nux Vom.

DIARRHOEA – GENERAL

Abdomen: distended, Aconite, Aloes, Apis; tender, Aconite, Apis; > pressure, Argentum Nit.
Air, craves fresh: Argentum Nit.
Anus: excoriation of, Arsenicum Alb.; redness of, Arsenicum Alb.

Babies, predominantly in: Aethusa
Colic, central, > bowel action: Aloes
Distress accompanied by tremulousness: Aconite
Disturbed, hates to be: Aloes
Eating, after: Aloes
Exhausted, extremely after stool, with tenesmus: Antimonium Crud.
Explosive: Aloes
Flatulence: gurgling, Aloes; without relief, Apis
Flatus: marked, Aloes; offensive, Apis
Irritable: Aloes, Apis
Knee, child unable to sit on adult's: Apis
Lips, dry: Argentum Nit.
Mentally fogged: Apis
Milk, intolerance of: Aethusa
Mouth, dry: Apis, Argentum Nit.
Movement, after: Aloes
Nausea: Aconite, Apis; intense, Antimonium Crud.
Pain: abdominal, Apis; burning in rectum, after stool, Arsenicum Alb.; burning in rectum, during stool, Arsenicum Alb.; cutting, before stool, Antimonium Crud.; intense, Apis; on passing water, Aloes
Rectum: excoriated, Aloes
Sickness, intense: Aethusa
Skin: dry, Aconite, Aloes; dusky, Aloes; dusky with intense heat, Aloes; hot, Aconite, Aloes
Speech, thick: Aconite
Stool: large, formed, hot, Apis; painless, Apis; profuse, offensive, Antimonium Crud.; scant, frequent, Capsicum; small, intensely green, Aconite; yellow, streaked with green, Aloes
Sudden onset: Aethusa
Sweat: Aconite
Taste: bitter, Aloes; horrible, Aconite
Tendency: to chronic conjunctivitis, Argentum Nit.; to cracks round nose, Antimonium Crud.; to snuffles, Antimonium Crud.
Tenesmus: after stool, Aconite; before stool, Aconite; before stool, Aloes; during stool, Aloes; relieved by bowel action, Aconite; with thirst, Capsicum
Thirst: Aloes; intense for sips, Arsenicum Alb.
Thirstless: Aethusa, Antimonium Crud., Apis
Tongue: intense red tip, Aloes; red, shiny, Apis; thickly coated, Antimonium Crud.
Vomiting: Aconite; burning, anything from mucus to blood, Arsenicum Alb.; violent, Antimonium Crud.
Water, difficulty in passing: Capsicum

DIARRHOEA – APPEARANCE

Collapsed: Aethusa
Depressed: Antimonium Crud.
Face: bright red, Capsicum; large, Graphites
Face and nose, red: Capsicum
Features, fattish: Graphites
Flabby: Antimonium Crud.
Frightened: Arsenicum Alb.
Head, large: Graphites
Lying position: with knees drawn up, Apis; with legs apart, Aloes
Lips: bluish, Arsenicum Alb.; dry, Arsenicum Alb.; pale, Arsenicum Alb.; puffy, Capsicum; tendency to bleed, Arsenicum Alb.
Nose, cold: Capsicum
Pale: Aethusa, Antimonium Crud., Kali Carb.; anaemic, Calc. Sil.
Restless: Arsenicum Alb.
Terror, look of: Aconite
Thin: Argentum Nit.
Tremulous: Argentum Nit.
Useless: Antimonium Crud.
Weak: Argentum Nit.
Wrinkled: Argentum Nit., Arsenicum Alb.

DIARRHOEA – CAUSATION

Alcohol: Arsenicum Alb.
Anger: Aloes
Children, recently weaned: Argentum Nit.
Chill: Antimonium Crud., Arsenicum Alb.
Cold: drinks, Arsenicum Alb.; exposure to, Aconite
Diarrhoea, patient chilly during: Argentum Nit.
Drinks, excessively cold, in warm weather: Antimonium Crud.
Fright: Aconite
Heat, excessive in summer: Aethusa
Homesick: Capsicum
Overeating in summer: Aconite
Teething: Aethusa, Arsenicum Alb.
Weather, hot: Aloes, Antimonium Crud., Apis, Argentum Nit.

URINARY TRACT INFECTION – GENERAL

Abdomen, tenderness of: Terebinthina
Alone, cannot bear being: Clematis
Appetite, poor: Sarsaparilla

Bowels, desires to open: Berberis
Cold, acute sensitiveness to: Causticum
Confused and cannot remember: Sabal Serr.
Constipation: Sabal Serr.
Danger, unknown, thinks some is ahead: Sabal Serr.
Distension: after very little food, Sarsaparilla; gurgling and tenderness in abdomen, Terebinthina
Drowsiness: Sarsaparilla
Epilepsy, fear of getting: Terebinthina
Food, disgust for: Cantharis; empty feeling immediately after: Sarsaparilla
Fretful: Clematis
Gouty diathesis: Berberis
Inflammation, burning: Berberis
Irritable, angry, fretful: Clematis
Language, frightful: Cantharis
Mental dejection: Berberis
Mouth, dry, sticky, with frothy saliva: Berberis
Night, has to get up during: Sabal Serr.
Pain, burning/cutting: before, during and after micturition, Cantharis
Pain: at root of nose, goes into head, Sabal Serr.; in head, Berberis; in kidney region, < pressure, Berberis; shooting in rectum, Causticum
Pains start in one spot and radiate: Berberis
Prostate, enlarged: Sabal Serr.
Restless: Causticum
Sleeps badly: Causticum
Stools, burning, light in colour, sticky: Berberis
Sweat: clammy in bed, Terebinthina; easily, Berberis
Testicles, painful, tightly drawn up: Sabal Serr.
Tinkling in ears: Terebinthina
Twilight, people and dogs look larger in: Sabal Serr.
Urinary organs, irritation of all: Cantharis
Urinate, spasm on attempt to: Terebinthina
Urination: painful, Sabal Serr.
Urine: cannot pass because of burning pain, Sarsaparilla; clay-like mucus, Berberis; diminished secretion of, Terebinthina; involuntary passage of, Causticum; pale, Sarsaparilla; pale yellow, gelatinous sediment, Berberis; passes frequently, Sarsaparilla; scalding to patient, Sabal Serr.; urging to pass, Causticum; wants to pass urgently, Sarsaparilla

URINARY TRACT INFECTION – AGGRAVATION

4 p.m. until night: Berberis
Afternoon: Cantharis
Walking, motion: Sarsaparilla

URINARY TRACT INFECTION – AMELIORATION

Pain, > sleep: Sabal Serr.

URINARY TRACT INFECTION – APPEARANCE

Anxiety: Causticum; extreme, Cantharis
Expression, sickly: Berberis
Lips, dry: Berberis
Look, half-intoxicated: Terebinthina
Melancholy: Causticum

URINARY TRACT INFECTION – SENSATIONS AS IF, AS OF

Afternoon, hot in: Berberis
Bladder, cannot empty properly: Cantharis
Cap, wearing a: Berberis
Head, cold in right side of: Berberis
Morning, creeping chillingness in: Berberis
Urethra, constriction in, with slow flow: Clematis
Urination, burning sensation at beginning of: Clematis

MENSTRUATION

Assurance, air of: Natrum Mur.
Backache: < waking, > moving, Natrum Mur.; > walking, Sting Ray; from lying on something hard, Natrum Mur.; from pressure, Natrum Mur.
Bright: Squid
Character, definite: Natrum Mur.
Chilly: Squid
Colouring: dark, sandy, Natrum Mur.
Discharges: acrid, pussy, yellow, Natrum Phos. white of egg, Natrum Mur.
Dysmenorrhoea, acute: Sepia
Excitement, sexual: Lilium Tig.
Expression, sullen: Sepia
Eye, shadow extending across nose to cheekbones: Sepia
Faints if stands too long: Sting Ray
Fair-skinned: Pulsatilla
Food >: Natrum Mur.
Happy one minute, tears the next: Pulsatilla
Headache: < noise, > evening, Sting Ray
Heat <: Sting Ray

Intelligent: Squid
Interested in other people: Squid
Menopausal patients: Squid
Menopause: Pulsatilla
Menses: irregular, Natrum Mur.; scanty, Lilium Tig., Sepia
Movement >: Natrum Mur.
Mucous membranes, dry: Natrum Mur.
Pelvic: congestion, Lilium Tig.; feeling of organs going to fall out, Sepia
Quick: Squid
Sallow: Natrum Mur., Sting Ray
Scraggy: Natrum Phos.
Sexual intercourse, prostrated by: Natrum Phos.
Sterility, of value in: Sepia
Tall: Natrum Phos.
Thin: Natrum Phos.
Tired: looks, Sting Ray; rings round eyes, Sting Ray
Underweight: Natrum Phos.
Uterus, anteverted with bowel irritation: Lilium Tig.
Weather changes, sensitive to: Sting Ray
Well-covered: Pulsatilla

RHEUMATISM – GENERAL

Alert, intellectually: Aluminium Ox.
Arms, weakness in: Natrum Phos.
Cold, irritable: Ferrum Phos.
Comfortable, cannot get: Drosera
Contented: Aluminium Ox.
Despairing: Aurum Met.
Dysentery, never well since: Dysenteriae Comp.
Eggs, desires: Calc. Carb.
Feet stick out of bed: Medorrhinum
Have to sit up in bed: Aurum Met.
Heaviness: Natrum Phos.
Irritable if talked to: Bryonia
Joints: red, Bryonia; swollen, Bryonia
Lumbago: Nux Vom.
Miserable: Aconite
Move suddenly, cannot: Causticum
Movement, worse for all: Bryonia
Muscles: stiffness, tightness, Natrum Phos.
Onset: and disappearance rapid, Kalmia Lat.; sudden, Aconite

Pain: acute, Nux Vom.; comes on suddenly, Pulsatilla; cramping,
Nux Vom.; crick in neck, Actea Rac.; down legs, Drosera; drawing,
Drosera; elbow, Natrum Phos.; goes from above downwards,
Rhododendron; goes gradually, Pulsatilla; jumps from joint to joint,
Aurum Met.; knee, Pulsatilla, Thuja; left elbow, Natrum Sulph.;
lumbar, Natrum Phos.; lumbosacral, Radium Brom.; moves from joint
to joint, Rhus Tox.; moves into fingers, Natrum Phos.; moves into
palm, Natrum Phos.; opposite side of body, Actea Rac.; right, Natrum
Phos.; right elbow, Natrum Phos.; sciatica to ball of foot,
Medorrhinum; settles in one joint, Medorrhinum; several joints,
Medorrhinum; shifts about, Rhododendron; from shin into ankle,
Drosera; shooting, Drosera; shoulder, Natrum Phos.; single joints,
Pulsatilla; spasmodic, Nux Vom.; stretching, Drosera; wandering,
Kalmia Lat.; wrist, Natrum Phos.

Palpitations: Kalmia Lat.

Periodicity, seven days: Sanguinaria

Restless: Aconite

Shivering when at rest: Drosera

Stiffness: forearm, Natrum Sulph.; left leg, Natrum Sulph.; single joint,
Bryonia

Sweats: Nux Vom.; all over, Drosera; at night, Drosera; on uncovered
part, Thuja

RHEUMATISM – AGGRAVATION

Cold: Calc. Carb., Nux Vomica; wind, Rhododendron

Draught: Nux Vom.

Heat: Pulsatilla

Initiating movement: Rhus Tox.

Keeping still: Rhus Tox.

Motion: Nux Vom.

Movement: Medorrhinum

Pressure: Nux Vom.

Rain: Rhododendron

Weather, dry, cold: Nux Vom.

RHEUMATISM – AMELIORATION

Movement, continuing: Rhus Tox.

Weather: damp, Nux Vom.

Warm dry application: Nux Vom.

RHEUMATISM – APPEARANCE

Bluish: Aurum Met.
Chilly: Nux Vom.
Face haggard, pale, inclined to vomit: Sanguinaria
Fat: Natrum Sulph.
Florid yellowness: Natrum Sulph.
Hair, fair: Thuja
Hands, chilly, clammy, cold: Calc. Carb.
Restless: Rhus Tox.
Scraggy: Natrum Phos.
Skin, fine: Thuja
Thin: Natrum Phos.
Undersized: Natrum Sulph.
Underweight: Natrum Phos.

RHEUMATISM – CAUSATION

Cold: Nux Vom., Rhus Tox.
Weather, wet: Rhus Tox.
Getting chilled: Medorrhinum

SLEEPLESSNESS

Abuse: of alcohol, coffee, tobacco, Nux Vom.
Afraid: at night, < 1–2 a.m., Arsenicum Alb.; he is going to die, Aconite; to go to sleep, Sabal Serr.
Ambitious boy's sleeping remedy: Lycopodium
Anxiety at night: Calc. Carb.
Asleep, cannot fall: Lycopodium
Asleep: falls, for an hour or two then wakes up, Chamomilla
Awake at 4 a.m.: Lycopodium
Carried, wanting to be: Chamomilla
Causation – missing someone for a long time: Cocculus
Chill, which brings on restlessness: Aconite
Coffee drinkers, after ordeal: Coffea Crud.
Coffee, from drinking: Coffea Crud.
Depressed, uncomfortable and restless: Gelsemium
Emotion, sensitive to: Coffea Crud.
Excitable: Aconite
Fear of dark: Calc. Carb.
Fearful at night: Rhus Tox.
Food, over-rich: Pulsatilla
Mental strain: Silicea; after, Nux Vom.

Mind, active: Lycopodium
Mottled-looking: Pulsatilla
Muttering delirium: at night, Bryonia; until morning, Baptisia
Physical strain: Silicea
Restless: makes tea, moves around, Arsenicum Alb.; talk, Thuja; uncomfortable, Causticum; walks, Arsenicum Alb.
Sleep: cannot, Silicea; cannot from planning and arranging things, Coffea Crud.; cannot if he lies down, Chamomilla; talks and groans in, Arnica
Sleeper, bad: Causticum
Sleeping: phases of not, Pulsatilla
Sleepless: early in night (in children), Chamomilla; from pain, < keeping still, Rhus Tox.; persistently, Thuja
Sleeps: arms above head, Pulsatilla; on back, Pulsatilla
Study, apt to, late at night: Nux Vom.
Talk to themselves in bed: Calc. Carb.
Tea, makes quantities of: Rhus Tox.
Thinks cold drink makes him feel better: Pulsatilla
Tired, too: Cocculus
Wakes between 3–4 a.m.: Nux Vom.
Walks about: Rhus Tox.
Warm room <: Bryonia, Pulsatilla
Worry, but not about themselves: Nux Vom.

DREAMS

Afraid of things: Lycopodium
Animals: Arnica
Anxious: Arnica
Arguments: < menses, Sepia; awful, Aurum Met.
Being: buried alive, Chelidonium; in a vice, Thuja; killed, Chelidonium; shut in dark, Arsenicum Alb.
Children's dream remedy: Calc. Carb.
Colour, dusky: Aurum Met.
Corpses: Aurum Met., Calc. Carb., Thuja
Danger, that he may be in: Arsenicum Alb.
Death: Arnica
Drowning: Arnica
Dying: Calc. Carb.
Faces: Calc. Carb.; red, Arnica
Falling: down, Chelidonium; from a great height, Thuja
Fears: all kinds of, Pulsatilla; cannot sleep because of, Pulsatilla
Fire: Arsenicum Alb.
Ghosts: Kali Sulph., Pulsatilla

Hungry, being: Aurum Met.
Ill: Calc. Carb.
Night terrors (children): Calc. Carb.
Odd: Pulsatilla
People standing round bed: Calc. Carb.
Robbers: Kali Sulph.
Sorrow, great: Arsenicum Alb.
Unpleasant: Pulsatilla
Wild animals: Lycopodium

MENTAL HANDICAP – BIRTH INJURIES

Blind, apparently: Baryta Carb.
Habits, unclean: Baryta Carb.
Legs, weak: Natrum Mur.
Nervous, acutely: Natrum Mur.
Swallowing solid food, difficulty in: Baryta Carb.
Talk, unable to: Natrum Mur.
Vomiting: < alone, Borax; being carried downstairs, Borax

MENTAL HANDICAP – CONGENITAL

Cough, wheezing: Kali Iod.
Discharge, greeny-yellow: Kali Iod.
Intelligence, limited: Kali Iod.
Mentally alert, not: Calc. Carb.
Snuffles, constant: Kali Iod.
Sweaty: Calc. Carb.
Talk: a little, Kali Iod.; unable to, Calc. Carb.
Unhealthy-looking: Calc. Carb.
Walk, unable to: Calc. Carb.
Wasserman, positive: Lueticum

MENTAL HANDICAP – INDUCED INJURIES

Grimaces: Thuja
Movements, clumsy: Thuja
Noise, terrified by sudden: Thuja

FOOD – AGGRAVATION

Alcohol: Arsenicum Alb., Calc. Carb., Calc. Sil., Natrum Ars., Natrum Phos.
Beer: Kali Bich.
Bread: all Natrum salts
Coffee: Cocculus, Natrum Sulph., Nux Vom.
Drinking: Carbo Veg.
Drinks: cold, Lycopodium; warm, Silicea
Eating: Calc. Sil., Carbo Veg.; muddle-headed after, Aesculus; warm food and drinks, Kali Carb.
Fat (after taking food): Nitric Acid
Food: Kali Bich.; after, Kali Sulph.; cold, Kali Iod.; warm, Silicea; warm, small quantity, Sarsaparilla
Foods: fatty, Natrum Ars., Natrum Carb., Natrum Phos., Natrum Sulph.; fruit: Natrum Ars., Natrum Carb., Natrum Phos., Natrum Sulph.; iced, in hot weather, Arsenicum Alb.; rich, Natrum Ars., Natrum Carb., Natrum Phos., Natrum Sulph.; sour and acid, Natrum Phos.; starchy, Natrum Sulph.
Fruits: juicy, Arsenicum Alb.; watery, Arsenicum Alb.
Meat: Nux Vom.
Milk: all Natrum salts, Nux Vom.; intolerance of, Aethusa
Smell of: cooking, Sepia; tobacco, Sepia
Starches: all Natrum salts
Sweets: Natrum Carb.
Tea: Nux Vom.
Tobacco: Nux Vom.
Vegetables: Natrum Sulph.
Vomits: after drink or food, Arsenicum Alb.

FOOD – AMELIORATION

Drinks: hot, Lycopodium; warm, Calc. Fluor.
Food: Graphites, Medusa; particularly hot soup, Kali Bich.; warm, Calc. Fluor.
Milk, warm: Graphites
Water, cold: Baryta Mur.

FOOD – APPETITE

Appetite: poor, Sarsaparilla; good, Sulphur
Fast eaters: Cuprum Met.
Hungry: Chininum Sulph., Kali Iod., Lac Can.; after a few mouthfuls will feel full, Lycopodium

Quickly satisfied: Kali Phos.
Varies, but usually good: Calc. Phos.

FOOD – AVERSIONS

Beer: Phosphorus
Bread: Kali Phos., Lilium Tig.
Coffee: Lilium Tig.
Eggs (in children): Ferrum Met.
Fat (but may also desire fat): Hepar Sulph.
Fish: Graphites
Food: Baryta Mur.; cold, Kali Iod.
Ice cream: Kali Iod.
Meat: Graphites, Kali Bich., Kali Carb., Kali Phos.
Milk: Guaiacum, Kali Iod., Lac Can.; milk puddings (in children),
  Phosphorus
Salt: Graphites, Natrum Mur., Natrum salts
Sweets: Graphites

FOOD – DESIRES

Bread: Natrum Ars.; (markedly), Natrum Mur.
Cocktails: Nux Vom.
Coffee: Arsenicum Alb.
Diet, cold: Sarsparilla
Drinks, hot: Lycopodium
Fat: Nitric Acid., Nux Vom.
Fluids: (in acute illness, but would not ask), Baptisia
Food: cold, Cuprum Met., Natrum Ars.; every two hours, Natrum Carb.;
  smell of good, Lycopus; sweet and sour, Kali Phos.
Foods: bitter, Natrum salts; cold, Silicea; farinaceous, Natrum Carb.; hot,
  Lycopodium; pungent, Sepia; seasoned, Phosphorus; spicy,
  Phosphorus; sweet (jam), Lycopodium
Ice cream: Phosphorus, Silicea
Lemon juice: Belladonna
Meat: Lilium Tig.
'Pick-me-ups': Nux Vom.
Pickles: Nitric Acid.
Refreshing things: Phosphorus
Salt: all Natrum salts, Phosphorus; (preferred as salt bacon or meat), Calc.
  Phos.
Savouries: Nitric Acid.
Soup: Sodium salts

Sour things: beer, Kali Bich.; hot lemon juice, Guaiacum; wines, Phosphorus
Starch: Silicea
Strong taste: herring, pickles, Hepar Sulph.
Sugar: Kali Carb.
Sweets: Kali Carb., Natrum Carb.
Vinegar: Kali Phos., Sepia
Wine: Sepia

FOOD – THIRST

Bitter: Sarsaparilla
Drinks: cold, Dulcamara, Merc.Cy., Natrum Ars., Natrum Carb., Natrum Sulph.
Liquids, sour: Kali Carb.
Milk: boiled, Natrum Sulph.
Taste: metallic (in febrile conditions), Rhus Tox.; metallic, bitter-sweet, Sarsaparilla; sweet, Nitric Acid.; water tastes unpleasant, Kali Bich.
Thirst: Kali Iod., Sarsaparilla; for cold drinks, Chininum Ars.
Thirstiest of remedies: Phosphorus
Thirstless: Lycopodium, Nitric Acid
Water: cold, Cuprum Met., Guaiacum, Sulphur; cold <, Cuprum Met.; iced, Kali Phos.

AGGRAVATION – GENERAL

Alcohol: Calc. Carb., Natrum Ars.
Anger: Calc. Sil.
Anytime: Calc. Sil.
Bath: Natrum Phos.
Breakfast, after: Calc. Sil.
Cold: Natrum Phos.
Damp cold: Natrum Ars., Rhus Tox.
Hot room: Bryonia
Hunger: Lac Can.
Motion: Calc. Sil., Calc. Sulph.
Movement: Bryonia
Noise: Calc. Sil.
Open air: Kali Bich.
Overheated: Calc. Sulph.
Rest: Calc. Fluor.
Sexual intercourse: all Kali salts, Natrum Phos.

Side of body: left, Croton Tig.; left to right, Terebinthina; right, Lycopus, Senega
Standing: Sulphur; in warm room, Sepia
Stuffy rooms: Aesculus, Sting Ray
Uncovered: Kali Carb.
Walking fast: Calc. Sulph.
Warmth of bed: Calc. Sulph.

AGGRAVATION – SEASONS

Spring: Natrum Sulph.
Summer: Natrum Mur., Kali Bich., Kali Carb.
Winter: Natrum Ars.

AGGRAVATION – TIME

1–2 a.m.: Arsenicum Alb.
2 a.m.: Kali Brom.
2–5 a.m.: Kali Bich., Kali Carb., Kali Iod.
4–8 a.m.: Lycopodium
10.30–11.30 a.m.: Natrum Mur.
11 a.m.: Sulphur
1–2 p.m.: Arsenicum Alb.
4 p.m. until sleep: Berberis
4–8 p.m.: Lycopodium
5 p.m.: Natrum Carb.
9 p.m., (acute illness): Bryonia
Afternoon: Cantharis
Anytime: Calc. Sil.
Darkness: Arsenicum Alb.
Early wakening: Kali Sulph.
Evening: Hepar Sulph., Kali Sulph.; dreads, Calc. Sil.
Midnight: Natrum Ars.
Morning: Aloes, Hepar Sulph., Sepia; on waking, Natrum Carb., Natrum Phos., Natrum Sulph.
Night: Ferrum Phos., Pulsatilla, Rhus Tox.
Noon, tails off early evening: Natrum Carb.

AGGRAVATION – WEATHER AND TEMPERATURE

Cold: Magnesia Phos., Natrum Carb., Nitric Acid; dry to warm, Sepia;
  dry weather, Hepar Sulph., Nux Vom.
Damp: Natrum Phos.; cold, Natrum Ars., Sepia; weather, Kali Carb.
Heat: Aloes, Apis, Kali Iod., Lachesis, Lilium Tig., Pulsatilla
Sun: hot, Natrum Carb.; at noon, Natrum Mur.
Throat, heat to : Calc. Sulph.
Warmth of bed: Calc. Sulph.
Weather: change in, Kali Bich., Natrum Phos.; warm, Sulphur

AMELIORATION – GENERAL

Cool: Aloes
Draught of air: Aesculus
Mental amelioration in open air: Natrum Ars.
Movement: Sting Ray, Tub. Bov.; general, Calc. Fluor.
Moving gently in open air: Ferrum Phos., Pulsatilla
Open air: Allium Cepa., Aurum Met., Kali Iod.
Rubbing: Calc. Fluor.
Sympathy: Lycopodium, Medusa
Warm evening: Graphites
Warmth: Calc. Fluor.
Weather: damp, Hepar Sulph., Nux Vom.; dry warm, Sulphur

Index of Remedies

361

Classical Homoeopathy, Dr Margery Blackie, 1986. The complete teaching legacy of one of the most important homoeopaths of our time.

0906584140

Everyday Homoeopathy, Dr David Gemmell, 1987. A practical handbook for using homoeopathy in the context of one's own personal and family health care, using readily available remedies.

0906584183

Homoeopathic Prescribing, Dr Noel Pratt, revised 1985. A compact reference book covering 161 common complaints and disorders, with guidance on the choice of the appropriate remedy.   0906584035

Homoeopathy as Art and Science, Dr Elizabeth Wright Hubbard, 1990. The selected writings of one of the foremost modern homoeopaths.   0906584264

Homoeopathy in Practice, Dr Douglas Borland, reprinted 1988 with Symptom Index. Detailed guidance on the observation of symptoms and the choice of remedies.   090658406X

Insights into Homoeopathy, Dr Frank Bodman, 1990. Homoeopathic approaches to common problems in general medicine and psychiatry.

0906584280

Introduction to Homoeopathic Medicine (2nd Edition), Dr Hamish Boyd, 1989. A formal introductory text, written in categories that are familiar to the medical practitioner.   0906584213

Materia Medica of New Homoeopathic Remedies, Dr O. A. Julian, paperback edition 1984. Full clinical coverage of 106 new homoeopathic remedies, for use in conjunction with the classical materia medicas.   0906584116

Studies of Homoeopathic Remedies, Dr Douglas Gibson, 1987. Detailed clinical studies of 100 major remedies. Well-known for the uniquely wide range of insights brought to bear on each remedy.

0906584175

Tutorials on Homoeopathy, Dr Donald Foubister, 1989. Detailed studies on a wide range of conditions and remedies.   0906584256

NOTES

NOTES

NOTES

NOTES

NOTES

NOTES

NOTES

NOTES